P9-DEO-358

ANNALS OF THE NEW YORK ACADEMY OF SCIENCES

VOLUME 263

September 19, 1975

DEVELOPMENTAL PSYCHOLINGUISTICS AND COMMUNICATION DISORDERS*

Editors and Conference Chairpersons

DORIS AARONSON AND ROBERT W. RIEBER

CONTENTS

*This series of papers is the result of a conference entitled Developmental Psycholinguistics and Communication Disorders, held by The New York Academy of Sciences on January 24 and 25, 1975.

Financial support was received from:

- THE GRANT FOUNDATION, INC.

LINCOLN CHRISTIAN COLLEGE

Lincoln Christian College

ANNALS OF THE NEW YORK ACADEMY OF SCIENCES

VOLUME 263

DEVELOPMENTAL PSYCHOLINGUISTICS AND COMMUNICATION DISORDERS

Edited by Doris Aaronson and Robert W. Rieber

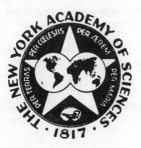

The New York Academy of Sciences
New York, New York
1975

Copyright, 1975, by The New York Academy of Sciences. All rights reserved. Except for brief quotations by reviewers, reproduction of this publication in whole or in part by any means whatever is strictly prohibited without written permission from the publisher.

Library of Congress Cataloging in Publication Data
Main entry under title:

Developmental psycholinguistics and communication disorders.

(Annals of The New York Academy of Sciences ; v. 263)
Includes bibliographical references.
1. Languages—Psychology—Addresses, essays, lectures. 2. Children—Languages—Addresses, essays, lectures. 3. Speech, Disorders of—Addresses, essays, lectures. I. Aaronson, Doris. II. Rieber, Robert W. III. Series: New York Academy of Sciences. Annals ; v. 263. [DNLM: 1. Language development—Congresses. 2. Language disorders—Congresses. 3. Psycholinguistics—Congresses. 4. Communication—Congresses. Wl NE538 v. 263 / WM475 D489 1975]
Q11.N5 vol. 263 [P37] 401'.9 75-28001
ISBN 0-89072-016-9

ACS/PCP
Printed in the United States of America
ISBN 0-89072-016-9

INTRODUCTION

Doris Aaronson

Department of Psychology
New York University
New York, New York 10003

Robert W. Rieber

Department of Psychology
John Jay College of Criminal Justice
The City University of New York
New York, New York 10019

The conference on which this volume is based was interdisciplinary in nature and included speakers from the following fields: psychology, linguistics, philosophy, anthropology, physiology, and medicine. The approaches of both basic laboratory research and research applications are represented.

The participants considered the major areas of progress in psycholinguistics during the past decades and the important issues for the next decade. Topics considered include the role of cognition in the acquisition and development of language, the influence of verbal and nonverbal factors in this process, methods of understanding better the notion of linguistic competence in order to account for linguistic performance; and an investigation of the physiological bases of language perception and production. In developing this conference, we formulated two basic issues that could permeate throughout all sessions of the conference. These issues are: (1) What relations exist between the building up and breaking down of the developmental language process? What can we learn from the study of one to tell us about the other? (2) What dimensions of individual differences are empirically and theoretically important? How can a knowledge of individual differences in language development help us understand and deal with cognitive and linguistic abilities and disabilities? The participants discuss the varying research methodologies and theoretical viewpoints as well as the conflicting empirical results in recent research.

The editors of this book, along with the conference speakers, prepared slightly edited versions of the discussion periods. In a very few cases the speakers expanded their responses to some questions, in order to provide a more complete and unambiguous reply. In all cases we tried to preserve both the content and the tone of the original interchange.

We would like to thank the Grant Foundation for so generously supporting this conference and the New York Academy of Sciences for its sponsorship. Also, we thank New York University* and John Jay College, CUNY, for supporting much of the secretarial, engineering, and communication costs. The conference was a joint endeavor of the Linguistics and Psychology Sections of the Academy. The chair and the vice-chair of these respective sections are Lawrence Raphael and Rosamond Gianutsos; Kurt Salzinger and Florence Denmark. We appreciate the help of the Academy staff: Ellen Marks, Ann Collins, Beatrice H. Radin, Bill Boland, Tom Houston, Renée Wilkerson, and Elvira Flores. We thank our secretaries and our

*Recipient of NSF University Science Development Program Grant GU-3186 (Psychology Department).

5

graduate students for technical help: Helen Snyder, Deanna Pattirane, and Susan Barbarisi; Edward Grupsmith, Doug Ohman, and Gail Levy. We were pleased to have the help of interpreters for the deaf during the conference: Gail Turney and Robert Battersby of the New York University Deafness Research Center. We thank Leo Schiff for running the audiovisual aids and Cyril Lichtensteiger for transcribing the proceedings.

We would like to thank the session chairpersons for organizational help before the conference, and for an excellent job of coordinating and moderating the sessions at the conference itself: Dr. Sam Glucksberg, Princeton University, Princeton, N. J.; Dr. Louis Gerstman, City College, CUNY, New York, N. Y.; and Dr. Lawrence Raphael, Lehman College, CUNY, New York, N. Y. Finally, and most important, we thank all of the conference participants who created the stimulating and important scientific content of the conference.

THE ROLE OF LANGUAGE AND THOUGHT IN DEVELOPMENTAL PSYCHOLINGUISTICS—AN HISTORICAL REVIEW

Robert W. Rieber

Department of Psychology
John Jay College of Criminal Justice
The City University of New York
New York, New York 10019

My words fly up, my thoughts remain below.
Words without thoughts never to heaven go.

Hamlet, III, iii, 97

A tree is my structure, I shall always want,
He leadeth me through the valley of a new science,
He restoreth my syntax and replenisheth faith in my intuition;
He anointeth my LAD with an infinite generative capacity,
He borroweth an old branch of cognitive psychology,
And gathereth converts without an apology:
Surely syntactics, semantics and pragmatics will follow me
All the days of my life,
And I will live in the house of abstractions forever.

R.W.R.

There is an old saying in psychology, stemming as far back as Aristotle,[1] that "as one thinks, so one speaks." It was not until the 1940s, with the promulgation of the Sapir-Whorf hypothesis, that the converse—"as one speaks, so one thinks"—received much consideration.[2] The reciprocal relationship between the two processes of thinking and speaking is still a basic enigma to the psycholinguist. Polemics centering on this issue weigh in at more pounds per paragraph than this writer would care to calculate, yet there is still a need for a careful study of the history of the various positions. I shall briefly cover some of the important aspects of the controversy, especially those related to communication disorders, as they developed from the seventeenth through the nineteenth centuries.

We begin at the end of the seventeenth century with Geraud de Cordemoy (d. 1684), a Cartesian scholar whom Chomsky designates in his *Cartesian Linguistics* as a Chomskian before Chomsky.[3] This may well be the case; nevertheless, in reading Cordemoy one can hardly fail to notice certain resemblances to both Locke and Hartley. Specifically, he seems to anticipate the two English philosophers by suggesting that in language development children will learn one thing rather than another according to the degree of pleasure or pain associated with the learning situation. One may also see here, in a more rudimentary form, an anticipation of learning theory.

Cordemoy goes on to discuss the idea of communication as a dialogue, and

7

stresses the notion that the speech act is the basis of all behavior, including individual creativity. His position on innate ideas is clear:

> But since I only look here after the princples, I am not to proceed so far to particulars. I desire only that by the way an important truth may be taken notice of, which this example of children evidently discovers to us, viz., that from their birth they have their reason entire, because indeed this way of learning to speak is the effect of so great a discerning and of so perfect reason that a more wonderful one cannot possibly be conceived.[4]

We now jump ahead nearly a century to another much more famous Frenchman, Denis Diderot (1713–1784), whose *Letter on the Deaf and Dumb* appeared in 1751. It was no particular interest in the problems of deaf people that prompted Diderot to write this book, but rather a desire to better understand how ordinary individuals develop knowledge about things in the real world, through an analysis of language and its natural development, as well as a communication disorder known as deafness.[6]

Diderot's *Letter* begins with the linguistic problem of inversions, but ranges widely over such topics as the origin and historical development of language, epistemology, rhetoric, and so on.

Through the example of an imaginary deaf person, Diderot attempts to determine the relationship between thought and language. The deaf person represents a hypothetical prelinguistic society. Here Diderot seems to anticipate modern Gestalt psychology:

> Mind is a moving scene, which we are perpetually copying. We spend a great deal of time in rendering it faithfully; but the original exists as a complete whole, for the mind does not proceed step by step, like expression. The brush takes time to represent what the artist's eye sees in an instant.

I find this statement as provocative today as it must have been at the time it was written. Neisser (1967) has suggested that the Gestalt school of psychology is the most direct ancestor of current psycholinguistics.[8] Others who follow the Chomskian point of view suggest Wundt, because of Wundt's emphasis upon the sentence as the basic unit of analysis. Those who think in terms of verbal behavior would probably not agree with Blumenthal (1970),[9] but would name Watson as the most likely candidate. No doubt all of the nominees have played an important part, one way or another, in setting the stage for the currently accepted version of the psychology of language.

Diderot, however, did not compromise any of his convictions regarding the psycholinguistic nature of man. He consistently assumed knowledge to be completely dependent upon the senses, and more specifically, to the number of senses actually operating. As an interacting hypothetical experiment he imagines a society made up of five persons, each having only one of the five senses; and he comes to the conclusion that each person in this society would have a view of the world determined by his own sensory modality, and that each individual would relate to the others as being senseless. This new and more innovative psychology was quite different from the older, more absolute way of approaching the problem.

During the latter part of the eighteenth century, scholars continued to struggle with this important issue. Two other men are worth mentioning before we go on to the next century: Erasmus Darwin (1731–1802) and John Horn Tooke (1736–1812). Darwin's two most important works in the area of language and thought are *Zoonomia* (1794–96) and *The Temple of Nature* (1803). The first was Darwin's best-received work; the second, containing among other things his theory of evolution and theory of languages, was not well appreciated in his time. Darwin points out carefully that "Mr. Tooke observes that the first aim of Language was to communicate thoughts, and the second to do it with dispatch, and hence he divides words into those which were necessary to express our thoughts, and those which are observations of the former."[10] As T. Verhave points out, Darwin's psychology is a variant of eighteenth century association theory, and is, in part, a restatement of views stated by David Hartley in his *Observations on Man* (1749). Rieber and Froeschels (1966) discussed Darwin's theory of stuttering, also deriving from the theory of association. This is very similar to Mendelssohn's (1783) viewpoint, which in turn was apparently influenced by a paper written by Spalding, in the Magazine *Erfahrungsseelenkunde*, an introspective report of a case of transitory sensory motor aphasia.[11, 11a]

We now pass over a hundred years more to the latter part of the nineteenth century. Here we will be concerned with the work of Wilhelm Preyer (1841–1897), a German professor of physiology at the University of Jena. Preyer, although not well known today, was quite influential during the late nineteenth century. His pioneering work helped to establish the field of developmental psychology, and he also wrote significant works on hypnosis and neurophysiology. His most important work, *The Mind of the Child* (1881) has recently been reprinted by Arno Press, unfortunately without an introduction.[12]

Originally written in Germany, *Die Seele des Kindes* was translated into many other languages, including English. It had a direct influence upon two of the most influential psychological theorists of our time, Jean Piaget and Sigmund Freud. Freud rarely quoted other writers, but it has been possible to establish the fact that he was familiar with Preyer's works; indeed, it is my contention that Freud was under the influence of Preyer's ideas when he established as part of his theoretical system, first, the notion that *the study of abnormal development will help us better understand normal development;* and second, *the value of using stages of development as a better means of understanding the psychological growth pattern of the child.* Preyer's probable influence upon Freud has not to my knowledge, been previously noted.[13]

Freud, of course, stressed the affective, psychosexual aspect of maturation, whereas Preyer gave emphasis to the cognitive and conative. Preyer devotes the second volume of his book almost exclusively to the linguistic and cognitive development of the child. A whole chapter deals with speech and language disturbances in adults, particularly aphasia. He then draws a parallel to speech and language disturbances in childhood, thus anticipating one of the major themes of our conference.[14]

Interest in the problem of the relationship between language and thought was quite strong in the 1880s and 1890s. Max Müller was the major advocate of the notion that thinking was not possible without language. The polemics on this issue were about as bad as the polemics of the last decade regarding competence and performance. Müller, a professor of linguistics (philology) at Oxford, engaged in active debate, mainly through the journal *Nature*, with such prominent psychologists as Sir Francis Galton and George Romanes.[15]

Galton vehemently denied Müller's contentions, arguing that a careful study of congenitally deaf individuals would prove him wrong. But Galton never carried out the study himself, and it was not until the twentieth century that experimental cognitive psychologists were able to demonstrate what Galton had anticipated. Galton's warning to Müller is worth quoting, for it is as pertinent now as when he wrote it in 1887: "Before a just knowledge can be attained concerning any faculty of the human race, we must inquire into its distribution among all sorts and conditions of men on a large scale, and not among those persons who belong to a highly specialized literary class." (Reference 15, p. 4.)

Romanes used an example of a disorder of communication, namely, aphasia, to challenge Müller's thesis. He pointed out that, once attained, symbolic concept formation afterwards continues to operate without the use of words. He continues: "This is not based on one's own personal introspection which no opponent can verify; it is a matter of objectively demonstratable fact. For when a man is suddenly afflicted with aphasia, he does not forthwith become as thoughtless as a brute. Admittedly he has lost all trace of words, but his reason may remain unimpaired." (Reference 15, p. 15.)

We see, then, even from this capsulized review, that the question of the relationship between thought and language is of long standing. In the seventeenth and eighteenth centuries, Cordemoy and Diderot were making a clear distinction between the processes of thought and language. While language was for them a magnificent extension of thought, thought was necessary before language acquisition could even begin, even where there was no possibility of language acquisition.

The homogenized, atomistic concepts of associationists such as Erasmus Darwin and Horn Tooke tended to blur distinctions between thought and language, just as they did for psychological and physiological processes.

In the nineteenth century tremendous progress in neurophysiology and the treatment of speech disorders gave a new impetus to investigations of the thought-language problem. The accumulated research, particularly on the comparison between speech development in children and adult communication disorders, points to the conclusion that language is indeed an extension of thought, rather than a prerequisite to it.

NOTES AND REFERENCES

1. HAMMOND, W. A., Ed. 1902. A treatise on the principle of life. *In* Aristotle's Psychology. London, England.
2. WHORF, B. L. 1956. Language, Thought and Reality. MIT Press. Cambridge, Mass.
3. CHOMSKY, N. 1966. Cartesian Linguistics. Harper & Row. New York, N.Y.
4. DE CORDEMOY, G. 1974. A Philosophical discourse concerning speech, together with a discourse written by a learned friar. *In* Language, Man and Society. R. W. Rieber, Ed. Reprint Series. AMS Press. New York, N.Y.
5. OSGOOD, C. This annal.
6. DIDEROT, D. 1973. Diderot's Early Philosophical Works. Reprint Series. Language, Man and Society. R. W. Rieber, Ed. AMS Press. New York, N.Y.
7. Similar to Condillac's "statue," which allowed the philosophers to hypothesize about developmental psychological mechanisms. (Condillac's Treatise on the Sensations.)
8. NEISSER, U. 1967. Cognitive Psychology. Appleton-Century-Crofts. New York, N.Y.
9. BLUMENTHAL, A. L. 1970. Language and Psychology; Historical Aspects of Psycholinguistics. John Wiley & Sons. New York, N.Y.
10. DARWIN, E. 1792. The Temple of Nature: 266. T. & J. Swords. London, England.
11. VERHAVE, T. 1974. A man of knowledge revisited. Preface to new edition of Darwin, E. Zoonomia, or The Laws of Organic Life. R. W. Rieber, Ed. Reprint Series, Language, Man and Society. AMS Press. New York, N.Y.
11a. 1966. *In* Speech Pathology. R. W. Rieber and R. S. Brubaker, Eds. North Holland Pub. Co. Amsterdam, The Netherlands.
12. PREYER, W. 1889–90. Parts I & II. Reprint Classics in Psychology. Arno Press. New York, N.Y. 1973. The original edition is Die Seele des Kindes, Leipzig. 1881; first Amer. edit. The Mind of the Child. 1896. D. Appleton & Co. New York, N.Y.
13. See FREUD, S. 1905. Drei Abhandlungen zur Sexualtheorie. Leipzig & Wien. We quote from the translation Three Contributions to the Sexual Theory. (Nervous and Mental Disease Monograph Series no. 7. 2nd edit, New York, N.Y., 1910): "No author has to my knowledge recognized the lawfulness of the sexual impulse in childhood, and in the numerous writings on the development of the child the chapter on Sexual Development

is usually passed over. [Freud's footnote: This assertion on revision seemed even to myself so bold that I decided to test its correctness by again reviewing the literature. The result of this second review did not warrant any change in my original statement. A chapter on the sexual life of children is not to be found in all the representative psychologies of this age which I have read. Among these works I can mention the following: Preyer, Baldwin, Perez . . .]")

An examination of the catalog of the Freud Library, part of which is now in a special collection at the New York State Psychiatric Institute, indicates that two other books by Preyer were in Freud's possession. These books are Fascination, 1895, Stuttgart, and Der Hypnotismus, 1890, Wien. In a personal communication, Dr. Kurt R. Eissler informed me that after the Second World War he interviewed Heinrich Hinterberger, the Vienna rare-book dealer who sold Freud's collection to the Psychiatric Institute in 1939, and checked his records, which indicated which of the books sold did not belong to Freud himself. From this we verify that the Preyer books did belong to Freud. (See EISSLER, K. R. Eine Berichtigung zur Geschichte Der Bibliothek Freuds. American Elsevier Pub. Co. New York, N.Y. In press.

14. FROESCHELS, E. Language Development and Aphasia in Children. R. W. Rieber, Ed. New York, N.Y. In press. A new translation of Kindersprache und Aphasie. 1918. Springer-Verlag. New York, N.Y., Vienna, Austria.
15. See Muller, M. 1909. Three Introductory Lectures on the Science of Thought. Open Court. Chicago, Ill.
16. See Ref. 15. Thought Without Words: 4.
17. See Ref. 15. Thought Without Words: 15.

PSYCHOLINGUISTICS SINCE THE TURN OF THE CENTURY*

Doris Aaronson

Department of Psychology
New York University
New York, New York 10003

I will continue where Dr. Rieber left off, and describe some of the highlights of psycholinguistics since the turn of the century. Since that time there have been two major theoretical approaches, and methodological approaches closely coupled with them, which were often at odds: empiricism and rationalism. At times one of these approaches attracted psychologists and the other attracted linguists. More frequently, however, interdisciplinary subgroups engaged in philosophical battles against each other. The empiricists postulated molecular components comprising language and thought. Their research was concerned with associations between verbal units, and with the translations of sensations of the enviornment into the muscular responses involved in speech. They ingeniously developed some of the most important experimental apparatus and methods, such as tachistoscopes to present linguistic segments, which were believed to be "molecules," for brief slices of time; and eye-movement recording equipment to provide indices of elemental processes during reading. The rationalists, on the other hand, were concerned with the innate properties giving rise to global events, with holistic ideas comprising entire sentences, and with internal mental states and processes. Their research tools were more generally those of logic and introspection, and they developed some of the more important theoretical ideas.

The leader of the rationalists from about 1880 to 1920 was Wilhelm Wundt. He might easily be called the father of the interdisciplinary study of language, as he himself contributed as a psychologist, linguist, philosopher, physiologist, philologist, and anthropologist. Although many consider him the father of modern experimental psychology, his tools for the study of language were mainly logic and intuition. He felt that language and other higher mental processes could not be studied by the experimental procedures of the natural sciences, but that knowledge of the mind must be inferred from theory. His theoretical ideas concerning higher mental processes are actively discussed today, and included concepts such as preattentive processes, attention span, creative synthesis, and rhythmical grouping. Complementing Wundt's research on the structure of language was his less-known work on congition and affect, which resulted in a three-dimensional classification of fundamental feelings: pleasantness-unpleasantness, stain-relaxation, and activity-passivity. This approach is strikingly similar to recent work of Osgood and his colleagues, who used the "semantic differential" to measure meaning.

Regarding language development, Wundt stated that the infant is born with psychological and physical traits favorable to the reception of language. Based on daily observations of his own two children for sixteen months, and on his studies of untrained deaf-mutes, he concluded that language acquistion involved a good deal of spontaneity and creativity within the child. Imitation and habit under environmental influence played a secondary role. In addition to his contributions in psychology, Wundt also initiated many of the ideas found in today's linguistic journals. For example, in 1880,

*Supported in part by grant MH16,496 from the National Institute of Mental Health to New York University, New York, N.Y.

his book *Logik* employed tree-diagrams to describe the relations among the components of words and sentences. Throughout his work he was concerned with the psychological reality of his more formally described linguistic components. He followed many of Humboldt's ideas that related the "inner linguistic form" or deep structure of ideas and ideals to the "outer linguistic form" or surface structure of phonemes and syntax. These psychological relations, according to Wundt's work on memory and concept formation, were based on mental principles or rules for regenerating past experiences. Indeed, Wundt's approach to linguistics and psycholinguistics shares much with that of Chomsky, and with many of the participants in this conference.

The empiricist opponents to Wundt included a group of neogrammarians (*Junggrammatiker*) at Leipzig. They emphasized data collection and empirical laws. They maintained that languages must be studied as "natural objects" and they opposed complex theory construction. One of their leaders was Hermann Paul, a follower of Herbart. In contrast to Wundt, Paul felt that linguistics should be descriptive and historical. Paul fought heatedly with Wundt over what we refer to today as the competence-performance distinction. Paul maintained that verbal expression was isomorphic to mental constructs; that sentences were produced as associations between individual words; and that children learned language by analogy and association. Paul antedated Skinner's reinforcement approach to language acqisition in suggesting that children's earliest utterances, even single-word utterances, are "demand" sentences in reference to their needs, and "command" sentences to interact with their environment.[1]

At about the same time, Clara and William Stern, students of Ebbinghaus, also leaned toward an empiricist approach, postulating that children have an environmentally influenced "speech need." However, along with Wundt, the Sterns felt that language acquisition involved a combination of spontaneity and imitation. Their book, *Die Kindersprache*, (1907) included descriptions of their daily observations of their two children for six years. As investigators are doing today, the Sterns noted the gestures and environmentally oriented responses that accompanied "one-word sentences." They also discussed some of the child's syntactic strutures, such as negations, questions, and clauses, as well as the development of word forms and semantic categories. The Sterns were concerned with individual differences in language development and with special linguistic problems of children such as phonetic distortions, sound development, elliptical constructions, and original creations.[2] The Sterns' work was more linguistically sophisticated than Pryer's earlier work discussed by Dr. Rieber, and was an important influence in Europe following Pryer's major initial contributions.

During this time period, an important trend toward empiricism and behaviorism was also developing in America. This trend dominated much of psychology, and linguistics until the 1950s. In the study of thought and language, the theoretical ideas of William James were often romantic and imprecise, and were presented in terms of specific concrete examples rather than formal logic. According to James, although the sentence as a whole is the appropriate psychological unit of analysis, its conscious processing is done in a set of time segments, with a serially ordered mapping between the thought stream and the stimulus words. Although he was willing to consider data from many methods of investigation, including introspection, experimentation, and comparisons across species, James was quick to point out flaws in these methods which he attributed to the theoretical biases of the experimenter. In his book, *Principles of Psychology* (1890), James referred to Wundt's formal psychophysical methods as "microscopic psychology ... asking of course every moment for introspective data." He stated critically, "This method taxes patience to the utmost, and could hardly have arisen in a country whose natives could be bored."[3] Wundt, in turn, criticized James' book by saying, "It is literature, it is beautiful, but it is not psychology."[4]

In other American laboratories, frequency counts of individual words and of speech categories proliferated in the study of vocabulary growth in children. During this time, E. L. Thorndike at Columbia provided massive word counts for the vocabularies of children and adults. G. K. Zipf, trained in part at Harvard, published a wide variety of word-frequency distributions in his book, *The Psycho-biology of Language* (1935), providing some of the groundwork for the mathematical information theory analyses of language and communication. Such frequency data were also used to plot empirical correlations between language development and other psychological and physiological functions. For example, in 1919 Clark and Bertha Hull wrote a paper on relations between increases in vocabulary and bladder control in children. In an empiricist tradition, Harvard's Floyd Henry Alport described language acquisition in his book *Social Psychology* (1924) as based on chained reflexes which develop from random articulation by conditioning, imitation, and practice, in response to environmental stimuli. He was concerned with language disabilities, for example, in deaf children, where ear-vocal reflexes could not develop, and were replaced by eye-vocal reflexes.

Within the behaviorist tradition, psychologists and educators intensely studied the learning of reading skills. Surprisingly, some of this empirical orientation stemmed directly from Wundt's students. For example, G. Stanley Hall, Wundt's first American student, established a laboratory for child development at Clark University. Then, Edmund Burke Huey, a student of Hall, developed much of the work on "automatization of function" in children's reading. Another student of Wundt, James McKeen Cattell, studied the perceptual units involved in reading tachistoscopically presented words and nonsense syllables.

The behaviorist orientation was most strongly and fully developed by B. F. Skinner at Harvard. He followed the lead set by Watson early in this century, in maintaining that human language behavior was based on the same stimulus-response principles as animal behavior. Skinner's work on *Verbal Behavior* (1957), which was begun in the 1930s, provides the foundation for important research on language learning in children that will be discussed by several of our conference participants today.

Simultaneously, a strong behaviorist orientation was also developing among the linguists. Leonard Bloomfield, who studied at Leipzig, developed the taxonomic study of language in his 1933 book *Language*. Zellig Harris continued the Bloomfield efforts at the University of Pennsylvania, putting forth important procedures for segmenting and classifying speech elements in his 1951 book, *Methods in Structural Linguistics*.

However, Harris' own student, Noam Chomsky, was responsible for a return to rationalism and mentalism and a major revolution in the trends of linguistic theories with his development of generative transformational grammars. His books, *Syntactic Structures* in 1957, and *Aspects of the Theory of Syntax* in 1965, provide the theoretical foundation for much of the research that our panelists will discuss at this conference. Simultaneously, and in close communication with Chomsky, George A. Miller, at Harvard, was developing psychological theories that incorporated hypotheses about complex mental operations in language perception and production. Miller's work included rich expansions of some of Karl Lashley's earlier notions on integrative processes in language comprehension. Miller and his students were responsible for developing many of the important experimental procedures used to test these cognitive theories of human language abilities.

Much of the research presented at our conference by both psychologists and linguists will concern the grounds on which the behavioral and mentalistic approaches can be fruitfully combined, and those areas in which there are still sharp conflicts.

ACKNOWLEDGMENTS

I thank Lloyd Kaufman for helpful comments on an earlier draft of this paper.

REFERENCES

1. Based on BLUMENTHAL, A. L. 1970. Language and Psychology: Historical Aspects of Psycho-linguistics. John Wiley & Sons Inc. New York, N.Y.
2. Based on excerpts from STERNS' *Die Kindersprache*. 1907. Translated by Jim Lyon and A. L. Blumenthal. Language and Psychology: Historical Aspects of Psycholinguistics. John Wiley & Sons Inc. New York, N.Y.
3. From JAMES, W. 1890. The Principles of Psychology. Chap. VII. Henry Holt and Co. New York, N.Y.
4. BLUMENTHAL, A. L. 1970. Language and Psychology: Historical Aspects of Psycholinguistics. John Wiley & Sons Inc. New York, N.Y.

A DINOSAUR CAPER:
PSYCHOLINGUISTICS PAST, PRESENT, AND FUTURE

Charles E. Osgood

Department of Psychology
University of Illinois
Urbana, Illinois 61801

My theme for pyscholinguistics over the past quarter-century is frankly *marital*—engagement, abduction, marriage, divorce, and reconciliation. Since interpretation of this history is inevitably personal, an introspective little dinosaur (there were little dinosaurs, you know) will, of necessity, be the main character. But first . . .

A Confession and an Awakening

The baby dinosaur was teethed on Meaning by a dentist grandfather who had always wanted to be a professor. This baby was fed rare words and then given pennies to buy other goodies when he used them correctly in sentences. Around the age of ten, his aunt gave him Roget's *Thesaurus*, and he vividly remembers having recursive dreams about multicolored, jellybean-like, word-points distributed in clusters all about an endless space.

The *Thesaurus* came in very handy, and after editing and writing for his high school newspaper and magazine, he went off to college convinced that he was destined to become, not a dinosaur, but a newspaper man and novelist. But under Ted Karwoski at Dartmouth, and later an old dinosaur at Yale named Clark Hull, he found what he wanted: a focus on meaning within a field, psychology, that seemed to offer the right balance between rigor and creativity. The year 1950 found him at Illinois, busily at work on both the (learning theory) nature of meaning and the (semantic differential technique) measurement of certain aspects of it.

Now the confession: at this time—except for the work of Charles Morris in semiotics—this young dinosaur didn't have the foggiest idea of what scholars in other fields were thinking and doing about language and meaning. Specifically, as to linguistics, he had only the vague notion that these were strange, bearded, bird-like creatures who inhabited the remoter regions of libraries, babbling away in many exotic languages and constructing dictionaries for them—hardly fit companions for a robust, rigorous, and objective young dinosaur! The a-linguistic state of his awareness is evident from a perusal of the last chapter (title, "Language Behavior") of his graduate text, *Method and Theory in Experimental Psychology* (1953);[1] it is devoid of reference to the works of linguistics (the possible exception being Benjamin Lee Whorf).

His awakening came in the summer of 1951 when—sparked by Jack Carroll (attuned to linguistics by virtue of his tutelage under Whorf) and supported by John W. Gardiner (a psychologist, then with the Carnegie Corporation of New York, and later to become secretary of HEW, and still later organizer of Common Cause)—the Social Science Research Council sponsored a summer conference of linguists and psychologists at Cornell University. By some fluke—perhaps because he had just been awarded an SSRC Research Fellowship for support of the semantic differential work—the youthful dinosaur was invited to participate and—frankly, in part because of the attractiveness of a summer in the hills and by the lakes of Ithaca—he

16

readily accepted. (I often wonder how the course of my own scientific life would have run if this "fluke," and all that followed from it, had not happened.) In any case, that summer was an eye-opener: not only were the linguistics there *neither* polyglots nor lexicographers, but they *were* robust, rigorous, and objective, maybe even a bit more so than the young dinosaur!

As a result of that summer's meeting, the SSRC established a new Committee on Linguistics and Psychology in October of 1952. The initial membership was as follows: Charles E. Osgood (psychologist and first of a series of rotating chairmen); John B. Carroll (psychologist, Harvard); Floyd Lounsbury (ethnolinguist, Yale); George A. Miller (psychologist, M.I.T.); and Thomas A. Sebeok (linguist, Indiana). Joseph H. Greenberg (ethnolinguist, Columbia) and James J. Jenkins (psychologist, Minnesota) were added in the fall of 1953. This turned out to be a very lively little committee.

THE ENGAGEMENT

One of the first steps taken by this new Committee was to plan and sponsor a research seminar on psycholinguistics, this being held during the summer of 1953 on the campus of Indiana University, when and where, not by chance, the Linguistic Institute was also having its summer session. In his foreword to the monograph that resulted from this seminar (*Psycholinguistics: A Survey of Theory and Research Problems*, 1954),[2] John Gardner says, correctly, that the seminar "... set itself to the task of examining three different approaches to the language process [and their relationships]: (1) the linguist's conception of language as a structure of systematically interrelated units, (2) the learning theorist's conception of language as a system of habits relating signs to behavior, and (3) the information theorist's conception of language as a means of transmitting information ... [as well as] to examine a variety of research problems in psycholinguistics with a view to developing possible experimental approaches to them." (p. x)

According to one impartial chronicler, A. Richard Diebold, Jr. (writing in 1965),[3] "within a year or two of its appearance, this monograph became the charter for psycholinguistics, firmly establishing the discipline's name. It so successfully piqued the interest of linguistics and other behavioral scientists that the volume itself was soon out of print, and also became notoriously difficult to obtain second-hand, or even in libraries." (p. 208) And he notes that one of the graduate-student participants, Sol Saporta, was in 1961 to edit the first "... long-awaited reader, *Psycholinguistics: A Book of Readings* ... [which was] also a testament to the fact that there [was] an ever-growing number of university courses variously titled 'psychology of language,' 'psycholinguistics,' 'linguistic psychology,' etc." (p. 208) According to another observer, Howard Maclay (1973),[4] "The Formative Period was characterized by extremely good relations between psychologists and linguists. This happy state of affairs had two major sources: a common commitment to an operationalist philosophy of science, and a division of labor that prevented a number of potential difficulties from becoming overt ... linguists were assigned the 'states of messages,' while psychologists assumed responsibility for the 'states of communicators' and also, by default, 'the processes of encoding and decoding.'" (pp. 570–71)

The thrust of the continuing SSRC Committee on Linguistics and Psychology is evident in the other projects and seminars it supported during the 1950's: a "Southwest Project on *Comparative Psycholinguistics*" (centered at the University of New Mexico, summer, 1954); a conference on *Bilingualism* (Columbia University, 1954); another conference on *Techniques of Content Analysis* (University of Illinois,

1955); yet another on *Associative Processes in Verbal Behavior* (University of Minnesota, 1955); yet another on *Dimensions of Meaning—Analytic and Experimental Approaches* (1956) (it was at this one that our dinosaur first met young Noam Chomsky and got the impression that he was brilliant, but, alas!, *not* convinced that meaning was the central problem for students of language); a very impressive, large-scale conference on *Style in Language* organized by Tom Sebeok (Indiana University, 1958); a summer seminar on *The Psycholinguistics of Aphasia* (Boston Veterans Administration Hospital, 1958); and a conference on *Language Universals* (Dobbs Ferry, N. Y., 1961).

Ah, happy, eager dinosaur! Now reaching maturity, he had participated in the full kaleidoscope of these SSRC activities, and Spring was turning into what *had* to be a Golden Summer. He was also very busy in his own daisy patch at Illinois. There was a series of theoretical papers elaborating his own version of Neobehaviorism and its relevance for understanding human perceptual, motivational and semantic processes, in general as well as in language behavior per se. There was a *Psychological Bulletin* article titled "The Nature and measurement of Meaning" (1952)[5]—which demonstrated the abject wrong-headedness, of course, of everything psychologists had previously done in trying to measure this elusive thing. And there was a rather well-kept secret, titled "Cognitive Dynamics in the Conduct of Human Affairs," published in the *Public Opinion Quarterly* (1960)[6]—which was an excursion into the dynamics of congruence and incongruence ("psycho-logic") in human thinking and sentencing.

In these days, when so much of research is "administered"—senior people like myself having practically nothing to do with it between original designing and terminal writing-up—it is a real pleasure to look back on those early days at Illinois when we literally lived and breathed our research from morning to night. I used to be my own first "guinea pig" in every experiment (not impossible for a *small* dinosaur!), to try to get a feel for what might go on in the heads of real subjects. In the midst of doing one experiment, others were always aborning—over coffee, over sandwiches and beer, and even over cocktails and dinner, much to the amusement, but never irritation, of our spice. I am minded of an enlarged photograph on the wall of my office which caught Percy Tennenbaum and myself, glasses in hand, in animated midflight over something or other—and a caption had been appended, reading "BUT THERE *MUST* BE A MEDIATION PROCESS!" Al Heyer and I spent an hilarious weekend, practically without sleep, constructing a monstrous three-dimensional distance model with colored balls and wooden dowels to represent the meaningful similarities among forty facial expressions of emotions. I still have that old model in my office, but ANGER and BITTERNESS have fallen off, and SURPRISE has somehow gotten attached to ADORATION—by a bemused janitor, no doubt.

Meanwhile, the little group of psycholinguistics at Illinois was busily pushing the developing Semantic Differential Technique (SD for short) into various nooks and crannies of the social sciences. In the summer of 1955 dinosaur and family took off on its first sabbatical, in Tucson, Arizona. Packed into the trunk of our second-hand Buick Roadmaster (freshly painted in Dartmouth Green) was everything psychological about meaning and the measurement thereof that he could put his hands on. The sabbatical job was to put all the SD work into one document. As each section was completed, it would be whipped off to George Suci and Percy Tannenbaum, now the dinosaur's closest colleagues in this exploration of semantic space. *The Measurement of Meaning*[7] was published in 1957. To the enduring amazement of Osgood, Suci, and Tannenbaum, this little book proved to be one of the best-sellers on the University of Illinois Press list. It also got some solid reviewing—by psycholinguist Roger Brown ("Is a Boulder Sweet or Sour?"), by linguist Uriel Weinreich ("Travels through Semantic Space"), by psycholinguist John Carroll, who at least concluded by asserting "it is *good*, it is *active*, it is *potent*"—thus plusses on all three affective factors!

But by the end of the 1950's the distant mutterings of a scientific revolution were in the air, impelled by Chomsky's generative and transformational grammar, certainly in linguistics and possibly in cognitive psychology, too. In the preface to his *Psycholinguistics* (1961),[8] Sol Saporta was to say: ". . . all attempts by psychologists to describe 'grammaticality' exclusively in terms of habit strength [etc.] . . . seem inadequate . . . to account for some of the most obvious facts of language." (p. v) In 1959 Chomsky[9] wrote a carefully documented and scathing review of Skinner's *Verbal Behavior* (1957)[10]—never responded to by Skinner himself—and this was to have cumulative impact on may psycholinguists. Perhaps because our dinosaur was confidently mature, had a much more complex behavior theory, and, indeed, had written a highly critical review of Skinner himself,[11] he was not particularly disturbed and kept right on nuzzling among and munching away at his semantic daisies.

THE MARRIAGE

While the mature dinosaur was at the Center in Palo Alto in 1958-59, George Miller, Eugene Galanter and Karl Pribram were also there and were working on their *Plans and the Structure of Behavior*, to be published in 1960;[12] it was heavily influenced by Chomsky and included a chapter on "Plans for Speaking." This was followed by Miller's important paper titled "Some Psychological Studies of Grammar" (1962)[13] and soon thereafter by a small flood of papers by Miller, his students, and others testing the psychological reality (in terms of effects upon processing time, memory and the like) of grammatical structures and transformations. The consumation of this intimate relation between linguistics and psychology was symbolized by two chapters in the *Handbook of Mathematical Psychology* (1963),[14] written jointly by Chomsky and Miller: "Introduction to the Formal Analysis of Natural Languages" (Chomsky and Miller) and "Finitary Models of Language Users" (Miller and Chomsky).

The distant mutterings of revolution were becoming heavy rumblings of immanent paradigm clash. In concluding their debate with Martin Braine over the learning of grammatical ordering of words in sentences, Bever, Fodor and Weksel (1965)[15] felt themselves able to say: "As the empirical basis for assuming an abstract underlying structure in language becomes broader and the explanatory power of that assumption becomes deeper, *we recommend to all psychologists that they seriously question the adequacy of any theory of learning that cannot account for the fact that such structures are acquired.*" (p. 500, italics theirs, not mine).

By the middle 1960's even the middle-aged dinosaur in his Illinois daisy patch was beginning to eye the ominous storm with some concern. But he was still eager and busy, and—as such things are measured—he was successful in his profession and therefore quite confident. So early in 1963 he began to worry about what he should say to his fellow psychologists in his presidential address. He went through a period of intense ambivalence about this: on the one hand, since his year at the Center at Palo Alto he'd been giving top priority to strategies of international relations in a nuclear age and he knew that most of his potential audience expected a tough policy speech on this major social issue; on the other hand, he felt a strong urge to follow the tradition of most past presidents of APA and talk about the most crucial scientific issues in his own specialty, even if to a much smaller audience as far as concern or comprehension were concerned. He took the latter course, and the title of his address,[16] "On Understanding and Creating Sentences," indicates what he thought was the most crucial issue for psycholinguistics at that time.

Oh, how the dinosaur worked on that APA address! By the middle of the summer of 1963 (and only a few weeks before the convention) he had pounded out a small book of 204 double-spaced pages—that had to be paired down to about 36 deliverable pages! The full version was never published—he was not really satisfied with it—but much of it was predictive of the path he would be following through the next decade.

By 1966 the conflict between competing psycholinguistic paradigms had reached what Thomas Kuhn (1962)[17] terms the "crisis" stage in scientific revolutions. Fodor (1965)[18] had published a paper titled "Could Meaning Be an r_m?", explicitly aimed at O. Hobart Mowrer but obviously including me, to which I replied (Osgood, 1966);[19] it claimed to reduce neobehaviorist two-stage mediation theories to single-stage Skinnerian theory, hence rendering them heir to all of the inadequacies claimed by Chomsky (1959).[9] In the spring of 1966, at the University of Kentucky, there was a conference with an innocent-enough sounding topic, *Verbal Behavior and General Behavior Theory*. This was published in 1968 under the same title (Dixon and Horton, editors).[20] Particularly in the session on Psycholinguistics, the prepared papers by "revolutionaries" Bever, Fodor, Garrett, and McNeill constituted a frontal attack on behaviorism and associationism generally. As discussant of these papers, I found myself in the unfamiliar and unenviable role of defending The Establishment. The title of my discussion, "Toward a Wedding of Insufficiencies," is indicative of my ambivalence in this role. And I was beginning to realize that I *was* a dinosaur!

There is not time here to go into any detailed analysis of scientific revolutions (however, see Volume III of my *Focus on Meaning* being published by Mouton),[21] but I have come to the conclusion that, although the impact of Chomsky on linguistics was certainly a revolution in Kuhnian terms, this has not been the case for his impact upon cognitive psychology (or even psycholinguistics). Why? Because it has not met the criteria that distinguish revolutions from mere pendula swings in the competition between viable paradigms: (1) there has been no attempt to incorporate solutions to problems successfully handled by the old paradigm; (2) the old paradigm has not been shown to be insufficient *in principle*;[21] (3) there has been no new paradigm to shift *to*—in the sense of a well-motivated, internally coherent alternative theory of language performance. There has been a shift *away from* behaviorism in any form, but in the absence of any alternative paradigm this would be better termed "revulsion" than "revolution."

Maclay (1973, p. 579)[4] notes that the responses of ". . . psychologists who had a vested interest in research on language . . . fell into the three familiar categories of AVOIDANCE, CONVERSION, and COMPROMISE . . . their overwhelming response was conversion . . . (*and*) the quasi-religious nature of scientific conversion required that those who had seen the light should condemn everything connected with the erroneous views they had previously held." Maclay also points out (pp. 579–80) that in a clash between paradigms the middle ground becomes very insecure, and he very kindly comments that "Osgood was the only major psychologist who continued to take linquistics seriously but who rejected some of its implications for psycholinguistics . . . (*particularly*) the assumption of the centrality of grammar. While acknowledging the success of transformationalism as a linguistic theory and insisting that his students be trained in linguistics, he continued to argue that a revised version of behavior theory was, at the least, an essential component of an adequate *psycho*linguistic theory."

But nevertheless it was a rather lonesome dinosaur who kept offering his daisies at the shrine of a near-deserted (even if still viable) paradigm in the late 1960's. The old fellow even sent some of his best students (after helping guide them to their Ph.D.'s) to serve at the shrine of the opposing paradigm at M.I.T.—Merle Garrett and then, for briefer periods, Ken Forster and John Limber. But this period was another busy one on the home grounds, and the dinosaur didn't have much time to brood about possible paradigms lost. For one thing, the extension of the SD technique cross-culturally had begun in 1960, and the number of communities involved around the world increased steadily from 6 to about 25 during that decade. Another major thrust was toward development of an objective semantic feature discovery-procedure other than the semantic differential—a "semantic interaction technique," in which the appositeness, permissibility, or anomaly of words in syntactic combination (e.g. $^!$*plead with humbly,* ^{o}*plead with sincerely,* **plead with tolerantly*) were judged by native speakers and the pattern of judgments analyzed factorially to infer the features operating (cf. Osgood, 1970a, 1970b).[22,23]

DISILLUSION AND DIVORCE

The marriage between linguistics and psycholinguistics in the 1960's might better have been called an *elopement*—or perhaps even an *abduction*—because it was a very one-sided affair. The intuitions of generative linguistics were to provide a theory of Competence and the wifely psychologists were to cook up experiments on Performance designed to demonstrate empirically the validity of such a theory of how the mind works in sentencing. This presumed a direct Correspondence Hypothesis—that the derivational history of a sentence corresponds step by step to the sequence of psychological operations executed when a person processes the sentence. (I might note that in an oft-quoted (recently) footnote, Chomsky himself (1961)[24] early stated that this is an "utterly mistaken view.") Learning a language was equated with the acquisition of its syntax, and semantics took a back seat. Since it seemed inconceivable that such an incredibly complex capability as a transformational grammar could be learned in the incredibly short period of three or four years, it was assumed that much of it must be innate—universal to humans and specific to language.

Although the early psycholinguistic studies of sentence processing by George Miller (1962)[13] and his students and associates seemed to give credence to such a Correspondence Hypothesis, even by the mid-60's sufficient contrary evidence had accumulated to lead Fodor and Garrett (1966, p. 162)[34] to say "... an acceptable theory of the relation between competence and performance models will have to represent that relation as abstract, the degree of abstractness being proportional to the failure of formal features of derivations to correspond to performance variables." In the absence of *any* characterization of this "abstract" relation, of course, all this does is to remove any competence grammar from the danger of being disconfirmed by performance data.

The denouement of the Competence/Performance distinction, in my opinion, came at a symposium on *Cognition and the Development of Language* held in 1968 at Carnegie-Mellon University, the papers being subsequently published under the same title in 1970 (Hayes, editor),[25] particularly in the contributions of William C. Watt ("On Two Hypotheses Concerning Psycholinguistics") and Thomas G. Bever ("The Cognitive Basis for Linguistic Structures"). Watt first demolished (to his satisfaction, as well as mine) the hypothesis that a Competence Grammar, derived from the intuitions of linguists, could be isomorphic with what he terms a deeper Mental Grammar—i.e., that Competence could describe how the mind works in understanding and creating sentences; he then proposes the hypothesis that what he terms an Abstract Performance Grammar (APG) must be isomorphic with the deeper Mental Grammar—and although he is rather vague about the nature of this APG, it is clear that a theory of "how the mind works in sentencing" is to come from abstracting about the performances of speakers, particularly children. The main theme of Bever's paper was that Performance, at least in part, determines ultimate linguistic Competence; "many aspects of adult language derive from the interaction of grammar with the child's processes of learning and using language," (p. 280), and after demonstrating this in a variety of language-processing situations, he concludes that we must ". . . reject the claim that a linguistic grammar is in any sense internal to such linguistic performances as talking and listening." (p. 344)

RECONCILIATION AND REENGAGEMENT

Needless to say, the elderly dinosaur was following these developments with great interest, and even the casual observer could see the brightening gleam in his eye and the increasing vigor with which he flicked his tail. By the early 1970's he had discovered a new field of semantic daisies—ones that grew in a wondrous variety of little bands made up of chains of linked blooms—and he fed upon them with relish while he refurbished and expanded the shrine for his paradigm. The denouement of the Competence/Performance distinction had paved the way (some might say, paradoxically) for a new, more balanced, and potentially very productive relation between linguists and psycholinguists in what Maclay (1973)[4] has called The Cognitive Period of the 1970's.

The Reengagement is along rather different lines than the earlier Engagement: Linguists are becoming more concerned with *semantics* (cf. papers by Lakoff, Fillmore, and Bierwisch in the Steinberg and Jakobovits collection, *Semantics*, 1971)[26]— in fact, one can say that the thrust of the new Generative Semantics is to put the semantic horse back in front of the syntactic cart—and concerned with the necessity of dealing with the cognitive processes underlying the *presuppositions* of sentences (cf. papers by Lakoff, Langendoen, and the Kiparskys in the same volume) and even with the role of *nonlinguistic, contextual factors* in the ordinary conversational use of language. Psycholinguists, while becoming more sophisticated about transformational grammar, are also shifting focus from the syntax to the semantics of sentencing, as well as beginning to recognize the basic fact that the strategies for cognizing sentences have their origins in prelinguistic perceptuomotor cognizing—as well-illustrated in papers by the Clarks (Eve and Herb), Samuel Fillenbaum, Charles Perfetti, and many others in the early 1970's.

These developments have been driven by the disconfirmation of the Correspondence Hypothesis, by the nonappearance of any alternative psychological paradigm for Performance, and by the appearance of a new breed of psycholinguist—one trained and about equally competent in both fields, rather than having the alter field "grafted" on like a second language (as was the case for dinosaurs of all subspecies).

And in the Midwest this old dinosaur and his companions have also been moving happily into the new relationship. He contributed a paper titled "Where Do Sentences Come From?" to the same Steinberg-Jakobovits collection;[26] his main point was to demonstrate that there is an intimate interaction between nonlinguistic and linguistic channels in the process of Simply Describing ordinary events, and hence that these channels must share some deeper cognitive level that cannot, in principle, be characterized by purely *linguistic* constructs and rules. With one of his friends, Meredith Richards, he even invaded the heartland of the linguistic domain by publishing an article in *Language* (Osgood & Richards, 1973)[27] titled "From Yang and Yin to *And* or *But*," in which laws of cognitive congruence and incongruence were used to predict the discriminative use of these conjunctions in simple conjoined sentences of the form X is ADJ₁ ___ ADJ₂ ___(e.g. X *is sweet* ___ *kind* or *X is cowardly* ___ *honest*)—frames which, linguistically speaking, will accept either *and* or *but*.

In the spring of 1972, back from several long trips around the world in connection with the continuing cross-cultural project—which is becoming something like a dinosaur having a bear by the tail!—what we call our Cog Group at Illinois began to hold regular idea-suggesting and critiquing sessions. We are trying to build a fresh conception of "where sentences come from and go to"—or, going back to Watt's notions, you could say that we are trying to build an Abstract Performance Grammar on psychological as well as linguistic bases. These Cog Group sessions have been exciting for the old dinosaur, downright rejuvenating, in fact. And they've been good intellectual fun for all—particularly, I guess, when the old fellow tries to put his baby booties back on and intuit how his prelinguistic world was structured cognitively!

A number of doctoral theses and other research papers have already been generated by the Cog Group sessions, but only a few examples must suffice. Rumjahn Hoosain's thesis (1973)[28] confirmed the prediction that cognitions ("cogs" for short) encoded from the perceptual channel (e.g. pairs of outline faces to be conjoined by *and* or *but*) as well as cogs *across* perceptual and linguistic channels (e.g. SMILING FACE *and*/*but* "I flunked the exam") will display the same processing dynamics as do conjoined sentential cogs—namely, that affectively positive signs will be easier to handle than negative (the Yang and Yin of things) and that congruent cogs will be easier than incongruent (Psychologic). In her thesis, Gordana Opačić (1973)[29] explored the dynamics of conjoining sentential cognitions in different modes (Simple Junction, Sequence, Cause, and Intention in various combinations) and verified predictions based on a "Naturalness" principle—that, in a production task, clauses will be ordered according to the usual sequences of perceived events in (intuited) *pre*linguistic experience.

Working with S-complement sentences, Richard Harris (1974)[30] compared Logicolinguistic predictions (cf. the Kiparskys' paper above)[26] with those from Invited Inference and psycho-logical Congruence theories (the latter two being essentially identical); wherever predictions differed (e.g. for Nonfactual S-complement sentences), the results clearly favored psycho-logical as against logical models. Putting on his prelinguistic booties also led the old dinosaur to the radical notion that what has traditionally been called the Indirect Object is in cognitive reality the underlying Direct Object (that is, what the young child *perceives* is THE BOY/GAVE-A-TOY-TO/THE GIRL), and with Chris Tanz and some assistance from Joseph Greenberg and Phil Sedlak at Stanford, he is busily exploring this hypothesis.

THE FUTURE OF PSYCHOLINGUISTICS?

Predicting the future of any field is eminently personal (note the *but-not* signal of incongruity in the sentence, *some say that psycholinguistics will become more firmly based upon logic, but that is not my expectation*), so I leave the doddering dinosaur contentedly weaving his daisy chains and take full credit for my own biases. As we move toward the Year 2000:

(1) *There will be a complete shift from emphasis upon Competence to emphasis upon Performance.* This is already well under way, in linguistics as well as psycholinguistics, and in my crystal ball I can see the point approaching in the not-too-

distant future where correspondence to Performance principles will be the prime criterion for selecting among alternative grammars.

(2) As part of this shift, *there will be an increasing avoidance of dealing with sentences-in-isolation* (whether in linguistic or psychological methodologies) *and increasing dependence upon sentences-in-context* (in discourse, in ordinary conversation, and so on). This is already heralded in the rapid development of sociolinguistics and in the work of Bransford et al.,[31] Brewer,[32] and others on "memory for ideas."

(3) *Semantics will be moving into the foreground as syntax moves, reciprocally, into the background.* There is already serious questioning of the need for any syntactic deep structure, and I think that, as generative semanticists in linguistics and generative cognitivists in psychology elaborate their positions, the semantic "component" will gradually replace syntactic deep structure and generative syntax will become pretty much restricted to transformations upon semantic information.

(4) As I have already hinted, *logical, rationalist models of language will be shown to be inappropriate for ordinary speakers and will be superceded by more gutsy, dynamic psycho-logical models.* Humans have always tried to deny their close affinity to animals, even their close primate relatives, but—as what's going on in the Middle East, in Ireland, in Boston (you name it!) should make obvious—we *are* a kind of animal and the basic dynamics of our thinking are not the logics a few among us have achieved but the primitive psycho-logics that we share with other animals. If we could accept this, and act accordingly, I think we'd have a better chance of survival.

(5) *There will be a shift from ethno-lingo-centrism toward what might appropriately be called anthropo-linguo-centrism.* Just as Latin dominated the formulation of most tradition grammars, so has American English dominated the formulation of modern generative grammars—even when the linguists may be native speakers of other languages. Questions about language universals, at all levels, require *cross-linguistic data matrices* for their answers and—congruently expressing my bias—our Center for Comparative Psycholinguistics is now working across a matrix of 30 human language-culture communities around the world. Of course, we are not alone by any means in this particular bias; witness the work of the Stanford Universals Project and of Dan Slobin and his group at Berkeley.[33]

Will there be a *re*-marriage of linguistics and cognitive psychology by the Year 2000? I rather think there will. It will probably take the form of new departments of, say, Psycho-linguistics and Socio-linguistics—*new* departments because the psychos in Linguistics and the Linguos in Psychology will find more in common with each other than with their own departmental colleagues. *But all this presupposes that there will be a Mankind 2000,* and I must confess that I am not too sanguine about the prospect.

But I see that our old dinosaur, wrapped in his daisy chains, has fallen sound asleep . . . .

REFERENCES

1. OSGOOD, C. E. 1953. Method and Theory in Experimental Psychology. Oxford University Press. New York, N.Y.
2. OSGOOD, C. E. & T. A. SEBEOK, Eds. 1954. Psycholinguistics: A Survey of Theory and Research Problems. J. Abn. Soc. Psychol. 49; Internat. J. Amer. Ling. Memoir 10.
3. DIEBOLD, A. R. Jr. 1965. A survey of psycholinguistic research, 1954–1964. *In* Psycholinguistics: A Survey of Theory and Research Problems. (Reissue). University of Indiana Press. Bloomington, Ind.

4. MACLAY, H. 1973. Linguistics and psycholinuistics. *In* Issues in Linguistics: Papers in Honor of Henry and Renée Kahane. B. Kachru *et al.*, Eds. University of Illinois Press. Urbana, Ill.

5. OSGOOD, E. C. 1952. The nature and measurement of meaning. Psychol. Bull. **49**: 197–237.

6. OSGOOD, C. E. 1960. Cognitive dynamics in the conduct of human affairs. Pub. Opin. Quart. **24**: 341–365.

7. OSGOOD, C. E., C. J. SUCI & P. H. TANNENBAUM. 1957. The Measurement of Meaning. University of Illinois Press. Urbana, Ill.

8. SAPORTA, S. 1961. Psycholinguistics: A Book of Readings. Holt, Rinehart & Winston. New York, N.Y.

9. CHOMSKY, N. 1959. Review of *Verbal Behavior* by B. F. Skinner. Lang. **35**: 26–58.

10. SKINNER, B. F. 1957. Verbal Behavior. Appleton-Century-Crofts. New York, N.Y.

11. OSGOOD, C. E. 1958. A question of sufficiency. Review of B. F. Skinner, *Verbal Behavior*. Contemp. Psychol. **3**: 209–212.

12. MILLER, G. A., E. GALANTER & K.H. PRIBRAM. 1960. Plans and the Structure of Behavior. Holt-Dryden. New York, N.Y.

13. MILLER, G. A. 1962. Some psychological studies of grammar. Amer. Psychol. **17**: 748–762.

14. LUCE, R. D., R. R. BUSH & E. GALANTER, Eds. 1963. Handbook of Mathematical Psychology. John Wiley & Sons Inc. New York, N.Y.

15. BEVER, T. G., J. A. FODOR & W. WEKSEL. 1965. Theoretical notes on the acquisition of syntax: a critique of "contextual generalization." Psychol. Rev. **72**: 467–482.

16. OSGOOD, C. E. 1963. On understanding and creating sentences. Amer. Psychol. **18**: 735–751.

17. KUHN, T. S. 1962. The Structure of Scientific Revolutions. University of Chicago Press. Chicago, Ill.

18. FODOR, J. A. 1965. Could meaning be an r_m? JVLVB **4**: 73–81.

19. OSGOOD, C. E. 1966. Meaning cannot be an r_m? JVLVB **5**: 402–407.

20. DIXON, T. R. & D. L. HORTON, Eds. 1968. Verbal Behavior and General Behavior Theory. Prentice-Hall Inc. Englewood Cliffs, N.J.

21. OSGOOD, C. E. Focus on Meaning. Vol. III. Cognizing and Sentencing. In preparation. Mouton Press. The Hague, The Netherlands.

22. OSGOOD, C. E. 1970a. Speculation on the structure of interpersonal intentions. Behav. Sci. **15**: 237–254.

23. OSGOOD, C. E. 1970b. Interpersonal verbs and interpersonal behavior. *In* Studies in Thought and Language. J. L. Cowan, Ed. University of Arizona Press. Tucson, Ariz.

24. CHOMSKY, N. 1961. On the notion 'rule of grammar.' Proc. Symposia Applied Mathematics. Amer. Math. Soc. **12**: 6–24.

25. HAYES, J. R., Ed. 1970. Cognition and the Development of Language. John Wiley & Sons Inc. New York, N.Y.

26. STEINBERG, D. D. & L. A. JAKOBOVITS, Eds. 1971. Semantics: An Interdisciplinary Reader in Philosophy, Linguistics and Psychology. Cambridge University Press. Cambridge, England.

27. OSGOOD, C. E. & M. M. RICHARDS. 1973. From yang and yin to *and* or *but*. Lang. **49**: 380–412.

28. HOOSAIN, R. 1973. Cognitive Processing Load as a Function of Embedding in Conjoined Cognitions. Doctoral dissertation. University of Illinois. Urbana, Ill.

29. OPAČIĆ, G. 1973. Natural Order in Cognizing and Clause Order in the Sentencing of Conjoined Expressions. Doctoral dissertation. University of Illinois. Urbana, Ill.

30. HARRIS, R. J. 1974. Memory and Comprehension of Truth-Value Information in S-complement Sentences. Doctoral dissertation. University of Illinois. Urbana, Ill.

31. BRANSFORD, J. D., J. R. BARCLAY & J. J. FRANKS. 1972. Sentence memory: a constructive versus interpretive approach. Cog. Psychol. **3**: 193–209.

32. BREWER, W. F. 1974. The problem of meaning and the interrelations of the higher mental processes. *In* Cognition and Symbolic Processes. W. B. Weimer & D. S. Palermo, Eds. Earlbaum (Wiley).

33. SLOBIN, D. I. 1973. Cognitive prerequisites for development of grammar. *In* Studies of Child Language Development. C. A. Ferguson & D. I. Slobin, Eds. Holt, Rinehart & Winston, New York, N.Y.
34. FODOR, J. A. & M. Garrett. 1966. Some reflections on competence and performance. *In* Psycholinguistic Papers: Proc. 1966 Edinburgh Conference. J. Lyons and R. J. Wales, Eds. Edinburgh University Press. Edinburgh, Scotland.

SPEECH ACTS AND RECENT LINGUISTICS*

John R. Searle

Department of Philosophy
University of California at Berkeley
Berkeley, California 94720

Until fairly recently it seemed possible to draw a boundary, however vague, between linguistics and the philosophy of language: linguistics dealt with the empirical facts of natural human languages; the philosophy of language dealt with the conceptual truths that underlie any possible language or system of communication. Within the terms of this distinction, the study of speech acts seemed to lie clearly on the side of the philosophy of language, and until the past few years most of the research on speech acts was done by philosophers and not by linguists. Lately, however, all this has changed. In the current period of expansion, linguists have simply moved into large territories where previously only philosophers worked, and the writings of such philosophers as Austin, Grice, and others have now been assimilated into the working tools of the contemporary linguist. The philosopher of language can only welcome this development, for the linguist brings to bear a knowledge of the facts of natural human languages, together with techniques of syntactical analysis which, at least in the past, have been absent from the purely philosophical writings on language. The collaboration between linguists and philosophers is especially fruitful in studying what to me is one of the most interesting questions in the study of language: how do structure and function interact? This question involves such questions as, for example, what is the relation between the various kinds of illocutionary acts and the syntactical forms in which they are realized in the various natural human languages?

However, not all of the contributions of linguists to the study of speech acts have been equally useful, and in this talk I want to discuss two well-known approaches, both of which seem to me to be mistaken. They are the so-called *performative deletion* analysis, deriving from the work of John R. Ross (especially his article, "On Declarative Sentences"[1]) and the Conversational Postulates approach to the study of indirect speech acts, the best-known exposition of which is in an article by David Gordon and George Lakoff entitled, "Conversational Postulates."[2] Both of these theories seem to me to be mistaken explanations of the data concerning speech acts, and both—though in their quite different ways—make the same mistake of postulating a much too powerful explanation to account for certain facts, when there already exists an independently motivated theory of speech acts that will account for these facts.

Let me say before I start that it is quite possible that none of the authors I will be discussing still accepts the theses they advanced in these articles. I keep hearing rumors that Haj Ross has abandoned the performative deletion analysis, and Lakoff has written a paper that might possibly be interpreted as an abandonment of the Conversational Postulates approach to indirect speech acts.[3] I simply do not know Gordon's current views. However, I am not interested in the biographies of these linguists, but rather in certain patterns of analysis that they have advanced. These patterns of analysis have proved influential, as a look at some of the linguistic literature will show, and it is important, I believe, to refute them, regardless of whether their original authors still adhere to them.

*I am indebted to Charles Fillmore and David Reier for discussion of these matters.

27

I begin with Ross's article on "Declarative Sentences." The thesis of this paper, Ross says, "is that declarative sentences, such as those in (1) ("Prices slumped.") must be analyzed as being implicit performatives, and must be derived from deep structures containing an explicitly represented performative main verb." (Ref. 1, p. 223.) Ross then gives us fourteen syntactic arguments to show that every delarative sentence must have a higher subject "I," must have an indirect object "you," and must have some performative verb, possibly abstract, as the main verb of the highest clause. The conclusion of his discussion, then, is that every declarative sentence of English has a deep structure of the form, "I say to you that S" or "I tell you that S," etc. Furthermore, it is easy to extend the types of arguments he presents to other sorts of sentences, and the conclusion that is eventually reached (though he does not state it in his original article) is that all English sentences have a performative main verb in the highest clause of their deep structure. A spectacular conclusion. Since the arguments in his original article seem to me to exhibit a common inferential pattern, I will consider only the first. If we consider examples like (all of these examples are from Ross's paper):

1. Tom believed that the paper had been written by Ann and him himself.
2. Tom believed that the paper had been written by Ann and himself.
3. *Tom believed that the paper had been written by Ann and themselves.

These (and many other examples) naturally lead us to the following rule formulation:

4. If an anaphoric pronoun precedes and emphatic reflexive, the former may be deleted, if it is commanded by the NP with which it stands in an anaphoric relationship.

He then goes on to consider examples like:

5. This paper was written by Ann and myself.

Furthermore, he then goes on to give a whole sequence of sentences on the model of 1 and on the model of 5, of which he says that "the acceptability spectra" match each other, exactly or nearly so. But if 4 is really a valid rule, and the examples certainly suggest it is, then in order to account for 5 we have to assume that its deep structure "will contain a higher performative clause which is obliterated by the rule of performative deletion, after the application of the rule stated in (4)." (Ref. 1, 228) Furthermore, he adds that whether or not the performative analysis is correct, all of these examples must be accounted for by the same rules or principles.

I must say that I find Ross's arguments very subtle and elegant. But what exactly is their logical form? They appear to be of the same logical form as some of the very early arguments used to prove the existence of a syntactic deep structure. For example, consider the sequence:

6. Hit him
7. *Hit you
8. Hit yourself
9. *She hit himself
10. He hit himself
11. You hit yourself
12. *He hit yourself

In these early discussions of syntactical deep structure it was claimed that in order to account for the occurrence of reflexives in imperative sentences, one has to postulate the occurrence of a second person pronoun "you" in the deep structure of all imperative sentences, in order that the same rule should account for the distribution of reflexives over declarative and imperative sentences. But again, what exactly is the logical form of these arguments?

It seems to be this: for any language L and any two forms F and G, if F and G generally occur together in the surface structure of sentences, and if facts about the form or presence of one are determined by the nature of the other, then for any sentence S in which F occurs in the surface structure, but G does not occur, there is some deep structure of S in which G occurs, but it is deleted in the surface structure.

Now as a general argument form that is certainly not valid; that is, it simply does not follow from the fact that F and G generally occur together and are related in certain ways in the surface structure that where one is absent, the other must exist in the deep structure. I don't suppose any linguist ever thought that it did follow logically, but nonetheless, this has been an extremely influential pattern of argument. Why? The pattern of inference, we are told, enables us to give a *simpler* account of the data. We require only one rule for the distribution of reflexives, whereas otherwise, if we did not postulate the occurrence of some element in the deep structure, we would require two rules. It is this appeal to an intuitive notion of simplicity that has made the inference pattern so attractive, but I believe the appearance of simplicity rests on an unexamined assumption, which I would like to challenge in the course of this paper.

The assumption is that *the rules which specify the distribution of syntactical elements must mention only syntactical categories.*

It may seem puzzling to accuse linguists who are famous for denying the autonomy of syntax of assuming such a principle, but unless they assume it, it is hard to see how they justify their acceptance of the performative deletion analysis or of the traditional (and, I believe, confused) arguments to show that imperative sentences have a deleted second person subject.

Before going on to challenge this assumption, I want to mention a couple of other arguments that were not in Ross's original article but which have subsequently been used to justify the performative analysis: consider sentences like:

13. Frankly, you're drunk.

"Frankly" in 13 does not seem to function as a sentence adverb as does "probably" in

14. Probably, it will rain.

Both syntactically and semantically, it has been argued, 13 requires us to postulate an underlying verb of saying in the deep structure. This is because, syntactically, "frankly" normally co-occurs with verbs of saying as in

15. John frankly admitted his guilt.

but not with other sorts of verbs, as in e.g.,

16. *It frankly rained.

and semantically, because there is nothing for "frankly" to modify in the surface structure of 13. The verb it modifies must be something other than what is in its surface structure. Therefore, the deep structure of 13, so the argument goes, must be the same as that of sentences of the form:

17. I verb you frankly: you're drunk.

Another class of arguments for performative deletion analysis concerns adverbial clauses. For example,

18. Since you know so much, why did John leave?

And here, it is argued, in order to account for the occurrence of the adverbial clause one has to postulate a deep structure similar to that of

19. Since you know so much, I ask you (am asking you) why did John leave?

These and many other arguments all lead to the same conclusion. Every sentence of English and presumably of every other language has a performative main verb in its deep structure. These arguments have been attacked in their details by various authors, especially Bruce Fraser, but I believe that so far no one has challenged the fundamental assumptions on which these arguments rest. Before doing that, I want to call your attention to what an intuitively implausible conclusion the performative deletion analysis leads to. It has the consequence that in an important sense of "saying" you can only perform an illocutionary act by saying that you are performing it, for the deep structure of every sentence you utter contains "an explicitly represented performative main verb." I find it hard to imagine that any arguments of the sort we have considered could convince one of such a counterintuitive conclusion.

I believe there is a much simpler explanation of the data, and the explanation contains only the assumption of elements that are "independently motivated" by the theory of speech acts. Ross almost considers this explanation, but he does not quite face it squarely. It is this:

In any speech situation there is a speaker, a hearer and a speech act being performed by the speaker. The speaker and the hearer share a mutual knowledge of those facts together with a mutual knowledge of the rules of performing the various kinds of speech acts. These facts and this knowledge enable us to account for certain syntactical forms without forcing us to assume that the facts themselves have some syntactical description or representation in the deep structure of sentences that they help to explain. For example, in 13, "frankly" is predicated of the speech act that is being performed in the utterance of the sentence. It is not necessary to assume that it also modifies a verb; rather, it characterizes the act which the speaker is performing, and that act need not be, and in this case is not, represented by a verb anywhere in the deep structure of the sentence, since the speaker and hearer already have mutual knowledge of the existence of that act. In the utterance of 18 we see the same phenomena at work. The speaker asks a question and in so doing gives a reason for asking it. This explanation is quite adequate without any further requirement that there must be some verb of asking which the adverbial clause modifies. This sort of phenomenon, where the speaker conjoins the peformance of a speech act with the giving of a reason for performing it, in the utterance of one and the same sentence, is very common in English. Consider:

20. He must be home by now, because I saw him on his way a half an hour ago.

Here the "because" clause does not give a reason or a cause for its being the case that he is home; my seeing him does not cause him to be home by now; rather, it gives a justification for my *saying* that he must be at home, by giving the evidentiary basis for my saying and believing it.

Ross almost considers this approach, but not quite. He considers what he calls "the pragmatic analysis." This analysis, says Ross, "claims that certain elements are present in the context of a speech act and that syntactic processes can refer to such elements." The context provides an "I," a "you," and a performative verb which are " 'in the air,' so to speak." (Ref. 1, p. 254 ff.) It is crucial to Ross's characterization of the pragmatic analysis that it postulates the presence not of speakers, hearers, and acts but of the words, "I," "you," and the performative verbs. But given that the pragmatic analysis postulates the presence of words, it would seem to differ only very slightly from the performative deletion analysis which Ross subscribes to; and indeed, he says, "Given this isomorphism [of the performative and pragmatic analyses], it may well be asked how the pragmatic analysis differs from the performative analysis: why are they not merely notational variants?" I believe that as he presents the two they are just notational variants of each other, but for that very reason he has missed the point of talking about the "context" in which the speech act is performed: the speaker, the hearer, and the speech act performed by the speaker are not in the air; they are very much on the ground. The "elements" in the analysis I am presenting are not the words "I," "you," and the performative verbs, but speakers, hearers, and acts performed by speakers. It is only if one accepts the so-far unjustified and unargued assumption that syntactical rules can only make mention of syntactical categories that one would ever want to construct a "pragmatic analysis" of the sort Ross considers. What I am arguing is that there is no need to postulate an "I," a "you," or a verb either in the air or in the deep structure, once that assumption is abandoned, since we already have an independent motivation for believing that in speech situations there are speakers, hearers, and speech acts, and it is these elements which are referred to in the statement of the relevant syntactic rules. It has been suggested to me (by David Reier) that perhaps Ross makes this confusion because he is committing a use-mention fallacy; that is, he is confusing the speaker and the "I" which refers to him, and the hearer and the "you" which refers to him, and the acts and the verbs which specify those acts. Of course, the formulation of the rules which mention speaker, hearer, and act will *use* expressions to refer to speaker, hearer, and act, but it will use and not mention those expressions. Under the analysis I am proposing, the statement of the rule will contain, for example, the use of an illocutionary verb, but it would be a simple use-mention confusion of the most egregious variety to suppose that the rule mentions (or refers to or is about) a verb. I find it hard to believe that Ross is guilty of so elementary a mistake; rather, it seems more plausible to assume that he is in the grip of the assumption that if the rules are to be adequate they must mention only syntactic elements. And that, I believe, is why when he presents the "pragmatic analysis" it is not a pragmatic analysis at all but a variant syntactical analysis.

But isn't the performative deletion analysis and the deleted subject analysis of imperatives simpler in some fairly clear sense of simpler than the alternative I have been proposing? I think these theories fail the test of simplicity provided by Occam's razor: a theory should not postulate the existence of more entities than is necessary to account for the facts. Since we already know that a speech situation contains a hearer, a speaker, and a speech act, it is an unnecessary complexity to introduce deleted syntactical elements corresponding to these entities. It appears simpler only if we insist on the principle that syntactical rules can mention only syntactical categories. Once we abandon this assumption, our alternative theory becomes simpler in two respects. First, we use independently motivated semantic and "pragmatic" knowledge; and second, we do not have to postulate any deleted syntactical elements. Consider how this would work for imperative sentences. There is an independently motivated propositional content rule on the directive class of speech acts to the effect that the propositional content of a directive predicates some future course of action of the hearer.[4] Now, since in English the imperative form is the standard illocutionary force indicating device for directives, the literal utterance of an imperative form necessarily involves a predication of the hearer. It is therefore not necessary to assume an additional syntactical representation of the hearer. Reference to the hearer is already contained in the relevant rules of speech acts. The reflexive rule does indeed involve a repeated element, but that element need not always be present in the syntax. In

He hit himself.

the repetition that permits the reflexive is present in the syntax because the subject and object are coreferential; but in

Hit yourself,

there is no repetition in the syntax, because there does not need to be. It follows from the theory of speech acts that in the utterance of this sentence the verb "hit" is predicated of the hearer. But it does not follow from that fact that the sentence has a syntactical subject "you." Rather, the sentence does not have a syntactical subject, because, being an English imperative, it doesn't need one. Of course, not all languages are like English in this regard. The point is not that the theory of speech acts forces the elimination of the subject expression in imperative sentences, but rather that the theory explains the possibility of that elimination.

I think that the forms of the argument we have been considering are not valid or even intuitively plausible forms of inference. I think that they have seemed appealing because of certain tacit assumptions about what syntactical rules should look like. As a further indication that something is fishy about the form of the argument, I want to call your attention to some counterintuitive results that a consistent adherence to the argument form would produce. Consider nonimperative sentences that can take a preverbal "please," e.g.,

21. Can you please pass the salt? or
22. Will you please leave us alone?

Now since "please" normally occurs with the imperative mood as in

23. Please pass the salt.

I suppose a consistent adherence to the Ross argument form would force us to say that each of these sentences has an imperative deep structure, and consequently, that sentences of the form

24. Can you plus vol verb

and

25. Will you plus vol verb

are really ambiguous, as they both have an imperative and a declarative deep structure. This seems to me a most implausible result, especially since there is a very simple explanation of the occurrence of "please" in nonimperative sentences like the above: these sentences are often used to perform indirect requests, and "please" makes the request more polite. It can be inserted before the verb that names the act being requested. A similar *reductio ad absurdum* argument can be constructed for sentences containing an anaphoric pronoun with no NP antecedent. In a sentence such as

26. He's drunk.

are we really to say that there is a deep structure NP that is an antecedent to "He"? It would seem that a consistent adherence to the traditional argument forms would force us to that conclusion.

Let me conclude this half of the paper by distinguishing what I am saying from what I am not saying. I am not saying that there are no good arguments for deleted syntactical elements in the deep structure of sentences. A sentence such as

27. I met a richer man than Rockefeller.

clearly seems to derive its ambiguity from the fact that there are two different possible deleted elements corresponding to

28. I met a richer man than Rockefeller met.
29. I met a richer man than Rockefeller is.

It is because of these two deletions that we can use 27 to say two quite different things, represented by 28 and 29. But in that sense of "say," when I say that prices slumped, I am not also saying that I am saying it. It is an intuitively implausible result to suppose that I can only perform an illocutionary act by using a sentence with an explicit performative verb in its deep structure, and the arguments that might incline one to this result are easily accounted for by a theory of speech acts which we already have some reason to believe is true.

I now turn to the second half of this paper, the discussion of the conversational postulates approach to the study of indirect speech acts, the most well-known version of which is in the article by Gordon and Lakoff.[2] For the sake of brevity, I will discuss their article under the following headings. (1) What is the problem? (2) What is their solution? (3) Why is it inadequate? and finally, (4) I will try to suggest an alternative approach from the point of view of the theory of speech acts. To anticipate a bit, my general criticism of their approach will be that they offer the phenomena that need to be explained as if they were themselves the explanation.

The problem is simply this. How is it possible for the speaker to say one thing, mean what he says, but also to mean something else. I say

30. Can you reach the salt?

or

31. I would appreciate it if you would get off my foot,

but I mean not only what I say but I also mean: *pass the salt*, and *get off my foot*. In such cases the primary illocutionary point of the utterance is that of a request to do something, but the literal and secondary illocutionary point is that of a question or statement. How is it possible for the speaker to mean the nonliteral primary illocutionary point and for the hearer to understand the nonliteral primary illocutionary point when all the speaker utters is a sentence expressing the literal secondary illocutionary point? A second aspect of the problem is this. Many of the sentences that are most commonly used in the performance of indirect speech acts seem to be systematically related to the primary illocutionary point that they are indirectly used to convey. Thus, for example, consider the sequence of sentences that concern the hearer's ability to perform the action.

Can you pass the salt?
Could you pass the salt?
Are you able to reach that book on the top shelf?
You can go now.
You could get off my foot.

All of these have a very natural use as indirect requests, and some of them will take "please." Furthermore, they seem to be systematically related to one of the preparatory rules on the performance of the directive class of illocutionary acts, the rule that says that the hearer must be able to perform the act and that the speaker and hearer must believe that he is so able.[4] Or consider the sequence of sentences such as

I would like you to go now.
I want you to leave the room.

> I would appreciate it if you would get off my foot.
> I should be most grateful if you could take off your hat.

All such examples concern the speaker's desire that the hearer do something; and in a theory of speech acts, the speaker's desire or want that the hearer should do an action is the sincerity condition on the directive class of speech acts. A third set of examples is provided by sentences such as

> Will you leave the room?
> Would you kindly go now?
> Are you going to continue to make so much noise?

and so on. All of these again relate to a condition on speech acts, namely, the propositional content condition that the speaker predicates a future course of action of the hearer. So we have both a general problem of accounting for the move from literal to primary illocutionary points and within that problem, there is a special problem of accounting for the fact that certain sets of sentences seem to be systematically related both to indirect speech acts and to our general theory of speech acts.† How should we account for these problems?

The solution that Gordon and Lakeoff propose is really quite simple. They claim that in addition to the rules such as those above for the performance of directive speech acts (the preparatory, sincerity, and propositional content rules), the speaker knows an additional set of rules called conversational postulates: and "it is by means of such postulates that we can get one speech act to entrail another speech act."[2] Thus, for example, the conversational postulate

$$\text{ASK (a,b, CAN (b,Q))}^* \longrightarrow \text{REQUEST (a,b,Q)}$$

tells us that if a asks b a defective question whether b can do the act specified in Q, then that question "entails"‡ a request from a to b to do that act. That is, these conversational postulates are supposed to be additional rules that the speaker-hearer knows which enable him to go through the alleged "entailments."

What exactly is the form of their solution to the problem? It seems to me that the form is something like this. They have described a fairly well-known pattern of indirect speech acts, at least within the directive class. They then suppose that the patterns are themselves the solution, for the conversational postulates that they use to explain the data derive directly from the patterns. That is, they discover a pattern to the effect that a speaker can ask a hearer to do something by asking the hearer if he is able to do it. In order to account for this, they simply redescribe it by saying that the speaker knows a rule, or rather, conversational postulate, to the effect that if you ask a hearer a (defective) question about his ability to do something, the utterance is ("entails") a request to him to do it. Furthermore, the mistake seems to me quite similar in form to the mistake that I am alleging against Ross. In both cases, an unnecessary supposition is made in order to account for the data. In this case we already have a theory of conversation of the Gricean type; and we have a theory of illocutionary acts of a sort outlined in *Speech Acts*, and we know certain things about speakers' and hearers' powers of inference and rationality. It is entirely *ad hoc* and unmotivated to claim that in addition to all of this knowledge, the speaker-hearer must have some extra knowledge of a set of conversational postulates. The hypostatization, in short, of

---

†A third problem is that in some sentences, e.g., "Are you going to continue to make so much noise?" the indirect request negates the propositional content.

‡Literally, it makes no sense to speak of one *act* entailing another act. Entailment is a relation between propositions, not between acts, whether speech acts or otherwise.

conversational postulates seems to me to be unnecessary and unsupported by the evidence and, indeed, the phenomena recorded by the postulates are precisely what we need to explain. They do not themselves provide the explanation.

I think these objections will become clearer after I have presented an alternative account of indirect speech acts.§ Consider the simplest sort of case: someone at a dinner table says to me

Can you pass the salt?

Now, it is quite clear that unless the circumstances are most peculiar, he is not just asking me whether I can pass the salt; he is asking me to pass him the salt.

Sure I can pass the salt.

is not an adequate answer. Now, how do I know that? How do I get from the knowledge that he has asked me whether I can pass the salt to the knowledge that he has asked me to pass him the salt? And that question, how do I understand the primary illocutionary act when all he says is the secondary illocutionary act, is part of the answer to the question: how is it possible for him to *mean* the primary illocutionary act when all that he actually says is the secondary illocutionary act? Two answers I am rejecting are: first, that the sentence is ambiguous, that it really has two different meanings, and second, that I must know an extra rule or conversational postulate to the effect that whenever somebody asks me a certain sort of question about whether I can do something, he is really asking me to do it. I think, indeed, that as a generalization, it is largely correct; that is, in our culture whenever somebody asks you certain sorts of questions, they are usually trying to get you to do something, but it is that generalization which our theory needs to explain; the mistake is to suppose that we have explained it or anything else by calling the generalization a "conversational postulate."

At the risk of pedantry, I will set out the steps necessary for the hearer to derive the primary indirect illocution from the literal secondary illocution. The apparatus necessary for the hearer to make the inference includes a theory of speech acts, a theory of conversation, factual background information, and general powers of rationality and inference. Each of these is independently motivated; that is, we have evidence quite independent of any theory of indirect speech acts that the speaker-hearer has these features of linguistic and cognitive competence.

Let us take the simplest sort of case; X at the dinner table says to Y

Can you pass the salt?

by way of asking Y to pass the salt. Notice that not anything X says about salt will do as a request to pass the salt. Thus, if X had said

Salt is made of sodium chloride.

or

Salt is mined in the Tatra mountains.

without some special stage setting, it is very unlikely that Y would take either of these utterances as a request to pass the salt. Notice further that in a normal conversational situation Y does not have to go through any conscious process of inference to derive the conclusion that the utterance of "Can you pass the salt" is a request to pass

§What follows is a shortened version of a longer account I have given of these matters entitled "Indirect Speech Acts."[5]

the salt. He simply hears it as a request. This fact is perhaps one of the main reasons why it is tempting to adopt the false conclusion that somehow these examples must have an imperative force as part of their meaning or that they are "ambiguous in context" or some such. A bare bones reconstruction of the steps necessary for Y to derive the conclusion from the utterance might go roughly as follows:

Step 1.   S has asked me a question as to whether I have the ability to pass the salt. (fact about the conversation)

Step 2.   I assume that he is cooperating in the conversation and that therefore, his utterance has some aim or point. (principles of conversational cooperation)

Step 3.   The conversational setting is not such as to indicate a theoretical interest in my salt-passing ability. (factual background information)

Step 4.   Furthermore, he probably already knows that the answer to the question is "yes." (factual background information)
          (This step facilitates the move to Step 5, but is not essential.)

Step 5.   Therefore, his utterance is probably not just a question. It probably has some ulterior illocutionary point. (inference from Steps 1, 2, 3, and 4) What can it be?

Step 6.   A preparatory condition on any directive illocutionary act is the ability of H to perform the act predicated in the propositional content condition. (theory of speech acts)

Step 7.   Therefore X has asked me a question the affirmative answer to which would entail that the preparatory condition on requesting me to pass the salt is satisfied. (inference from Steps 1 and 6)

Step 8.   We are now at dinner, and people normally use salt at dinner; they pass it back and forth, try to get others to pass it back and forth, etc. (background information)

Step 9.   He has therefore alluded to the satisfaction of a preparatory condition on a request whose obedience conditions it is quite likely he wants me to bring about. (inference from Steps 7 and 8)

Step 10.   Therefore, in the absence of any other plausible illocutionary point, he is probably requesting me to pass him the salt. (inference from Steps 5 and 9)

The hypothesis being put forth in this paper is that all the cases can be analyzed, using this apparatus, without involving any "conversational postulates." According to this analysis the reason why I can ask you to pass the salt by saying "Can you pass the salt?" but not by saying "Salt is made of sodium chloride" or "Salt is mined in the Tatra mountains" is that your ability to pass the salt is a preparatory condition on requesting you to pass the salt in a way that the other sentences are not related to requesting you to pass the salt. But obviously that answer is not by itself sufficient, because not all questions about your abilities are requests. The hearer therefore needs some way of finding out when the utterance is just a question about his abilities and when it is a request made by way of asking a question about his abilities. It is at this point that the general principles of conversation (together with factual background information) come into play.

The two features that are crucial, or so I am suggesting, are first a strategy for establishing the existence of an ulterior illocutionary point beyond the illocutionary point contained in the meaning of the sentence, and second, a device for finding out what the ulterior illocutionary point is. The first is established by the principles of conversation operating on the information of the hearer and the speaker, and the second is derived from the theory of speech acts together with background information. The generalizations are to be explained by the fact that each of them records a strategy by means of which the hearer can find out how a primary illocutionary point differs from a secondary illocutionary point.

The chief motivation—though not the only motivation—for using these indirect forms is politeness. Notice that in the above example the "Can you" form is polite in at least two respects. Firstly, X does not presume to know about Y's abilities, as he would if he issued an imperative sentence, and secondly, the form gives—or at least appears to give—Y the option of refusing, since a yes-no question allows "no" as a possible answer. Hence, compliance can be made to appear a free act rather than that of obeying a command.

Let me summarize the difference between my approach and the Conversational Postulates approach. Both agree that there are sets of generalizations that one can make about indirect speech acts, for example, generalizations such as that one can make an indirect request to a hearer to do something by asking him if he is able to do it. On my account these generalizations are to be explained by a theory of speech acts, including a theory of conversation, and by the assumption that speakers and hearers know certain general things about the world and have certain general powers of rationality. On the conversational postulates approach, each generalization is elevated to the status of a rule or conversational postulate, and we are asked to suppose that people understand indirect speech acts because they know these rules ("it is by means of such postulates that we can get one speech act to entail another speech act.") On my account there is no reason to believe in the existence of any such rules, because our existing theories will already account for the existence of indirect speech acts, and indeed, the rules have no explanatory power, since they are mere reformulations of the material we need to explain.

Incidentally, the actual rules that they propose don't work. Consider, for example, the one just mentioned. Stripped of its "formalization," it says that whenever you ask somebody a defective question about whether he can do something, you are asking him to do that thing. By "defective" they mean that a question is not intended to be conveyed, and the hearer assumes it is not intended to be conveyed. But such a claim is, I believe, simply false. Thus, if I say

Can you eat the square root of Mount Everest?

I have certainly asked a defective question in their sense because I know that the final noun phrase contains a category mistake and hence I do not intend to convey a genuine question, and I assume you know that. But it simply does not follow from this, nor is it the case that, my utterance conveys, implies, or "entails" a request. Such counter-examples will work for all of their conversational postulates. It is also worth noting that the actual cases of successful indirect speech acts are, in general, cases where the literal secondary illocution is conveyed, and the primary illocutionary act is successful only because the secondary illocutionary act is conveyed.

I now want to draw some general conclusions from the discussion of these two patterns of analysis. Both of them seem to me to exhibit a mistaken conception of the place of a theory of speech acts within a general account of language.

It is common to hear people say, following Chomsky, that the task of linguistics is to specify the set of rules that relate sound and meanings. Each language provides a set, presumably infinite, of possible sound sequences and another set, presumably infinite, of possible meanings. The phonological, syntactical, and semantic components of the grammar are supposed to provide the finite sets of rules which the speaker knows will enable him to go from sound to meaning and back again. I don't think that this picture is false, so much as it is extremely misleading and misleading in ways that have had unfortunate consequences for research. A more accurate picture seems to me this. The purpose of language is communication. The unit of human communication in language is the speech act, of the type called *illocutionary act*. The problem (or at least an important problem) of the theory of language is to describe how we get from the sounds to the illocutionary acts. What, so to speak, has to be added to the noises that come out of my mouth in order that their production should be a performance of the act of asking a question, or making a statement, or giving an order, etc.? The rules enable us to get from the brute facts of the making of noises to the institutional facts of the performance of illocutionary acts of human communication. Now, if that is the case, then the role of a theory of speech acts in a grammar will be quite different from what either the proponents of generative syntax or even most of the proponents of generative semantics have considered. The theory of speech acts is not an adjunct to our theory of language, something to be consigned to the realm of "pragmatics," or performance; rather, the theory of speech acts will necessarily occupy a central role in our grammar, since it will include all of what used to be called semantics as well as pragmatics.

Furthermore, the theory will provide us with a set of rules for performing illocutionary acts, which rules may have consequences in other parts of our linguistic theory, such as syntax. It is not at all surprising that the theory of speech acts should have syntactical consequences, since, after all, that is what sentences are for. A sentence is to talk with. My objection to the two theories I have discussed in this paper is that they both fail to use the resources of existing theories of speech acts. Both, when confronted with puzzling data, postulate a solution that requires the introduction of extra and unnecessary elements. In each, a proper understanding of the role of speech acts would enable us to account for the data without introducing these extra elements.

REFERENCES

1. Ross, J. R. 1970. On declarative sentences. *In* Readings in English Transformational Grammar. R. A. Jacobs & P. S. Rosenbaum, Eds. Ginn & Co. Waltham, Mass.
2. Gordon, D. & G. Lakoff. 1971. Conversational postulates. Papers of the Chicago Linguistic Soc. no. 7.
3. Lakoff, G. 1975. Pragmatics in natural logic. *In* Berkeley Studies in Syntax and Semantics. Vol. 1. Univ. Calif. Berkeley, Calif.
4. Searle, J. R. 1969. Speech Acts.: 66. Cambridge Univ. Press. Cambridge, England.
5. Searle, J. R. 1975. Indirect speech acts. *In* Studies in Syntax and Semantics. Vol. 3. Speech Acts. J. Morgan & P. Cole, Eds. Seminar Press. New York, N.Y.

DISCUSSION

Sam Glucksberg, *Chairperson*

Department of Psychology
Princeton University
Princeton, New Jersey 08540

DR. BEVER: I want to ask a question in the form of an assertion to be responded to by each of the speakers. Dr. Osgood characterized the current situation as one in which we do not have a "paradigm," and therefore the field will resubside back into the former swamp, or forest primeval. Yet, I detect in what Dr. Searle said an example of an appropriate paradigm to get out of the forest and past the trees. What Dr. Searle said is the following. The purpose of a grammar, a cognitive theory, and an illocutionary theory is not determined a priori, but is decided in part as a function of what the theory does. As we construct the theories of syntax, semantics, and illocutionary acts, we find out certain kinds of facts about sentences as a function of what the theories tell us. That seems to me to be a common point from any area of science.

The paradigm that comes out of this perspective is one in which one views language behavior as the result of internally interacting mental structures. One such mental structure we might call "syntax," another "the system of illocutionary acts," another "the system of cognizing certain aspects of the world." Different kinds of facts are explained by each structure; to argue that all facts are described by the same kind of structure might distort the nature of the mind. Dr. Searle took an example of such linguistic imperialism in which some linguists had proposed that a particular kind of fact ought to be described within linguistic theory. He pointed out that there was an independently motivated theory of illocutionary acts, a theory which one needs for other purposes anyway, that could account for this phenomenon. Therefore, insofar as the linguistic devices that are needed to account for the phenomena in a "grammar" are unnecessarily strong (in the mathematical sense), one should avoid them, in order to make more interesting the nature of syntax. At the same time, we can account for the phenomenon as due to an interaction with an extrasyntactic system. So, the way we interpret certain kinds of questions as requests for action is itself a function of the literal meaning of the sentence (specified by the syntax) and of a system of illocutionary interpretation. That interaction of systems exemplifies the paradigm. We view behavior in general and language in particular as the result of interacting systems of knowledge and behavior. This is admittedly a very difficult paradigm to pursue because one doesn't know ahead of time for any given phenomena what kind of phenomenon it is going to turn out to be, what kind of structure underlies it. But it does offer us a way to avoid the pitfalls of treating every human mental phenomenon as ultimately "linguistic," or "mental." Linguistic imperialism is no better or worse than cognitive imperialism. I think that the answer lies in their interaction. This is not really a question, but you could respond to it if you like.

DR. OSGOOD: I wasn't talking, by any means, about going back into the swamp, and if you mean going back into a simple-minded behaviorism, for example, then certainly that was not what I had in mind. In fact, I would say the same thing, but not quite so strongly, about my going back even to the views that I held about the time (1966) we were at the Kentucky Conference together. I had essentially a lexicon, a semantic system of bipolar, mediator components in behavioral terms, without any

39

structure whatsoever, without any dynamics or interactions, etc., among these components. The Cog Group I've been working with is essentially trying to go beyond this.

By saying that there is not, at this point, as far as I can see, an alternative paradigm for a *performance* grammar, a theory, if you will, of language performance, I mean that there is none that meets the criteria of being an integrated and highly generalized kind of theory that handles semantic relations, problems of entailment, of metaphor (you were mentioning) and things like that. It must also include the dynamics of congruence and incongruence of whole cognitions, insertions and deletions, memory for ideas (what happens in the Bransford et. al. experiments) and so forth. I mean a *general* performance theory, and I have no illusions that this particular dinosaur is ever going to last that long. But at least I am thinking of the direction one could go in trying to develop a well-motivated (as the phrase goes), generalizable theory of performance. I agree that what Dr. Searle has been talking about is very relevant to such a thing.

DR. SEARLE: I'm very grateful for Prof. Bever's remarks. It won't surprise you that I agree with them, but let me underline a couple of aspects. The "paradigm," as he calls it, really isn't so much like one of Kuhn's paradigms, because it is almost a methodological paradigm. What it says is: try to account for the maximum amount of data with the minimal number of general principles. Where you have independently motivated principles, use them to account for as much data as you can without having to suppose additional principles, unless you absolutely need to.

Pursuing the methodological paradigm, I would like to add a couple of elements to it. I found it very useful in philosophy not to keep looking over my shoulder all the time at the great classical battles. We should try to forget what Kant said about the categorical imperative, and get on with whatever it is we're working on. That's how I feel about many of the Titanic struggles that go on in linguistics.

I'll mention briefly the generative syntax and generative semantics hassle. Sometimes it seems to me rather like the following. Suppose somebody had formed the syntax of tic-tac-toe. You draw these marks on the blackboard and some will be grammatical and others won't. You have one matrix that's all "O's"; every slot is filled by an O. Star that one. That's ungrammatical. Now you have another one that has the proper distribution of O's and X's. All right, there will be grammatical and ungrammatical tic-tac-toe games. You can then get a generative theory of tic-tac-toe where you'd have formal rules that will generate all and only the grammatical tic-tac-toe games. Now suppose there was a tremendous hassle that grew up over whether the rules had to keep it secret that it was a game, or whether the rules could explicitly state that it was a game. Now I would say it really wouldn't much matter who won that hassle, because we all know it's a game and we all know what it's for. Incidentally, the generative syntax people would win that battle hands down because you could specify those rules independently of the fact that it's a game, and independently even of the fact that the X has to precede, and has to be followed by an O in the spots. That is, you could have a rule that never mentioned the fact that players had to take turns. It seems to me that much of the disputes are like that. Why avoid what we already know, namely, that we use these things to communicate with each other? So, I really don't find anything to disagree with in Tom's remarks. In fact, I'd like to underscore them.

DR. PHILIP PETERSON: Since we lost the elm trees on my street, I have this nostalgia for trees. Maybe that will explain this question, because I have this nostalgia for Ross trees, perhaps. I don't see much difference between what you say in general and the sort of thing Ross is doing. Let me suggest that instead of going right to Ross, consider Zeno Vendler's views of Austin's Speech Acts Extended to Mental Acts. He's engaged in enumerating a lot of them. This is directed to Prof. Searle. One could point out various subclasses of form and make up, very simply and clearly, abbreviational rules for generating these. I'm not sure whether you would need any transformations for representing anything about mental acts for speech acts; it would seem you would—I mean the very simple transformations that Vendler uses that don't get into any arguments about generative semantics or the standard model. So one could fully formalize a speech act theory with the tools of what we might call a "formal transformational grammar," as an extension of a mathematical theory of formal grammar.

Now, you seem to state a great antipathy for this. But, I don't see that you've given any reason why we should go ahead and do that, particularly if we're sort of mathematically and abbreviationally minded.

DR. SEARLE: Allow me to make the position clear. I have no objection to the study of syntax, nor to the representation of syntactical facts in trees. If I had to say one thing only about Zeno Vendler, I would say that the trees aren't rich enough. I think his trees don't have enough leaves on them; they're too denuded.

DR. PETERSON: Further, I think the Harris model is beside the point.

DR. SEARLE: It could be. But, I am not objecting to the representation of syntactic facts in tree structures, nor am I objecting to trying to get properly formalized statements of our theory. Now, the syntactical facts that Vendler records are not a theory of speech acts. They are an attempt to find syntactical correlates to a speech act taxonomy. I think that that's a useful project; I've worked on that a bit myself. What I was objecting to was the methodological assumption that all of the interesting facts about language somehow or other have to be fit into a tree. One of the interesting things about them—about Bever's recent research that he did out in Berkeley—was to show that some of the unexplainable facts of language had to do with perceptual strategies, and are not properly parts of the syntactical tree. So my objection was not to the enterprise of investigating syntax; far from it. To me, one of the most interesting questions in language is how form and function interact. You have all of these speech acts. How do they get realized in sentences of real live languages? Why do you use gerunds, and why the "to" form in the infinitive, or others for other kinds of illocutionary acts? I'm all for that, and I want to go beyond what Vendler does. I think his trees aren't nearly rich enough.

DR. OSGOOD: Although you didn't ask me a question, I'd like to ask you a question. Something puzzles me about these hypersentences, superhypersentences. You can go on and on, and that is the simple case that John gave of the implicit "I say to you that it's raining." My question is this: Isn't the essence of the methodology of linguists, in terms of finding out or developing what could be called a competence grammar, really relying on their intuitions about the language? Now, if there is anything that is completely beyond any intuitions that I have—maybe it's just because I'm not a linguist—is that I have something in my head which is saying that "I tell you that...," or "I say to you that...," or any of the more elaborate ones that have been proposed. How can one put into such a linguistic explanation something which is counter intuitive? Do you have such intuitions when *you* make such an assertion? I ask you that.

DR. PETERSON: That strikes me as a very strange question, because what you might enter into it is what, in fact, is not supposed to be at all available to introspection and intuition. Intuitive data is what people say, and they may do fantastic things in principle to relate what they say to each other. That is, we have to do fantastic things to form a representation. To speak English, you need not know any formal grammar of English, you just have to know English. It's another sense of knowing the grammar of English, in terms of the theoretical formulation of grammarians. There's just a tremendous gap between those two.

DR. SEARLE: I think I'd like to state a point which is very similar to Prof. Osgood's, and maybe even the same. What is so puzzling, what I find so fantastic about the performative hypothesis, is that it has the consequence that you can perform an illocutionary act only by saying that you are performing it. It does have that consequence if you take it in conjunction with the theory that deletions don't change meanings, and that the meaning is contained in the deep structure. Ross accepts both of these points, or at least accepted them at the time of publication of the papers. That has the consequence that when I say "it's raining" in the important sense of "say," I can only perform a speech act by saying that I'm performing it, and that seems to be very implausible.

DR. OSGOOD: I'd like to add one point, too, i.e. another reason. If the claim is that the underlying structure of assertion, "it's raining out," is "I tell you that it's raining out," then wouldn't it have to follow that the meaning of the two segments "It's raining out" and "I tell you that it's raining out" should be interchangeable? They should have the same meaning. I claim that I will only say "I tell you that it's raining out" when you have in some way implied that I do not know what I am talking about or that you don't believe me. Then I'll say "I tell you that it's raining out."

DR. PETERSON: There is a clear answer to that right from Austin, and I think Austin certainly mistakes some of the grammatical forms here. Consider giving a warning, to say the bull is going to charge. If I say "I warn you, the bull is going to charge," I submit that's somewhat odd, as a warning. If I'm going to warn you that the bull is going to charge, I say: "That bull is going to charge." I don't say "I warn you." Similarly, if I'm issuing an order, I issue an order. I say: "Everybody line up." If I say "I order everybody to line up," it's taken as slightly odd, except in the military context, where utterance of the verb "order" is in line. But I suggest that in most ordinary conversations where imperatives like orders are given, it's odd to say "I order." Similarly, to ask a question, you don't say "I ask you." That's some kind of extra emphasis added on. Such emphasis usually manifests itself in other ways: by intonation and by reversing the order of the words. To say "I ask you something or other" is slightly odd. That's an ordinary question, so I give it right back to you.

DR. SEARLE: We thought that was our point.

DR. MENYUK: Dr. Searle has suggested that we come down to the ground, and I'd like to bring him even lower and think a little bit about the child who is acquiring language. You raised the following question: why postulate rules of discourse as separate kinds of rules? It struck me that at an early stage of development the child's statements and questions might have implications that are beyond what the child meant to say. "Can you pass the salt" is like a set. But "Can you close the door" or "Can you open the window" might require additional rules that have to be acquired. A very interesting issue, especially concerning kids with language problems, is whether or not this is an almost insurmountable task.

DR. SEARLE: Well, to give a really adequate response to that would take more time than we have, so let me make the following inadequate remarks. I think that it's an empirical question how children learn these forms. I get many papers in the mail of an empirical kind, and some of them even suggest that certain of these forms are learned first, as requests, and later on have to be factored out into their literal meanings. But that supports the hypothesis that a lot of developmental people have held for a long time: namely, that we shouldn't just view children's grammar as a kind of small version of the grown-up grammar. It may have its own structure. But now you raised a difficult question, and that is, what about rules? What's a rule and what's a regularity? My methodological assumption would be that you're going to need rules anyhow, so try to get on with as few as possible. I think there are general rules of conversation like "Be relevant." If you go around deliberately saying a lot of irrelevant things, you can wreck any number of conversations, and people just don't know how to respond to that. That seems to me a rule or something very much like a rule, but a lot of things that people call "rules," I'm inclined not to call rules. I think that I don't need those conversational postulates in order to account for the data. They are generalizations. It's a true generalization about English and other languages that you can ask somebody to do something by asking him if he is able to do it in a certain kind of context. But that's not a rule. That is to be *explained* by means of rules.

I don't know if he still says it, but Michael Argyle used to identify a lot of things as rules that I think are probably not rules. We have the eye-contact regularities that he discovered, some of which we talked about earlier today. I am disinclined to say that I'm breaking a rule if I don't follow those eye-contact regularities. It's an open question: what are the features something has to have in order for it to be a rule? It not only has to be a regularity, but it has to be projectable, it has to cover all kinds of new cases, and it has to be normative.

My methodological program would be the following. Get as far as you can with as few rules as you can, and then if something really does have the features of a rule, it's a rule. But don't assume that every regularity you find is a rule, because you can account for a lot of those regularities in terms of other rules or simply other features of the speech situation.

MASTERING THE INTANGIBLE THROUGH LANGUAGE*

Marion Blank

Rutgers Medical School
College of Medicine and Dentistry of New Jersey
Piscataway, New Jersey 08854

For many years, psychological research in the area of language and cognition was guided by the idea that language, in particular the language of labeling, was a key tool in the child's acquisition of concepts.[1-4] Recently, there has been a dramatic reversal of this view. Influenced strongly by the Piagetian model, researchers have increasingly adopted the idea that language does not determine the formation of concepts. Instead, language is seen to reflect the concepts that the child has acquired prior to, and hence independent of, the acquisition of language.[5-10] The current view is captured in the statement by Nelson[11] that "a new approach . . . is necessary because current and traditional models of concept formation are not designed to solve the problem at issue: How does the child match words to his concepts? They are, rather, designed to answer a different question: How does the child form a concept to fit the word?" The latter conceptualization of the problem has been deemed inadequate because it supposes that "the child learns meaning from his encounters with the language rather than from encounters with the physical and social world" (p. 268).

This new formulation has been of value in redressing a long imbalance in the language-thought controversy. In its turn, however, it stands in danger of recreating the imbalance, albeit in the opposite direction. Specifically, many current statements are worded so as to suggest that this view is applicable to almost all of language functioning. In this form, it represents a major overextension of an idea that evolved in the context of studying the young child's earliest linguistic performance. During this initial period of language mastery, the child does seem to direct his efforts toward finding the semantic equivalents of relationships he has long since mastered on the preverbal, sensorimotor level. As Brown[12] has pointed out, these include relations such as "the nominative (e.g., "That ball"), expressions of recurrence (e.g., "More ball") . . . expressions of disappearance or nonexistence (e.g., "All gone ball") . . . the possessive (e.g., "Daddy chair"), two sorts of locative (e.g., "Book table" and "Go store"), and the attributive (e.g., "Big house") (p. 101).

A significant feature of analyses such as these is that they are confined largely to words that denote clear perceptual referents—i.e., to terms that McNeill[13] has described as representing "portrayable correlates." Essential to the notion of a portrayable correlate is the idea that the referent in question can be perceived through the sense of vision, touch, and hearing, with vision playing an almost overwhelmingly dominant role. Given the known proficiency of even the very young child in the visual sphere,[14] it seems reasonable to accept the idea that the child's mastery of the protrayable can proceed well, without language, and accord-

*This work was supported by the Grant Foundation and USPHS grants 5K2MH10749 and MH21051.

ingly, that the language associated with such material merely reflects and does not determine the child's knowledge in this sphere.

Language, however, contains many terms that have no "portrayable correlates." In fact, the presence of such terms—terms that denote intangible, but nonetheless meaningful properties—may be one of the unique characteristics of language. It is this line of reasoning that has led me to feel that one cannot easily dismiss the idea that language may make a major contribution to thought, even to the thought of the young child. If it is to be meaningful, however, any search for the contribution of language to thinking should be carried out not in realm where other modalities do an equal, or even better, job, but in the realm where language may have unique properties for organizing our experiences. Some terms that exemplify, but that far from exhaust, the phenomenon to which I am referring, are found in question words referring to cause (i.e., *why*), manner (i.e., *how*) and time (i.e., *when*). Largely because the question word *why* occurs more frequently and earlier than these other terms, and also because it has played a major role in the analysis of children's early thinking,[16, 17] the discussion that follows will largely be confined to the child's mastery of this term.

My thoughts in this area were stimulated not so much by theoretical considerations as by practical ones. For many years, I have been involved in developing a tutorial program to facilitate learning in poorly functioning, preschool-age children.[15] In the main, these are children with low IQ scores who come from what are commonly termed "disadvantaged backgrounds." The children have numerous difficulties in school-based material. What seems to epitomize their difficulties, in the tutorial dialogue at least, are their responses to questions of *why, when,* and *how do you know?* It is not simply that the children fail to display causal reasoning. Such reasoning would not be expected in children of this age.[16] Rather, it is that such questions frequently lead to an abandonment or disruption of the dialogue, even when the children are as old as six years. For example, if such a child is asked, "Why does this cup" (a bigger one) "hold more than this one?", he might well reply, "I got that in my house." The confusion and failure in the children stand in marked contrast to the ease and accuracy with which well-functioning children respond to the same material at the same ages.

The role of *why, how,* and *when* as critical indicators of the child's ability in cognitively demanding exchanges is, upon reflection, not surprising. Even a most preliminary analysis of such questions indicates that they entail demands that are of a different order or magnitude from other question words such as *where, what,* and *who.* For example, most *where* questions posed to a young child are of two types and can be handled by two simple strategies. The first involves pointing to the object named (e.g., "Where is your nose?"); the second involves offering a label when 1) no object is named (e.g., "Where are you going?") or 2) the object named is not present (e.g., "Where is the ball?"). By contrast, *why* questions cover a much wider, and more complex, range of possibilities. These include *why's* of action (e.g., "Why did he lie down?"), *why's* of function (e.g., "Why doesn't the pen write?"), *why's* of justification (e.g., "Why do you think" ["How did you know"] "he was angry?") and *why's* of causal relations (e.g., "Why do heavy things sink?") (see N. Isaacs' discussion[17] on the range of *why's* relevant to the preschool age child).

The complexity of the range of *why* questions that may be asked is mirrored on the response side in the number of strategies required for appropriate answers. For example, *why's* of action may require a statement of motivation (e.g., "He lay down because he wanted to rest") or a statement of condition (e.g., "He lay down because his back hurt"), while *why's* of function may require a statement of attribute (e.g., "The pen doesn't work because the point is broken"). Further, unlike the situation of *where* or *what*, nothing cited in the question and nothing present in the context need offer a clue as to what might be an appropriate response. For example, in the question "Why does that cup hold more?" there is no hint as to what feature in the situation should be named in the answer: should it be the color, the texture, the size, the location, or the function of the object? The situation becomes even more difficult when the question is such that no perceptible feature in the situation can serve as an answer (e.g., "Why is he packing the valise?"). In these cases, any possible answer (e.g., "He is going on a trip") is often disconnected, in both time and space, from the situation that the child can see at the moment.

Given this complex situation, one wonders how the child ultimately achieves mastery over the term. Having become intrigued with the problem, I began to review the literature that dealt with the acquisition of *why*. Several investigators[18-20] report the appearance of this word by two years of age, but generally they give little further information, apparently because for some time the word is used in ways that are judged "meaningless" by the adult. Significantly, the very meaningless of *why* reinforces the idea that this word is different from most other words used by the child, for implicit in the concept of meaningless is the idea that the word is being produced without being comprehended. As a result, it stands in opposition to the new theoretical formulation (outlined above), which states that meaning precedes language and does not follow it.

These scattered reports indirectly lent support to the notion that *why* may occupy a unique position in the child's early learning. However, the reports failed to provide a solid picture of the precise sequence by which this term was mastered. For such an understanding to be achieved, it was necessary to have additional data. Given the fact that the child's earliest uses of *why* were meaningless, it was clear that any such additional data could not be gained from a formal test situation, since formal testing would only reveal the child's lack of comprehension. Instead, it seemed essential to have a naturalistic situation where the child might spontaneously produce or respond to this question in normal interchange.

At the time that my thoughts on this issue were evolving, I was fortunate to begin working with Doris Allen, a linguist who, for quite different purposes, had collected bimonthly data on the linguistic performance of a middle-class child named Dusty.[21] The sessions took place when Dusty was between 18 and 31 months old, and they averaged about one hour each in duration. In all the sessions, the major participants were Dusty and her adult "playmate," Dr. Allen.

Given the impetus provided by the issues discussed above, we began to examine the data in order to extract all the interchanges in which this term occurred. This included the child's use of the term and the adult's response, as well as the adult's use of the term and the child's response. This section of the paper will be concerned with some of the findings that our search yielded. A fuller presentation of the results can be obtained elsewhere.[23]

Our analysis indicated that Dusty's production and reception† of *why* could be categorized into three basic strategies. The key features of each strategy are outlined in TABLE 1. As can be seen there, in the first strategy (which took place when Dusty was 18 to 25 months), one might be somewhat hard pressed to consider her reception of *why* as representative of a true strategy. She was rarely asked such questions by the adult, but when she was (as in "Why is the dolly going to sleep?"), almost invariably, she either ignored the *why*, tentatively touched the object named, or else changed the subject. Ervin-Tripp[24] noted similar behavior on the part of

---

†The term "reception" is used, rather than the more traditional term of comprehension, because the child's responses to *why* could not be said to indicate understanding on her part.

young children when *why* questions are put to them. This behavior contrasted strongly to the near universal and nearly always appropriate answers she gave to *what*, *where*, and *yes-no* questions.

Although Dusty seemed unable to answer adult-asked *why*'s, she did have a production strategy for this term even when she was only 18 months. (This state of affairs is, of course, the one responsible for the generalization that the production of *why* precedes its comprehension.) Her first use of this word was not frequent, but it was consistent. First, it occurred only in response to an adult statement; never as a means of describing or questioning perceived events. In other words, from the beginning, *why* was tied to the linguistic and not to the physical world. Second, the preceding adult utterance always contained a negative, such as *no* or *not*. Thus, a typical exchange in which it occurred went as follows. The object of

TABLE 1
HIGHLIGHTS IN A CHILD'S INITIAL DEVELOPMENT OF "WHY"

Strategy	Age (months)	Production	Reception
I	18–25	a) Asked, without apparent meaning, in response to negative statement by adult b) Limited to single-word utterance	Ignores the question or attends to item named in question
II	26–27	Continues Strategy I, but a) embeds *why* in multiple-word utterance b) occasionally asks *why* to initiate dialogue c) marked increase in number of *why* questions asked	Says "I don't know"
III	28–31	Asks why a) in response to both negative and affirmative statements by adult b) to initiate discourse about observed events	a) cites some feature in the environment associated with the objects named in the question. b) "appropriate" and inappropriate responses almost equally likely.

play was a toy cat who had "lost" its head. The adult commented, "The cat has a body, but no head." Dusty replied, "Why?" The adult responded "Why? I don't know why. Did someone break it?" Dusty's response was to turn away and go to the toy box.

Dusty's pairing of *why* and negation does not seem unreasonable in that it is probably based on her observation that adults themselves frequently ask "Why?" when they hear a negative statement (e.g., when someone says, "I don't want to...", a common reply is to ask "Why?" or "Why not?"). What seems of greater interest than the connection between *why* and negation is the fact that the child's *why*'s rarely led the adult to offer a response that provided any significant feedback about the meaning of the term other than the feedback that it has been used inappropriately. Typically, the adult might haltingly say, "I don't know why," or "Why do you think it is?" In fact, of the first 19 *why*'s that Dusty asked, only five received replies that might suggest to her that a meaningful response can be offered to this question (e.g., once, when told not to put a toy in her mouth, she responded by asking, "Why?", and the adult replied " 'Cause that would hurt you.").

Given the generally frustrating nature of such a situation, one wonders why Dusty, and other children, bother to produce the number of *why*'s that they do. No clear answer is possible, but it seems likely that a central element is the fact that the child's linguistic development at this stage is sufficiently advanced to permit her to recognize the existence of this word when she hears it used by others. But that is all her development allows her, for it is a word lacking a physical referent and there-fore it is unavailable for exploration through the child's oft-used sensorimotor repertoire (i.e., she cannot stare at it, pick it up, mouth it, kick it, etc.). Given the success that the child has had with her sensorimotor repertoire, it is likely that she will try its techniques on terms such as *why*. And, in fact, this characterizes one pattern of Dusty's initial response (e.g., touching the object named when asked a question such as "Why is the dolly lying down?"). From the response of the adult, specifically the break in the dialogue, the child soon learns that this approach is inadequate.

This situation contrasts sharply with that confronting the child when she hears unknown words referring to portrayable correlates. For example, if a child is asked to "touch her nose" she may do nothing because she is unfamiliar with the word "nose." In all likelihood, the adult will then point to the intended referent, and the child will imitate this action and also pair the label she has heard with the object she has long known. The child's ability to rely in this way on her sensorimotor skills (e.g., observation, imitation, and association) may be responsible for the common finding that the comprehension of language precedes its production.[13] Meaning can be gleaned by the child through trying one or more of her sensorimotor techniques. Hence understanding is possible for the child without her having to attempt any verbal formulation.

Not only are sensorimotor techniques closed off to the child in connection with comprehending *why*, but they are also closed off in producing the word, in that the child's much-used gesture system is rendered useless in this situation. For instance, question words such as *what* can be represented in many situations by pointing (e.g., "What is this called?") or by a furrowed brow (e.g., "What do you want?"). No comparable gestures exist, however, for a word such as *why*. Its expression seems dependent upon a verbal system.

This constellation of circumstances—namely, the inability to derive the meaning of *why* by sensorimotor techniques and the inability to express this term through nonverbal means—leaves the young child in a situation in which her preferred avenues of behavior are closed off. She is forced to derive the meaning through a different process. Specifically, she is led to produce the term before she compre-hends it. She must adopt this approach because it is the only way in which she can get sufficient feedback to figure out the meaning of the word. But, as indicated by the adult response to Strategy I (see TABLE 1), production is insufficient to give the child the information she needs in order to understand and use the term appropri-ately. It is probably for this reason that she embarks on a second type of strategy.

In the second strategy, which began when Dusty was 26 months old, she began to use *why* not simply as a single word utterance, but combined with strings of words. In addition, even though her questions were still "meaningless," she pursued the exchange, almost as if she were intent upon getting an answer. For example, in one exchange, the adult said, "That's the garage door." Dusty replied "Why the garage door? Why?" The adult answered "Hmm?" and Dusty repeated, "Why the garage door?"

The changes in the production of *why* were paralleled by changes in the child's response to *why*'s asked by adults. In place of the avoidance that Dusty previously demonstrated when asked *why*, at this stage she now answered, "I don't know." Even though this latter phrase had been in her repertoire since 21 months of age and had been used freely in answer to other WH questions, it was not until she was 26 months that she used it in response to *why*.

This second strategy in handling *why* was replaced two months later by a third strategy, in which Dusty took the whole of an affirmative, not negative, statement by the adult and repeated it, prefacing it by *why*. For example, in one exchange, Dusty asked "Where's Bobby?" The adult replied, "He's home reading a book." Dusty responded, "Why he reading a book?" As this example indicates, the words placed after the *why* were almost always imitations of what the adult had just said. (See Clark[25] for similar strategies in another child when faced with the mastery of new, complex verbal material.) Significantly, the child's attention to the whole of the adult sentence is almost a prerequisite if the child is to achieve mastery of this term. *Why* almost always refers to either predicates or whole sentences. Thus, *what*, *where*, and *who* can be meaningfully used when the focus is solely on the nominal phrase (e.g., "Where ball?"). By contrast, *why* with a nominal phrase is usually meaningless (e.g., "Why ball?"). It takes on meaning only when it goes beyond the single object focused on in the nominal and encompasses an entire event.

Her recognition of the importance of the information contained in the predicate was reflected in another use of *why*. Dusty now no longer limited *why* to being a response to a statement by the adult. Instead, she used it to initiate discourse about an observable change in the environment. For example, at one point the adult folded up a piece of paper and placed it in her pocket, and Dusty said, "Why you put this in your pocket?" Although Dusty's use of *why* in this manner was not common, it was ultimately much more productive for her. Almost always, the adult interpreted this type of question as meaningful and comfortably gave a relevant answer.

Although the *why*'s of Strategy III (TABLE 1) are frequently interpreted as meaningful by the adult listener, it is clear that the child still does not have a full grasp of the term, for she was as likely to ask meaningless *why*'s as to ask meaningful ones. For example, at one point, the adult said, "You're stepping on the wash cloth," and Dusty replied, "Why?"

Strategy III was also marked by changes in Dusty's response to the adult's *why* questions. In contrast to her earlier avoidance of the term and her later use of "I don't know," Dusty now began to maintain the exchange after the question was posed. For example, one exchange at 29 months went as follows: The adult asked, "Why are you putting the tissue in the closet?" and Dusty answered, "So be cool."

It seems clear that Dusty was beginning to grasp the idea that a feature associated with the event or situation should be cited in answer to a *why* question (e.g., placing of the tissues in the closet will result in a change of state). It seems equally clear, however, that as Piaget[16] has demonstrated, she had no real understanding of the causal or logical relationships that might be involved. For example, at one point, Dusty said (of a blanket), "I can't wash this." The adult asked, "Why not?" and Dusty replied, "In here."

From these examples it is evident that the child's task of understanding *why* is far from finished. She has still not determined which of several possible attributes may be selected for the answer, nor has she determined how different features relate to different *why*'s. Nevertheless, the child's preliminary acquisition of *why* represents a major achievement. Over a period of months, she has steadfastly pursued the meaning of this elusive term through a course of hypothesis testing. In essence, the child had to form a concept that ultimately matched the word she was struggling to comprehend. Arguments have been raised against such a concept-formation view in early language development on the grounds that its achievement would place "an enormous strain on memory and cognitive processing ability in that the child must hold in memory not only all the instances of word but all of the relevant attributes of these instances, until he has extracted the invariance common to all. Although there are common strategies for solving the problem, their use implies a sophistication in and capacity for the use of problem-solving skills that have never been attributed to the infant" (Ref. 22, p. 100).

Despite the intuitive appeal of this argument, the analysis of the child's behavior presented here suggests that these types of complex problem-solving strategies are, in fact, the ones that the child did adopt in mastering the word *why*. What I would further like to suggest is the idea that this type of cognitive activity may be uniquely demanded, and thereby uniquely fostered, by certain aspects of language acquisition. Rarely, in any other situation, does the very young child encounter tasks demanding this type of critical, sustained thinking. In other words, while the cognitive skills employed by the child may be potentially available for use in all situations, I believe that they may rarely be mobilized except to meet the demands of certain kinds of language tasks. This position does not state that the presence of words such as *why* automatically leads to the possession of particular concepts; rather, it states that these words are central in leading the child to use conceptual and problem-solving skills that would otherwise remain undeveloped.

From a single case, such as the one presented here, it is not possible to determine whether the sequence described above is characteristic of the learning of *why* in most children. But there is enough comparability between Dusty's handling of *why* and those of other children reported in the literature to suggest that the sequence reported here is typical of at least one common pattern by which this word is mastered. Most of the reports, however, including that on Dusty, concern children from middle-class backgrounds. We have almost no information on how this type of language task is handled by children of lower-class backgrounds.

Some doubts might be aroused by the suggestion that differences could be expected in this area; however, reasons for expecting such differences derive from at least two sources. First, as stated earlier, my interest in this problem developed largely because of the difficulties that many children of lower-class backgrounds experience with words of this type in the teaching setting. It seems likely that difficulties expressed at the preschool period have their origins in the children's experiences with these words at an earlier period. Second, a feature that could easily be overlooked in the analysis of the child's acquisition of *why* is the role that the adult must play if the child is to gain the information she is seeking. The presence of a responsive adult is not sufficient, since *the child must take an active part in initiating and sustaining the various exchanges.* But the presence of a more mature speaker is essential if the child is to get the feedback she needs for rejecting inadequate strategies. From a number of sources,[26-28] there is evidence to suggest that the nature of the dialogue in middle-class and lower-class homes may be different in ways that are critical for the mastery of terms such as *why.* It would seem productive, in light of the issues discussed above, to collect dialogues between adults and very young children of different backgrounds in order to see the nature of the exchange with regard to such terms as why.

Although such data would be valuable, they are presently not available. Therefore, rather than conjecture as to what the possible findings might be, I should prefer at this point to pursue related but somewhat different data on the mastery of *why;* in particular, the development of *why* that follows the achievements attained by Dusty. For a number of reasons, the data are based upon a different methodology and sampling procedure from that used with Dusty. These differences derive from the fact that by the time Dusty was 31 months old, she was beginning to offer responses that had characteristics of what would be appropriate answers to *why*. This achievement meant that in studying the continuing development of *why*, there was no reason to rely on the long and cumbersome procedure of recording spontaneous language in naturalistic situations. Instead, because the older child is capable of responding to adult imposed *why*'s, more traditional formal testing can be carried out on relatively large numbers of children in a short period of time. This testing method does not yield information about the spontaneous *why*'s produced by children past the level achieved by Dusty. (The reports of Isaacs[17] offer a considerable amount of information in that area with reference to the functioning of bright children.) The testing method, however, can yield a great deal of information about children's ability to deal with *why*'s asked of them by others.

The information that will be presented below is part of a much broader assessment of the cognitive skills in children of three to six years of age. The material to be discussed here specifically concerns a set of 44 items designed to tap the child's ability to deal with problem-solving questions. The questions, though largely based on *why* and *how*, were not confined to these terms. For example, some problems had to be included in order to present the "data base" necessary before one can pose a reasonable *why* question. For example, the child might first observe the workings of a balance scale, after which he would be asked, "What will happen if I put another paper clip on the scale?" Only after he has made a prediction would he then be asked to justify it through the question "Why" (will it go down?).‡

In general, the 44 items fell into four categories. These were:

a) Multiple choice. The child had to select which of several would be appropriate, given the conditions stated. (For example, a paper cup, with the bottom missing, is shown to the child. He is told, "Water won't stay in this cup." An array of six objects is presented, including one that is the actual bottom of the cup, one that is a similar piece of material but too small for the cup, and one that also involves a comparable piece of material but that contains holes throughout, etc. The child is asked, "Which of these should I use to fix the cup?") These items were included to assess the child's skill on problem-solving tasks that required no overt verbalization on his part. There were four such problems.

b) Predicting an event or reporting the reasons responsible for an observed event. (For example, the child is shown four blocks, one stacked upon the other. The examiner points to the blocks at the bottom of the pile and asks, "What will happen to the pile of blocks if I take this one away?") There were 16 such items.

c) Rationale for an observation concerning objects or events. (For example, the child is shown a mirror and is told, "We look into mirrors." The examiner then shows the child a piece of clear, reflecting metal and a piece of cardboard. The child is then told, "Mirrors are made of shiny material like this and not of cardboard like this." "Why do you think mirrors are made of things like this," [the tester points to the metal] "and not things like this?" [The tester points to the cardboard.] There were 18 such questions.

d) Rationale for inability to achieve a specified action. (For example, the

‡The children would be asked to justify a prediction, regardless of whether or not it was correct. The example above is given only for illustrative purposes.

TABLE 2
CRITERIA FOR "CORRECTNESS" OF RESPONSE

Sample Problem: Child is shown a balance scale: he observes paper clips being placed on each side. The examiner holds up another clip and asks "What will happen to the scale if I put another clip in?"

Score	Rating	Criterion
Fully Correct	3	child describes focal result: e.g., "that side" (pointing) "will go down"
Part Correct	2	
a		child gives correct but vague or poorly formulated answer: e.g., (points) "down"
b		child gives technically correct but not focal result: e.g., "there'll be three clips on it"
c		child gives correct answer, but adds detracting irrelevant information: e.g., "It will go down 'cos it's white"
Ambiguous	1	it is not possible to determine if answer is correct or incorrect: e.g., "It'll move"
Incorrect	0	child does not offer any correct response: e.g., "It has two cups"

child is shown a completed puzzle. He is then shown one piece that is a duplicate of a piece in the puzzle and is asked, "Why can't we fit this piece in the puzzle?") This category was separated from the category above because it was felt that the identification of "inappropriate" attributes demanded in *why not* questions might be somewhat easier than the identification of "appropriate" attributes demanded in a *why* question. There were six such questions.

Aside from the multiple choice items, the children's responses were scored on two major parameters. The first, shown in TABLE 2, rated the response on a correct-to-incorrect scale, with a score of 3 for correct and 0 for incorrect. The second, shown in TABLE 3, used a five-point scale to rate the pattern of thinking underlying any incorrect response that was offered.

This aspect of the test, like the full test, was administered to 300 children from three to six years of age. The results on all the children are too extensive to be

TABLE 3
CRITERIA FOR INCORRECT RESPONSE

Rating	Criterion
Invalid	Child's response shows an understanding of the question, but the answer is incorrect e.g., "it will go up"
Association	Child's response indicates no understanding of the question, but it is focused on the material, e.g., "the cups are white"
Irrelevant	Child's response shows no understanding of the question nor of the material
	a) "Personalizes" the task, e.g., "I got one of those at home"
	b) Imitation, e.g., "It will happen"
	c) Denial e.g., "You won't put it on"
Don't Know	Child states he cannot answer the problem e.g., "I don't know what'll happen"
No Response	Child offers no verbal response to problem e.g., shrugs

reported here. Instead, in line with the issues outlined earlier, the major focus was on a comparison of well and poorly functioning children's response to *why*-based problem-solving questions. For this purpose, a subsection of the total sample was studied. Specifically, it included those children in the sample who fit the criterion of well and poorly functioning at each chronological age (3, 4, and 5 years).

The history of research in this area is replete with criticisms that any assessment of children along these lines is frequently inaccurate because the poorly functioning children are mainly from the lower socioeconomic groups, whereas the well functioning ones are mainly from the middle-class groups. Hence, any comparison of the groups implicitly judges lower-class children according to a middle-class standard. In an effort to avoid the difficulties inherent in such a comparison, all the children involved here were from lower-class backgrounds, lived in the same neighborhoods, and attended the same schools. The comparison is therefore between lower-class children who are well-functioning and those who are poorly functioning. To arrive at the selection of these two groupings, children were selected on the criterion that they be between one and two standard scores above, and below, the mean IQ of their group at each age. The mean IQ of the well-functioning group was 116 and of the poorly functioning group was 89. The distribution of each group

TABLE 4

MEAN CORRECT SCORES TO PROBLEM-SOLVING QUESTIONS*

Age (years)	Group							
	Well-Functioning				Poorly Functioning			
	M.C.	Pred.	Rat.	Rat.	M.C.	Pred.	Rat.	Rat.
5	2.4	2.2	1.6	1.7	1.3	1.1	0.7	0.6
7	2.7	2.2	1.8	2.0	2.0	2.0	1.3	1.9
9	2.7	2.5	2.4	2.4	2.1	2.1	1.5	1.7
11	2.8	2.6	2.6	2.5	2.3	2.2	2.1	2.1

*M.C. = multiple choice; Pred. = prediction and observation; Rat. = rationale question (why and why not, respectively).

was approximately 35% Puerto Rican, 55% Black, and 10% White. This type of subject selection yielded six to ten children in each of the two groups at each age (3, 4, 5 years).

Initial examination of the data indicated dramatic differences in performance between the groups at each age; i.e., the mean scores on the 0–3 "correct" scale were 0.9, 1.6, and 1.9 for the well-funtioning group at three, four, and five years, respectively, and 0.2, 0.4, and 0.9 for the comparable poorly functioning groups. These findings indicate a not-surprising two-year lag[30] in that the performance of the five-year-old poorly functioning child was equivalent to that of the three-year-old well-functioning one. What is more significant, however, is the fact that the performance of the three and four-year-old poorly functioning children was so low on these tasks that it was not profitable to analyze their data further; their responses were comparable to those of Dusty when she was in Stages I and II of her mastery of *why*.

In view of these findings, it seemed to be more productive to begin the analysis by concentrating on the performance of the five-year-olds. (In that age range, there were 8 children in each of the two IQ groups.) As shown in the top line of TABLE 4, there were marked differences in all the categories between the two groups. On all the items considered together, the well-functioning 5-year-old children, on the average, achieved some level of correct response on 68% of the 44 problems, while the same age poorly functioning children achieved such responses on only 30% of the problems. These data indicate that these types of questions resulted in the former group enjoying, for the most part, a success experience, while for the latter group in the same situation, the experience was one of overwhelming failure. This pattern was maintained even on the Rationale questions, where the comparable figures were 63% and 22%, respectively.

Although the general pattern of the results was not unexpected, the magnitude of the difference had not been anticipated. It was as if the two groups of children were functioning on what effectively were qualitatively different levels. In the light of these findings, it seemed essential to study the outcomes of these different levels of performance in order to gain some insight into when the poorly functioning child could begin to cope with this type of material. Because a longitudinal follow-up of these children was not possible, it was decided instead to study the counterparts of these children at seven, nine, and eleven years of age. The term "counterparts" refers to the selection of children who, on the basis of reading performance, were either succeeding or failing at the same neighborhood schools that the five-year-olds would eventually attend. At each of these three age groups, eight well-functioning and eight poorly functioning children were tested on the 44 items described earlier.§

The results, shown in TABLE 4, indicate improving performance for all the children as they matured. There was, however, a sustained difference between the two "ability" groupings. As assessed in a 2 (group) × 4 (age) × 4 (type of task) repeated measures analyses of variance, the findings indicated a significant difference for all the main effects—groups ($F = 41.36$, df 1/56, p <.001) age ($F = 16.57$, df 3/56, p <.001) and type of problem ($F = 32.92$, df 3/168, p <.001). None of the interaction terms were significant, indicating that the patterns of growth in the two groups were not different at the different ages. The most striking feature of the findings is that it is not until the poorly functioning children are between nine and eleven years of age that their performance equals that of the five-year-old well-functioning child. This result suggests a developmental lag not of the usual two to three years, but rather a lag extending for a period of five years. What is more, the lag is one that has occurred on tasks that the well-functioning child has mastered in the preschool years.

The data suggest one additional finding that may be of significance. The well-functioning children showed steady progress at each of the ages tested. The poorly functioning children showed a spurt from five to seven years and then essentially no change until about ten years of age. It remains to be determined whether these results are characeristic of broader patterns of performance and, in particular, whether they are characteristic of a fairly rigid plateau of functioning in poorly functioning children in the latency period. If such findings were obtained, they would be of major relevance to the design of curriculum in the early school years.

The analysis of the quality of the errors, shown in TABLE 5, corroborates and extends the findings reported above. As was implicit in the definition of the various types of errors, their quality varies, with an Invalid Response being considered the

---

§Because of school regulations, it was not possible to obtain IQ measures on these children. Instead, reading performance was used as the criterion. Children who read at, or above, grade level were placed in the well-functioning group, and those reading one year or more below grade level were placed in the poorly functioning group. The actual reading scores at 7, 9, and 11 years, respectively, were 2.5, 5.0, and 7.4 for the former group, and 1.1, 2.0, and 2.7 for the latter group.

highest level and No Response the lowest. These *a priori* ratings received some validation from the results themselves, in that as performance improves (in terms of the number of items correct), the quality of the wrong response is also seen to improve. For example, Invalid Responses account for 30% of the wrong responses of well-functioning children at five years, but for 70% of their wrong responses at 11 years. Similarly, the comparable figures for the poorly functioning children rise from 9% to 42%. Nevertheless, at all ages, the poorly functioning children have a much higher percentage of their wrong responses in the "Poorer" categories. Just as occurred with the total number of items correct, it is not until the poorly functioning children are between nine and eleven years that their pattern of wrong responses begins to approximate that of the five-year-old well-functioning child.

In an effort to evaluate the results more systematically, the wrong responses were grouped into one of two categories—"teachable" or "unteachable." These categories, which are derived from the clinical experience with the children, refer to the fact that with certain types of wrong response, it is possible for the teacher to lead the child to overcome his error; hence, these are termed "teachable" errors. On the other hand, certain kinds of wrong responses indicate that the child is so at a loss that it is extremely difficult, if at all possible, to help him understand the problem

TABLE 5
PERCENTAGE DISTRIBUTIONS OF THE TYPES OF ERRORS*

Age (years)	Group									
	Well-Functioning					Poorly Functioning				
	Inv.	Ass.	Irrel.	D.K.	N.R.	Inv.	Ass.	Irrel.	D.K.	N.R.
5	29.7	41.0	12.0	7.6	9.5	8.6	37.8	26.8	3.4	22.1
7	22.0	60.9	5.7	5.4	5.4	14.0	37.8	19.3	0.0	28.8
9	34.5	26.7	9.9	14.6	4.1	19.9	40.2	15.4	0.0	24.1
11	71.4	12.4	9.4	0.0	0.0	41.5	32.2	15.6	7.6	3.1

*Inv. = invalid; Ass. = associated; Irrel. = irrelevant; D.K. = I don't know; N.R. = no response.

posed.[15] For example, if when asked the question what will happen to the balance scale when a clip is added, the child offers an Invalid Response such as "It will not move," the teacher has open possibility of saying, "Let's see," followed by a demonstration of the phenomenon. On the other hand, if the child offers an Irrelevant Response such as "My friend can do it," there is little the teacher can do at that moment to help the child recognize the solution to the problem posed. Although there are exceptions, the categories of Invalid, Associated, and I Don't Know are considered "teachable" responses, while Irrelevant and No Response answers are deemed "unteachable."¶ The percentages of each child in each category were converted by an arc sine transformation[31] and the results analyzed in a 2 (group) × 4 (age) repeated measures analysis of variance. The results indicated a significant effect for groups ($F = 21.91$, df 1/53, p < .001). There was no effect for

¶It may seem surprising to separate "I don't know" responses from "No response." Clinically, however, they are different behaviors. As Dusty's responses indicated, she gave "No response" when her understanding of the question *why* was minimal. As her knowledge and confidence grew, however, even though her mastery was far from complete, she began to offer "I don't know" responses and these responses served as a signal that she was willing to maintain the dialogue.

age, nor was there any significant interaction. These results indicate that across all ages, poorly functioning children gave a much greater percentage of "unteachable" responses, and until eleven years of age, the proportion was close to half of all their errors. Thus, not only did the poorly functioning child fail significantly more problems than the well-functioning one, but when he failed he was much more likely to offer a response that would be difficult for the teacher to cope with.

The picture conveyed by these data support the clinical observations that led to this research; namely, that the mastery of a term such as *why* is a long and difficult process for the child and that an initial delay in its early acquisition is associated with an unexpectedly long period of retardation in its ultimate mastery. As a result, poor performance in this sphere in the preschool years is almost a diagnostic sign that the child will experience difficulty in the academic setting.

But the picture is far from simple. As the data indicate, the poorly functioning children's difficulties were not confined to *why* questions. They also performed less effectively on the multiple choice items that did not seem to require any knowledge of *why* and that did not even require any overt verbalization on the part of the children. This type of result brings us back to the ever-present chicken-egg dilemma in conceptualizing the relationship between thought and language. Since the children's difficulties were not confined to *why* questions but occurred in all the problem-solving items, it could well be argued that their lack was not in the understanding of *why*, but rather in the averbal conceptual thought processes necessary if one were to deal effectively with the problems posed.

This line of reasoning, however, overlooks an important fact; that is, the problems all concerned concrete, sensorimotor-based events—events that are part of the everyday experience of all human beings. And indeed, all the children, regardless of whether they were well-functioning or poorly functioning, coped more than adequately when they had to respond directly to such events: (e.g., reaching to catch an object in anticipation that it might fall). It seems likely that regular encounters with the physical and social world are sufficient to lead to this level of adaptation, even in the absence of language. But the questions did not require this type of immediate, physical, appropriate response. Rather, they required the child to reflect upon his world and consider hypothetical, albeit potentially real, events. As a result, the child could not act upon the objects; instead, he had to accept the imposed problem and call upon skills whereby he could isolate attributes, reject inappropriate possibilities, discount salient but irrelevant features, and be attentive to subtle words in the statement of the problem. Many of the skills are similar, even identical, to the skills that Dusty had to employ in seeking the meaning of *why*. I should therefore like to propose that the development of these conceptual skills flows not from encounters with the physical world but rather from encounters with certain forms of complex dialogue. If children have not had the opportunity or need to engage in such dialogue (i.e., the dialogue necessary for the mastery of *why* and for the mastery of the many other words referring to intangible phenomena), then it follows that a wide range of their problem-solving skills will be adversely affected. In this view, failure to master readily certain types of language does lead to difficulties in conceptualization, but the difficulties do not bear a simple one-to-one correspondence between the word and the concept. Instead, the difficulties manifest themselves indirectly in those qualities of thinking that are fostered by particular types of linguistic mastery.

It is evident that there are weaknesses in this approach. The limited findings presented here certainly do not provide the broad data base necessary to make this hypothesis intellectually compelling. Further, it seems unlikely that any single set of data could be strong enough to provide unequivocal evidence in this area. The ultimate fate of this orientation can therefore be determined not by "the critical experiment," but rather by the study of the broad range of phenomena that may be involved in the language-cognition network. In this context, it is clear that the present data represent no more than a beginning attempt to tap into this enormously complex network. Nevertheless, despite these limitations, the data do seem strong enough to indicate that our understanding of the child's search for semantic mastery will not be complete if we limit ourselves to the increasingly prevalent assumption that his nonverbal knowledge is, in all cases, sufficient to explain his cognitive and linguistic achievements.

ACKNOWLEDGMENTS

Appreciation is extended to the many nursery schools in the New York City area and to the Divisions of Day Care and the Board of Education of New York City for their cooperation in this research, and to Laura Berlin, Francis Goldenberg, Marilyn Markowitz, and Rita Rapp for assisting in the collection of the data.

REFERENCES

1. WHORF, B. L. 1956. Language, Thought and Reality. John Wiley & Sons Inc. New York, N.Y.
2. LURIA, A. R. 1961. The Role of Speech in the Regulation of Normal and Abnormal Behavior. Liveright Publishing Corp. New York, N.Y.
3. KUENNE, E. R. 1946. Experimental investigation of the relation of language to transposition behavior in young children. J. Exp. Psych. 36: 471–490.
4. KENDLER, T. S. & H. W. KENDLER. 1959. Reversal and nonreversal shifts in kindergarten children. J. Exp. Psych. 58: 56–60.
5. BLOOM, L. 1970. Language Development: Form and Function in Emerging Grammars. MIT Res. Monogr. 59.
6. BROWN, R. 1973. A First Language: The Early Stages. Harvard University Press. Cambridge, Mass.
7. CLARK, E. V. 1974. Some aspects of the conceptual bases for first language acquisition. In Language Perspectives: Acquisition, Retardation, and Intervention. R. L. Schiefelbusch & L. L. Lloyd, Eds. University Park Press. Baltimore, Md.
8. OLSON, D. R. 1974. From utterance to text: The bias of language in speech and writing. Paper presented at the Epistemics meeting. Vanderbilt University, Nashville, Tenn.
9. SCHLESINGER, I. M. 1971. Production of utterances and language acquisition. In The Ontogenesis of Grammar. D. I. Slobin, Ed. Academic Press. New York, N.Y.
10. SLOBIN, D. I. 1973. Cognitive prerequisites for the development of grammar. In Studies of Child Language Development. C. A. Ferguson & D. I. Slobin, Eds. Holt Rinehart & Winston Inc. New York, N.Y.
11. NELSON, K. 1974. Concept, word, and sentence: interrelations in acquisition and development. Psychol. Rev. 81: 267–285.
12. BROWN, R. 1973. Development of the first language in the human species. Amer. Psychol. 28: 97–106.
13. McNEILL, D. 1966. The development of language. In Carmichael's Manual of Child Psychology. Vol. 1. P. H. Mussen, Ed. John Wiley & Sons Inc. New York, N.Y.
14. KAGAN, J. 1971. Change and Continuity in Infancy. John Wiley & Sons Inc. New York, N.Y.
15. BLANK, M. 1973. Teaching Learning in the Preschool: A Dialogue Approach. Charles E. Merrill Publishing Co. Columbus, Ohio.
16. PIAGET, J. 1959. The Language and Thought of the Child. Routledge & Kegan Paul. London, England. (First published 1926)
17. ISAACS, S. 1930. Intellectual Growth in Young Children. Routledge & Kegan Paul. London, England.

18. BROWN, R. 1968. The development of WH questions in child speech. J. Verb. Learn. Behav.
    7: 279-290.
19. FAHEY, G. L. 1942. The questioning activity of children. J. Genet. Psychol. 60: 337-357.
20. WEIR, R. 1962. Language in the Crib. Mouton. The Hague, The Netherlands.
21. ALLEN, D. 1973. The Development of Predication in Child Language. Unpublished doctoral
    dissertation. Teachers College, Columbia University. New York, N.Y.
22. NELSON, K. 1973. Structure and strategy in learning to talk. Monogr. Soc. Res. Child Dev.
    38 (1-2, Serial no. 149).
23. BLANK, M. & D. ALLEN. 1975. Understanding "Why": Its significance in early intelligence.
    In Infant Intelligence. M. Lewis, Ed. Plenum Press. New York, N.Y.
24. ERVIN-TRIPP, S. 1970. Discourse agreement: How children answer questions. In Cognition
    and the Development of Language. J. R. Hayes, Ed. John Wiley & Sons Inc. New York,
    N.Y.
25. CLARK, R. 1974. Performing without competence. J. Child Lang. 1: 1-10.
26. BERNSTEIN, B. 1971. Class, Codes and Control. Vol. 1. Routledge & Kegan Paul. London,
    England.
27. NEWSON, J. & E. NEWSON. 1968. Four Year Olds in an Urban Community. George Allen &
    Unwin. London, England.
28. WOOTTON, A. J. 1974. Talk in the home of young children. Sociology 8: 277-295.
29. LABOV, W. 1968. A Study of the Nonstandard English of Negro and Puerto Rican Speakers
    in New York City. Vol. 2. Columbia University. New York, N.Y.
30. DEUTSCH, M. & B. BROWN. 1964. Social influences in Negro-white intelligence differences.
    J. Soc. Issues. 10: 249-263.
31. WINER, B. J. 1971. Statistical Principles in Experimental Design. McGraw-Hill Inc. New
    York, N. Y.

THE LANGUAGE-IMPAIRED CHILD: LINGUISTIC OR COGNITIVE IMPAIRMENT?

Paula Menyuk

Boston University School of Education
Boston, Massachusetts 02215

An appropriate response to the question posed in the title of this paper might be a resounding "Both!" However, the conclusions that might be drawn from such a response do not lead to any clarification of the state of the language-impaired child. One might assume from this response that the distinctions and/or similarities between the terms *linguistic* and *cognitive* have been clearly defined and described, and that in every instance of a fully described language impairment, a cognitive impairment, also fully described, exists as well. This is not the case.

Language impairment usually appears in conjunction with certain conditions of developmental impairment. Children who are mentally retarded, brain damaged, or both, or who are suspected of having brain damage, do not develop language at a rate or in a manner similar to their normally developing peers. It might be hypothesized that blind children, as well, may display differences in language development because of delay in development of sensorimotor schema,[1] whereas deaf children do not display them in the acquisition of sign language.[2] These developmental differences have been attributed to either delay in cognitive development and therefore a delay in language development, or to specific problems in organizing, analyzing, storing, and retrieving both linguistic and nonlinguistic information. These differing opinions appear to stem from varying interpretations of what is meant by cognitive and linguistic development and from varying interpretation of sequential events. We will examine these presumptions by 1) reviewing what is meant by early linguistic and cognitive development and the relations proposed between these developments, and 2) reviewing the findings of some studies concerning the linguistic behavior and intellectual development of children who are not developing language normally. Finally, the implications of these findings for the content of remedial programs designed to aid the "communicatively disordered" child will be discussed.

EARLY LINGUISTIC AND NONLINGUISTIC DEVELOPMENTS

It has often been stated that during the first year of life the child is prelinguistic[3] but that the infant is obviously thinking during this period and before he uses language. If one accepts a definition such as Hockett's,[4] that every human language has a grammar containing a discrete repertory of meaningful elements (words and sentences) that are mapped into meaningless but differentiating elements (a discrete repertory of such sounds), then clearly the infant's vocalization behavior is nonlinguistic in structure. It is equally clear, however, that the vocalization behavior of the infant does serve a communicative function; that is, the expression of needs and feelings, and socialization. Vocal behavior during this period does not appear yet to serve the function of representing objects and events in the environment either for the child himself or for communicating these representations to others.

Marshall[5] discusses Buhler's theory of three stages in the language-acquisition process. At each stage language serves different functions. First there is the stage at which language has an indicative (or expressive) function, then the stage where language has a stimulative (or communicative) function, and then, finally, the stage where language has a representational (or descriptive) function. It is primarily this last stage, in Buhler's view, that differentiates man's communicative system from that of other animals. This latter stage also appears to be the one described by Vygotsky[6] as the point at which thought and speech meet. What is being described are the stages that occur once language, as defined previously, has begun. If, however, this is a reasonable description of stages in the language acquisition process, then during the so-called prelinguistic period the infant's vocalizations serve the functions of both stage one (indicative) and stage two (stimulative), but not yet stage three (representational). In addition, we have, thus far, only comments that have been made about vocalization production during this period, but not about what is understood. The constraints that operate on production may not be an exact reflection of either the child's categorizations of the structure of language or his conception of the functions of language, but, rather, his programming abilities in carrying out the motor task of articulating his linguistic thoughts within the limits of a certain time.

During the so-called prelinguistic stage, several observations have been made about the child's perceptual and productive vocal behavior.[7] Productively, both cry and noncry utterances are observed from birth. Noncry utterances are, during the first four or five months of life, largely vocalic in structure, and both cry and noncry vocalizations become more differentiated and controlled during this period. So-called conversational behavior on the part of the infant has been observed from two to three months of life. The infant appears to be listening to and responding to the vocalization behavior of his caretaker. At about five months, babbling (defined as syllabic or consonant-vowel utterances) becomes established. This behavior increases in frequency, variety, and length until the period at which first words appear; however, the frequency with which certain sounds are vocalized changes during this developmental period, and the pattern of change in the sound composition of babbled utterances is similar for children from the varying linguistic environments that have been observed. The prosodic features of these babbled utterances vary in that they can be either statementlike, demandlike, or requestlike in intonational contour. Just before recognizable words appear consistently, these utterances become much shorter (word length). These word-length utterances do not yet resemble lexical items sufficiently to be recognized as such with any great frequency. As lexical items are acquired, it has been observed that different phonological sequences are used to indicate or communicate about the same object or event (for example, "papa," "tata," "baba," or even "lala" for father) and that the same phonological sequence is used to indicate or communicate about different objects and events (for example, "papa" for father, mother, nurse, dog). Prosodic features, gesture, and contextual information are used in accompaniment with utterances. Both limitations on the degree of phonological variation from the target word and a reduction in the use of gesture occur over the "holophrastic" period.

Perceptually, during the first two months of life the infant shows evidence of discriminating between acoustic features that mark speech-sound differences between syllables and between rising and falling fundamental frequency patterns of syllables. Shortly thereafter, the infant has been observed to respond differentially to prosodic features that mark the difference between friendly and unfriendly, male and female voices and the voice of the mother versus other female voices. In the last quarter of the first year there is evidence that the infant discriminates between sentences with statement and question intonational contours, prefers to listen to word-length utterances, and understands the meaning of some words and phrases. The extent of the infant's understanding of language during the holophrastic period has yet to be fully explored. Most studies thus far have been observational, and it is difficult to determine the bases of the child's seeming understanding; that is, it is not clear whether the utterance heard is being understood in part or in full, or, rather, the situation and the gestures of the speaker. It seems likely that at this stage linguistic, paralinguistic, and situational cues are all used to understand utterances and that little "displacement" has occurred at this point. Systematic changes in the child's responses to questions, from mere repetition of final word to direct reply, have been observed during the end of the holophrastic period.[8] It has been stated with a great deal of regularity that the child's comprehension of language (phonologically, syntactically, and semantically) exceeds his productive abilities to some degree. The exact parameters of this difference have been explored only in some few specific instances,[9] and at a somewhat later stage of development.

Both productively and perceptually, the infant has achieved the ability to discriminate between and categorize at least syllabic segments or word-length utterances, and to discriminate between and categorize prosodic features that signal communicative intent during the period before two-word utterances appear. It has also been suggested that the child comprehends certain relations expressed in sentences (such as action-object, actor-action, possessor-possessed, object-location, attribution-object) before he expresses the two-part relationship.[8]

Nonlinguistically, during the first year and a half of life two accomplishments have been referred to as playing a crucial role in the acquisition of language. The first is the acquisition of the permanency of objects and the second is the development of symbolization.[10] The concept of permanency of objects develops between approximately six and eighteen months, and symbolization develops during the period of 19 to 26 months. Object-permanency is deemed a necessary prerequisite to the development of a lexicon. The development of symbolization is simultaneous with the production of "language" or the use of words to express relationships. This latter development has been described as representations of thought: first as signals and symbols, and then as signs. That is, a change occurs in the use of signifiers in that they first function as a property of the object or event, and are linked to or are a part of the object or event (symbols). Later, signifiers are distinct from the object or event (signs) to the user. This description of the development of signifiers appears to resemble quite closely Buhler's description of stages in language acquisition: from indicative to stimulative to representational.

Explanations of what object permanence "is" and what symbolization "is" and descriptions of how they develop are still matters of both speculation and argument. The Piagetians suggest that object-permanence is the search for an object that has disappeared. The notion of "out of sight, out of mind" at earlier stages, however, has been challenged by some recent research.[11] Symbolization has been described as an interiorization of (or mental image of) action schema. Both accomplishments are said to evolve through the processes of organized reflexes and differentiation of objects, consolidation and repetition of motor habits, and imitation, first immediate and then deferred. The development of these sensorimotor schema to the point at which they become internalized is a product of physiological maturation and the consequences of the behavior (success for the child and reward from the environment). There is, however, presumably no explanation of how and why symbolization develops.[12] Observations indicate only that there are behaviors that precede this development and are therefore deemed prerequisites. These prerequisites are knowledge about the properties of objects and the coordination of action patterns. The development of symbolization is said to be one mechanism by which signifiers that have no organic resemblance to reality (for example, phonological sequences) are linked to the real world (objects and events). This development seems to be attributed, in essence, to the nature of the human organism. There are, of course, other explanations of the perceptual-motor developments during this period that point to the establishment of S-R-R chains or associations and generalizations from these to account for the behavior observed.[13] However, most of the recent psycholinguistic discussions attribute language acquisition in the normally developing child[14, 15] and the failure or difficulty of language development in the nonnormally developing child[16] to the presence or absence of the cognitive accomplishments of object-permanence and/or symbolization.

Both verbal and nonverbal discrimination and categorization and the use of these categorizations over a limited domain (within the immediate presence of the child and with a limited amount of information) occur during the first year and a half of life. The use of both verbal and nonverbal categorizations in a symbolic or representational manner occurs after this period. TABLE 1 indicates the verbal

TABLE 1

SOME LINGUISTIC AND NONLINGUISTIC BEHAVIORS DURING THE
FIRST TWO YEARS OF LIFE

Linguistic Perception-Production	Nonlinguistic Visual-Motor	Approx. Age (mos.)
Segmental and suprasegmental differentiation between syllables Differentiation of friendly-unfriendly, male-female, mother-other voices Vocalic utterances, unmarked and marked Vocalization interchange	Surprise at object disappearance Object tracking Organized reflexes Hand-mouth coordination	1–4
Differentiation of question and statement sentences Consonant vowel utterances Statement, emphatic, and requestlike utterances	Properties of objects identified Consolidation and repetition of motor habits Motor recognition Procedures for making interesting things last	4–8
Attention to word-length utterances Appropriate response to some words Reduction of babbling to word-length utterances	Use of signs and symbols to anticipate events Observation of causality	8–12
Comprehension of two-term relations Holophrastic utterances	Object permanence	12–18
Comprehension of three-term relations Development of two-term utterances from performative to reportative	Spatial or functional arrangements Logical classification or ordering Use of objects symbolically	12–24

and nonverbal behaviors that have been observed during the first two years of life, and the approximate ages at which they are observed. Imitation and "deferred" imitation have deliberately not been mentioned in either category of behavior. There is sufficient controversy about the exact nature of this behavior (a copy or a transformation), and its appearance in the sequence of development of behaviors in either area (perception, imitation, production, or imitation, perception, production) to suggest that much further research is needed before one can even comfortably speculate about its position in the sequence of development.

It is not obvious from the observations that have been made during this early period that the verbal discriminations and categorizations are dependent on the nonverbal ones or vice versa. Rather, the development of each system of behavior seems to be dependent on the infant's increasing ability to observe differences between "objects" within each class of objects, to observe the use of these different objects, and to observe the consquences of the use of these objects. Finally, both verbal and nonverbal categorizations presumably become interiorized and are used in a symbolic or representational manner. Those maturing capacities leading to certain kinds of discriminations and categorizations in both the verbal and nonverbal domain have just begun to be experimentally explored. The possibility of feature detectors in auditory and visual perception that are part of the biological repertoire of the infant and the changing structure of memory during this period are just some of the questions currently being investigated. Certainly the "what" of what becomes known verbally and nonverbally by the infant during the period will become more fully explicated by these studies, as well as the sequential dependencies of these behaviors. Thus far, however, the cognitive psychologist's and the linguist's descriptions of early development do not clarify the underlying structures that are the basis for either verbal or nonverbal accomplishments during this period.

At later stages of development there have been increasing efforts to determine what cognitive accomplishments precede linguistic accomplishments, as if priority indicates dependency. Thus, there has been a number of studies examining the child's ability to classify, seriate, conserve, and so on, and his ability to acquire the properties of lexical items, to observe ordering rules in sentences, and to understand transformed sentences. The presupposition has been that the abilities required by the nonlinguistic and linguistic tasks are somehow similar, although the processes involved in carrying out either type of tasks have not been clearly described, and that the nonlinguistic abilities must be acquired in order that the linguistic abilities be acquired. The notion of similarity is clearly open to quesiton, as is the notion of dependency simply because one accomplishment occurs before another.

In a study designed to determine whether or not language is a condition either necessary or sufficient for the achievement of a cognitive accomplishment, de Zwart[10] compared the abilities of children who were conservers (of liquid), nonconservers, and "intermediate" to produce and understand quantitative and dimensional terms and comparatives. It was found that all three groups of children understood coordinated sentences containing these terms and could carry out manipulations involving the terms. There were distinct difficulties, however, in conservers' and nonconservers' production of these terms. An attempt was made to teach nonconservers to use the terms in a manner similar to that of conservers. Of those who succeeded in learning to produce the terms in a manner similar to that of conservers, very few succeeded in the conservation task. The experimenter concludes that operational structuring and linguistic restructuring *parallel* each other, and that both behaviors examined, linguistic and nonlinguistic, are dependent on decentration and coordination. Decentration and coordination abilities, of course, must also depend on processing factors that are at present undescribed. This experiment indicates that having the possibly appropriate linguistic structures is not a condition necessary or sufficient for the achievement of liquid conservation, but it indicates equally well that achievement of liquid conservation is not a necessary or sufficient condition for either the comprehension or production of quantitative and dimensional and comparative terms in coordinated sentences.

In summary, both at the early and later stages of development the relation between cognitive development and linguistic development, as described, remains undefined. Conclusions that certain cognitive accomplishments are necessary prerequisites to certain linguistic accomplishments and certainly that these accomplishments are a sufficient condition are not supported by the data. The conclusion that language schemes are a necessary prerequisite to generalization, abstraction, planning, and problem-solving in every instance because of studies indicating that language is important in some motor, recall, and problem-solving tasks is equally untenable. As has been pointed out by other experimenters, the nature of the specific task requirements may render language useful, nonuseful, or interfering in carrying out these tasks.[17]

LINGUISTIC AND NONLINGUISTIC BEHAIOR OF CHILDREN WITH LANGUAGE DISORDERS

The populations of children most frequently referred to when arguing that cognitive development is not dependent on language development are the deaf and the blind. The findings that deaf children who are in most instances (but not all) severely retarded in oral language development when compared to hearing children but who nevertheless display the same cognitive accomplishments at approximately the same ages as hearing children, have led to the conclusion that the acquisition of cognitive accomplishments is not dependent on language development. There are some exceptions to this overall pattern of similarity in cognitive development, primarily in the area of conservation.[18] The findings that blind children may be retarded in some cognitive accomplishments[10] but not in all,[19,20] while they appear to develop language normally except for some isolated instances of difference,[21] again lead to the conclusion that the acquisition of cognitive accomplishments cannot be dependent on language development. These latter findings also, of course, lead to the equally logical conclusion that linguistic development is not dependent on the acquisition of certain cognitive accomplishments. These experimental findings simply reinforce the conclusion that overall dependency relations between cognitive and linguistic accomplishments as described do not exist.

Other populations of children who are most germane to this discussion are those who have been labeled as mentally retarded, aphasic, and autistic. These children do not develop language at the same rate or, possibly, in the same manner as their normally developing peers. In these instances there may be suspected neurological abnormalities or hard signs of lesions. Aphasic children have been described as those children who are *not* generally intellectually retarded. That is, their measured intelligence on performance scales of standard tests falls within the range of average to superior. The findings with autistic children concerning intellectual development as measured on standard tests indicate that well over half the children so labeled have intelligence quotients in the subnormal range, but one quarter to one third of this population score in the normal range.[22] Thus, the children in these populations appear to fall into three categories. The aphasic children display normal intellectual development but nonnormal language development, the autistic children display either normal or nonnormal intellectual development and nonnormal language development, and the mentally retarded children display both nonnormal intellectual and language development. These populations, therefore, should provide important data concerning the relations between cognitive and linguistic development, but they do not do so because neither their cognitive nor linguistic development has been studied in a manner that might reveal relations. Despite these limitations in the data there are some findings that provide some clues to the relations or, at least, indicate the kinds of questions that should be raised.

Studies of the language development of mentally retarded children either indicate that they develop language in a manner similar to normally developing children but at a slower rate, or that there are distinct differences in the way in which they acquire language.[23] It is possible that both types of development might occur, depending on the particular aspect of language examined or the surface behavior observed. Lenneberg reports in a longitudinal study over a three-year period of 54 mongoloid children, ranging in age from 6 months to 22 years, that 75% of the children were found to reach at least the first stage of language (defined as having a small vocabulary and executing simple commands). Further, a graphic illustration of the data indicates that all children with IQs at 50 or above had "language fully established" by 14 years or less. These data might indicate that the language-acquisition process is similar to that of normally developing children and that to some extent the level of language maturation reached is a function of both the level of measured intelligence and what is acquired during the language learning period (before puberty). It is difficulit, however, to determine from this study the exact nature of the language used by these children. Widely different performances are found within this population in various linguistic tasks, and in comparisons of their measured intelligence with their performance on various tests of language behavior or with the language they produce. Widely different results in levels of correlation are obtained when comparing phonological or syntactic or semantic performance with measured intelligence.[25] Even within presumably the same component of the grammar, striking differences in results are found. These variations may be due to differences in the populations examined (institutionalized versus noninstitutionalized or different etiological factors causing retardation), or the nature of the particular linguistic tasks given these children that were supposedly all testing the same language behavior. There is sufficient variation in the findings on the language behavior of these children and its relation to measured intelligence to cause us to reexamine both the structure of the linguistic and nonlinguistic behavior being tested and the relations between the two types of behavior.

A fairly sizable comparative and longitudinal study of the linguistic and nonlinguistic performance of autistic and mentally retarded children has been carried out.[26] The results of standard intelligence tests indicated that 94% of the 115 autistic children had IQs of 67 or below, and 75% were below 51. This is contradictory to the previous finding cited[22] (that one quarter to one third of these children are within the range of norm on standard tests), and the findings concerning the language behavior of these children differ somewhat from that of other studies.[22] Again, we are confronted with the possibility of variation in both linguistic and nonlinguistic behavior within a categorical population, or sufficient variation in how the behaviors are being examined, to account for differing results. Low verbal IQs accounted most for the low scores of the autistic children. The scores of the population of mentally retarded children were significantly higher on verbal scales (55 vs. 35), and on performance scales (70 vs. 54). The overall finding of the study was that measured intelligence was a good predictor of eventual functioning of the child. Testing some six years later, and after an educational intervention program, indicated that children with general intelligence scores of 55–60 used some communicative speech and had some "splinter skills," whereas the lowest scoring group, with scores of 25–35, were still severely withdrawn and noncommunicative in speech, and displayed no splinter skills. The one exception to this overall finding was that mentally retarded children, who had scores similar to those of the high-scoring autistic children, nevertheless exceeded them in relating to other people, using speech communicatively, and demonstrating functional object use. In an effort to explain this exception, the experimenter suggested that there may be a difference in the type or extent of affected neurolgical modalities. Indeed, this may be the case. There were differences found between the "high" autistic children and the mentally retarded children in the specific verbal and nonverbal abilities tested. The high autistic children's scores in tested verbal abilities were lower than those of the mentally retarded children except for "number concepts." All groups of autistic children performed more poorly than the mentally retarded children on all the visual-motor tasks given except for color match and form board completion (middle autistic children performed better), fine motor movements with scissors and stringing beads (middle and high autistic children performed better), and gross motor imitation (high autistic children performed better). Although one would like to obtain clearer categorizations of both linguistic and nonlinguistic accomplishments, this study nevertheless indicates that, at least for those children whose intelligence scores range from 55 to 60, there are in all likelihood particular neurological involvements that in turn affect the manner in which they structure input information. This possibility seems to account better for the differences observed than does IQ alone.

Research on the language behavior of children with suspected neurological abnormalities indicates that there are important differences among them and between them and normally developing children in their ability to carry out linguistic tasks. It has long been known that within this population there are those who appear to

TABLE 2

DIFFERENT LANGUAGE BEHAVIORS OBSERVED WITHIN A POPULATION OF CHILDREN
WITH SUSPECTED NEUROLOGICAL ABNORMALITIES

Behavior Examined	Groupings of Behavior		Age Range (years)
Spontaneous Production	One Group Presentence S V O		3–6
Repetition of Sentences Expansion S V O	Two Groups Nonexpansion S V O		4–11
Repetition of Words Delayed Phonologically	Two Groups Different Phonologically		4–11
Perceptual Categorization Sounds Accurate	Three Groups Some Errors	Many Errors	4–11
Productive Categorization Sounds Many Errors	Three Groups Some Errors	Many Errors	4–11

have difficulty only in producing language and those who have difficulty in both perceiving and producing language, but it is not clear from these descriptions what effect this overall difference in functioning has on language development and processing. These children's language production in various settings has been examined.[27] Their ability to reproduce sentences[28] and morphemes and phonological units[29] and their ability to perceive and reproduce distinctions among members of speech sound sets[30] have also been examined. It has been found that within this group of children, diagnostically categorized as being alike, there are distinct differences in their ability to carry out specific linguistic tasks and in the level of linguistic maturation they appear to have achieved by their performance in these tasks, even though a structural analysis of the language they produce indicates great similarity between them. These differences in linguistic performance are neither a reflection of age differences nor particular scores of measured intelligence.

TABLE 2 indicates the distinctions in language-processing observed within this population. Over an age range of three to six years, little development was observed in the use of syntactic structures in spontaneous language production. Declarative utterances were unmarked as to tense and number, and negative and question sentences contained negative and question morphemes (or intonational markers) but were untransformed. Little conjunction or embedding was observed. In sentence and word-in-sentence repetition two distinct groups were observed: those who expanded the verb phrase into auxiliary and modal and whose phonological reproductions were similar to those of much younger children, and those who did not expand and whose phonological reproductions were unique in category and structure. In differentiation of members of speech sound sets, three distinct groups were observed: those who perceptually categorized differences accurately but had great difficulty productively, those whose perceptual and productive performance was quite similar to that of much younger children, and those who had great difficulty and made many errors in both tasks.

Not only are there differences in the language-processing behavior of these children and children developing language normally, but there also appear to be differences in their nonlinguistic processing behaviors. Despite the fact that the former achieve performance scores on standard tests indicating that they are equal to normally developing children in nonlinguistic tasks, some recent studies show that they differ in their auditory processing abilities[31] and in their motor imitation abilities.[30]

There does not seem to be some overall factor such as general cognitive retardation that completely accounts for the language problems of mentally retarded, autistic, and aphasic children. The distinctions among them in the performance of particular linguistic tasks suggest that there are also distinctions among them in their processing abilities and that these processing limitations affect both their ability to acquire linguistic and nonlinguistic structures. These processing limitations, in conjunction with the function and complexity of the linguistic and nonlinguistic structures to be acquired, affects the level of difficulty with which these structures are acquired by particular children. Our research should therefore be addressed to determining what these processing limitations are in any given instance.

IMPLICATIONS FOR REHABILITATION PROCESS

The child with a disability may be delayed or different in both his linguistic and nonlinguistic development because of the state of the child in processing abilities and the experiences he has been exposed to. Each of the children, despite a diagnostic categorization that assumes similarity within a category may possess distinct processing abilities. Selections of what they should be taught and the manner in which it is taught are either conducive to further development or are arbitrary decisions and therefore unhelpful.

The implications of various positions concerning the relations between cognition and language can obviously have a great effect on educational programs designed to aid these children. If the position is that language development is dependent on the acquisition of certain cognitive accomplishments, a great deal of time will be spent on teaching performance in cognitive tasks in the hope that language development will naturally follow from this. It has been suggested that the possibility may exist that processes that are not linguistic constitute the necessary basis for the development of functional language (in this instance, the achievement of object-permanence is suggested),[33] or that some manipulation of nonlinguistic symbols is prerequisite to language (in this instance symbolic play, role-playing imagery, and drawing are pointed to).[16] The inverse has long been suggested; that is, that acquisition of language structures will automatically lead to the acquisition of cognitive accomplishments. The position that accomplishments in one domain are a necessary prerequisite to accomplishments in the other domain often, unhappily, also leads to the notion that they are a sufficient condition. The data obtained with normally developing children and those with developmental disabilities do not support this position, and there is some evidence that the position can lead to poor, if not disastrous results. For example, a great deal of time has been spent in perceptual and perceptual-motor training with handicapped children in an effort to help them acquire primary school and reading skills with little educational effect.[34] It is to be hoped that programs will be developed that will take into account the processing capacities of these children in particular domains, the task requirements of accomplishments in the domains, and also what appears to be functionally important to these children. In both the linguistic and nonlinguistic domain appropriate and effective behaviors are the desired goals, and not merely the acquisition of particular structures.

REFERENCES

1. DeZwart, H. S. 1971. Sensorimotor action patterns as a condition for the acquisition of syntax. *In* Language Acquisition: Models and Methods. R. Huxley & E. Ingram, Eds. Academic Press. New York, N.Y.
2. Bellugi, U. & S. Fischer. 1972. Cognition 1: 173–200.
3. Jakobson, R. 1968. Child Language, Aphasia and Phonological Universals. Mouton. The Hague, The Netherlands.
4. Hockett, C. F. 1963. The problem of universals in language. *In* Universals in Language. J. H. Greenberg, Ed. M.I.T. Press. Cambridge, Mass.
5. Marshall, J. C. 1970. Can humans talk? *In* Biological and Social Factors in Psycholinguistics. J. Morton, Ed. Univ. Illinois Press. Urbana, Ill.
6. Vygotsky, L. S. 1962. Thought and Language. M.I.T. Press. Cambridge, Mass.
7. Menyuk, P. 1974. Early development of receptive language: from babbling to words. *In* Language Perspectives-Acquisition, Retardation and Intervention. R. L. Schiefelbusch & L. L. Lloyd, Eds. University Park Press. Baltimore, Md.
8. Greenfield, P. M., J. H. Smith & B. Laufer. 1972. Communication and the beginning of language. Harvard University. Circulated Paper.
9. Shipley, E. F., C. S. Smith & L. R. Gleitman. 1969. Language 45: 322–342.
10. deZwart, H. S. Developmental psycholinguistics. *In* Studies in Cognitive Development. D. Elkind & J. H. Flavell, Eds. Oxford Univ. Press. New York, N.Y.
11. Bower, T. G. R. 1971. Scientific American 225: 30–38.
12. Lezine, I. 1973. The transition from sensorimotor to earliest symbolic function in early development. *In* Biological and Environmental Determinants of Early Development. J. Y. Nurnberger, Ed. Williams & Wilkins Co. Baltimore, Md.
13. White, S. 1970. The learning theory approach. *In* Carmichael's Manual of Child Psychology. P. H. Mussen, Ed. Vol. 1: 657–703. John Wiley & Sons, Inc. New York, N.Y.
14. Bloom, L. 1973. One Word at a Time. Mouton. The Hague, The Netherlands.
15. Brown, R. 1973. A First Language. Harvard Univ. Press. Cambridge, Mass.
16. Morehead, D. M. & A. Morehead. 1974. From signal to sign. *In* Language Perspectives-Acquisition, Retardation and Intervention. R. L. Schiefelbusch & L. L. Lloyd, Eds. University Park Press. Baltimore, Md.
17. Menyuk, P. The Acquisition and Development of Language. Prentice-Hall Inc. Englewood Cliffs, N.J.
18. Furth, H. G. 1966. Thinking Without Language. Free Press. New York, N.Y.
19. Gottesman, M. 1973. Child Development 44: 824–827.
20. Gottesman, M. 1971. Child Development 42: 573–580.
21. Bartholomess, B. 1971. Perceptual and Motor Skills 33: 1289–1290.
22. Rutter, M. 1968. J. Child Psychol. Psychiat. 9: 1–25.
23. Cromer, R. F. 1974. Receptive language in the mentally retarded. *In* Language Perspectives-Acquisition Retardation and Intervention. R. L. Schiefelbusch & L. L. Lloyd, Eds. University Park Press, Baltimore, Md.
24. Lenneberg, E. H. 1966. The natural history of language. *In* The Genesis of Language. F. S. Smith & G. Miller, Eds. M.I.T. Press, Cambridge.

25. YODER, D. E. & J. F. MILLER. 1972. What we may know and what we can do. *In* Language Intervention with the Retarded. J. E. McLean, D. E. Yoder & R. L. Schiefelbusch, Eds. University Park Press. Baltimore, Md.
26. DE MYER, M. K. 1973. The measured intelligence of autistic children. Paper presented at First Intern. Leo Kanner Symposium on Child Development, Deviation and Treatment. Univ. North Carolina. Chapel Hill, N.C.
27. MENYUK, P. 1964. J. Speech and Hearing Research 7: 109–121.
28. MENYUK, P. & P. LOONEY. 1972. J. Speech Hearing Res. 15: 264–279.
29. MENYUK, P. & P. LOONEY. 1972. J. Speech Hearing Res. 15: 395–406.
30. MENYUK, P. 1974. Relations between acquisition of phonology and reading. Paper presented at the Hyman Blumberg Symposium Aspects of Reading Acquisition. Johns Hopkins University. Baltimore, Md.
31. TALLAL, P. & M. PIERCY. 1973. Neuropsychologia 11: 389–398.
32. LEVY, C. & P. MENYUK. 1974. Relations between certain cognitive skills and sentence comprehension. Paper presented at American Speech and Hearing Assoc. Las Vegas, Nev.
33. BRICKER, W. A. & D. D. BRICKER. 1974. An early language training strategy. *In* Language Perspectives-Acquisition, Retardation and Intervention. R. L. Schiefelbusch & L. L. Lloyd, Eds. University Park Press. Baltimore, Md.
34. MANN, L. & L. GOODMAN. 1973. Perceptual motor training: a critical retrospect. Paper presented at First Intern. Leo Kanner Colloquium on Child Development, Deviations and Treatment. Univ. North Carolina. Chapel Hill, N.C.

ON THE NATURE OF LANGUAGE FROM THE PERSPECTIVE
OF RESEARCH WITH PROFOUNDLY DEAF CHILDREN

H. G. Furth

Department of Psychology
The Catholic University of America
Washington, D.C. 20064

This presentation should fit well into current interest in investigating the pre-linguistic determinants of a child's speech, and it expands some specific points about the communicative function in general to which previous and subsequent speakers refer. Indeed, the principal message I would like to convey derives clearly from research results with deaf children. It is the overriding fact that many important, if not all, aspects that go under the name of linguistic universals are not uniquely peculiar to language; rather, they are characteristic of the development of human cognition and communication in general. I hasten to add that this perspective in no way diminishes the value of linguistic research; it merely stresses that the source of cognition and communication must be searched for in roots deeper than those in the verbal language of society, since the use of this language is itself dependent on the development of these more general human capacities.

Above all, if we claim to be behavioral scientists, we cannot continue using a terminology that is as ambiguous as many words in ordinary language. We owe it to ourselves and to the public to adhere to a circumscribed use of words. If we include in our presentation words like *language, speech, communication, symbols, representations, cognition, learning,* etc., we must first decide in what sense these words are understood by us, and then keep religiously to this preliminary taxonomy. One author, for example, may elect to include in the meaning of "language" what others call "speech" and "communication." In this case the three words become interchangeable, and to refer to the relationship between communication and language would be meaningless. Another may extend the connotation of the word language to any kind of representational thinking, in which case the phrase "thinking without language" becomes absolutely senseless, as would, for that matter, any investigation into the relation of thinking and language.

Further, our human capacity to shift subtly the meaning of words within an argument is quite uncanny and needs constant scrutiny. I have proposed that many profoundly deaf youngsters have no knowledge of language; they do not know the language of society, e.g., English, in any adequate sense, or the so-called "Sign language" of the deaf community of which they are not yet a part; therefore, they provide a unique opportunity to observe what, if any, influence the absence of a language has on the development of intelligent thinking. Even those who readily accept this premise frequently reject my conclusion on the ground that these deaf children may have acquired a different language, a mysterious "inner language," through which their thinking develops. These persons can therefore still reasonably continue to hold and to act on the assumption that language is of primary importance in the development of thinking.

This is a curious way of shifting the meaning of the word "language." When researchers or teachers propose that language importantly affects thinking, they understand by "language" a quite precise and circumscribed knowledge and behavior, namely, the use of the English language. They do not include in it the use of

70

spontaneous gestures or images or the intelligent handling of a concrete situation. But when it comes to deaf children, they suddenly extend the meaning of language to include all these extralinguistic behaviors, so that they can reject the logical conclusion to which a narrow definition of the word "language" could have forced them. And then, completing the cycle, they quite readily return to the narrow definition when they talk about language interacting with and furthering the intelligence of a child.

When I characterize deaf children as having no language, I use the word "language" in the narrow—but quite usual—sense of knowing; that is, of having a developed competence in the conventional symbol system of society through which its members communicate their everyday experiences. This definition would accept the gestural sign language of the deaf community as a language, but the overwhelming majority of deaf children are born to hearing parents and, at least until recently, are kept away from contact with signing deaf adults; at the same time, these deaf children are barely able to comprehend and express the simplest syntax of English. While they therefore do not have a conventional language, they can be observed to symbolize, communicate, memorize, and think. In fact, this is the main theme I want to present: if these children do acquire symbols, communication, intelligence, personality, it cannot be due to the external influence of a language society. Rather, it is due to the spontaneous development of their persons, a development that is much more than language can provide, whether one considers this from an empirical or theoretical evolutionary perspective.

I shall present my theme in three points. First, I will discuss and interpret psychological research on the development of profoundly deaf children. Second, I will consider the communication and language of deaf children and adults. Last, I will present some theoretical and practical conclusions derived from the evidence presented earlier.

DEVELOPMENT OF DEAF CHILDREN

This brief summary of research with deaf persons primarily pertains to intellectual functioning, but a few words will also be said about their social and emotional development. From a wide variety of more than 100 separate investigations, there is as yet no evidence whatsoever that language-deprived deaf children have any overall or any specific cognitive deficit that justifiably could be attributed to their specific linguistic deficit.

We are familiar with the range of individual differences observed in practically all types of behavior. Even where we cannot adequately measure the range of possible performances, we have a reasonable clear picture of what is considered typical and what is definitely atypical. The linguistic deficit of deaf children is not within the normal range of knowing a language. They are deficient in a sense that is quite different from that in which they may be called deficient in a particular classificatory problem because it could have taken them an average of 38 trials to reach a criterion whereas hearing children acquired the criterion on an average of 32 trials. When we say two groups are different, we often fail to acknowledge the immense area of communality that is tacitly presupposed. For example, in this hypothetical case of classification, both the hearing and deaf children had in common eventual success on classification, and there was a large overlap between the distributions of scores in the two groups. By contrast, the difference between the two groups in the knowledge of a language is almost absolute: on the one hand, a comfortable being at home in a language that is constantly used for all kinds of purposes, and on the other hand a meager knowledge of a few words and a few simple sentence constructions.

Consider the evidence. There are a few studies in which developmental differences were observed, deaf children showing a slight lag in comparison with hearing children, but the majority of studies did not yield any differences whatsoever. Regarding the first group of studies, one can point out that the poorer performance of deaf children falls fully within the range of hearing children. In other words, there are many groups of hearing children who perform comparably to deaf children such as children from different environments or cultures. But these hearing children certainly have language, and one cannot therefore clearly link the lowered performance to language. I suggest that an occasional lowered performance of deaf children can be readily attributed to slight environmental disadvantages that are only quite indirectly, if at all, related to language. These are disadvantages that spring from an inadequate or inappropriate emotional acceptance of the disability on the part of parents, or of an educational program that constantly stresses what is weakest in the child and neglects intellectually challenging occasions.

Studies that show no differences, however, are potentially quite clear in their interpretation; knowledge of a language cannot be a necessary or even facilitative influence in the emergence of these behaviors. The areas studied were quite diverse, such as rule learning, discrimination, and classification tasks, combinatorial and probability thinking, spatial concepts, logical symbols, memory recall, and some Piagetian conservation problems. There is just no evidence of any clear-cut deficit in any specific intelligent behavior that could be empirically and theoretically related to the clear-cut deficit in knowledge of a language.

When one considers the linguistic ignorance of young deaf children, it seems plausible to expect social and emotional deficiences in these children, even more than intellectual defects. However, one is again struck by the basic similarity of individual differences that fall fully within the normal developmental range. One observes disturbances similar to those of hearing children. The percentage of severe psychoses is certainly not greater. When it comes to neuroses and adjustment disorders, data are so poor and definitions so differently determined by prevailing cultural biases that it is very hard to reach any firm conclusions.

COMMUNICATION AND LANGUAGE IN DEAF PERSONS

Turning now from the personality and intelligence of deaf children to their language and communication, it is apparent that—unless prohibited by a quite unusual environment—all deaf children spontaneously use gestures and pantomime for the purpose of communication. Careful observations of these gestures demonstrate that they are used and function analogously to what is often called "linguistic universals." Developmental stages described in connection with verbal language can be found in the use of these gestures. For example, at first the gestures point to present objects; later on, they refer to absent objects or events. An even more important insight comes from ongoing research that looks for grammatical rules that deaf children adopt in their spontaneous gestures, rules that cannot possibly be related to an outside model, since no gesture language is used in those particular deaf children's environment. This evidence is, of course, germane to much current research on the prelinguistic roots of human communication. The presence of profoundly deaf children without the benefit of acquiring the verbal language of the hearing society or the visual language of the deaf society allows us to extend this study of human communication far beyond the prelinguistic period, yet without having to worry about the potential contamination of our data and theories on communicative development by the learning and modeling from the language of the social environment.

Concerning the Sign language of American deaf adults, it is quite remarkable and symptomatic of a deep-seated prejudice, which is only slowly disappearing, that a serious investigation into the nature of this language has only recently been attempted. Previously, one only looked at signing in order to compare it unfavorably to the spoken language and relegate it to a lower form of animal communication. Suffice it to point out that today nobody would seriously suggest that the Sign language as used by deaf persons is not truly a human language, even though one can still argue whether or not the chimpanzee Washoe has acquired the use of human language.

Why is the learning of the English language so difficult for deaf children? Is it because their first way of communicating by spontaneously developed gestures is not a fully articulated conventional symbol system, and in its medium is so radically different, that learning English is not like learning a second language? By contrast, as the deaf adolescents come in contact with deaf adults who use the Sign language, they unfailingly acquire it, even though they are at an age far beyond the normal age of first-language acquisition. Moreover, if the spoken language of a society, such as English, were a system with clear logical rules of semantics and syntax, deaf children would be able to learn it easily. They have no difficulties with logic or intelligent reasoning. Unfortunately, language and logic overlap only to a limited degree. Remenber also that many attempts have been made to teach English to deaf children according to a planned curriculum. These attempts have not been overly fruitful, and the teaching of language to deaf children today remains what it has always been, an unpredictable endeavour that is educationally extremely challenging, with a few mysterious successes and many more dismal failures. Our past psychological understanding of language acquisition has been of no appreciable benefit to the teaching of English to deaf children. However, it is my fond hope that the more radical insights gleaned from the observation of deaf children's spontaneous communication and intelligent development could lead to an educational environment for deaf children that would promise a greater likelihood of teaching the verbal language of society.

CONCLUSIONS

From the foregoing we can draw some theoretical and practical conclusions. First of all, one can, and it seems to me one must, distinguish very clearly between intelligence and conventional language. Many deaf children are intelligent persons who do not have a language, if language is taken to be the knowledge of an overall communication system of a society. Moreover, if one accepts the primacy of thinking vis-a-vis language, this has to be understood in a framework where symbolization is regarded as a spontaneous psychological consequence of an intellectual development that has proceeded beyond practical regulations to the threshold of theoretical thinking. At this point symbolization becomes the means for making present what is absent, that is, "representation." All symbols are representation and refer directly to the person's theoretical knowledge. Some symbols are external, such as play or gestures, some are internalized, such as internal movements or images. In this framework speech is a system of symbolization that the child acquires and uses analogous to the way he or she acquires and uses other symbols such as gestures and imagery. Such a perspective—and you realize this is effectively a summary of Piaget's theory—turns our usual view in these matters upside down. Instead of taking language as primary in intellectual development and inferring mind from language, we posit intelligence as primary and then derive representation from it and finally acknowledge speech and language as symbolic behavior that functions as other symbols do.

If this position on language and intelligent thinking is considered an extreme against a moderate, middle view that stresses the contributions and interaction of both intelligence and language, this can be due only to a misunderstanding of the words. It is no more reasonable to treat language and intelligence as two independent modalities that interact than it is to propose that life and the nuclear family relations interact in the growth of a person. More precisely, one can conceive of intelligence without language, but not of language without intelligence.

Roger Brown, who certainly cannot be accused of neglecting language, remarked in his recent book, *A First Language*, that next to nothing is known about what language has done for thought, and he continues, "we cannot even be sure that language has importantly affected the power of thought" (p. 38). He cites one solitary empirical finding for the proposition that language aids cognition; namely, the use of labels as a technique for extending short-term memory. He admits that this is a comparatively unimportant cognitive strategy: "It did not get us to the moon." In spite of this minimal yield from a field that has been labored over and harvested continuously since the days of the Whorfian Hypothesis and Skinner's Verbal Learning, Brown still does not abandon the plow, and speculates that "possibly very much more important reasoning processes are dependent on sentence construction, and especially the powerful processes of embedding and coordination." He believes that no one has even attempted to determine whether this is true. On this point, I think he is wrong. Those who have studied deaf persons have done so in the expectation of verifying these speculations. But these expectations were not confirmed. We have observed deaf adolescents who cannot construct embedded sentences but who show understanding of logical connectives, so that, for example, they distinguish a disjunction of two negations from a negated disjunction of two assertions. I fail to see how one can disregard these empirical results for the benefit of an inadequate theoretical position.

Quite rightly, Brown emphasizes the communicative social function of language. There is ample empirical evidence that many aspects of social behavior are peculiarly tied to language and speech even though they are grounded in a more general symbolic and communicative capacity. Quite probably, language has evolved for the purpose of persuasion, rhetoric, war-making, poetry, myth, religion, politics, and power over persons. That is what language is for. The hearing child will use it in the service of these functions. If the child does not use language, this is usually an indication that there is something wrong with his or her social-emotional development. But even here, it is not language that is at the base of these developments; rather, it is language behavior which indicates these developments. Deaf children without language also acquire adequate social-emotional skills.

Finally, as a practical conclusion in this all too compressed presentation, I would urge that we do not distort the evolutionary biological function of language by prematurely stressing the role of language in intelligent thinking. According to Piaget's theory, language in itself is an inappropriate medium for stimulating intellectual development as long as the child has not yet acquired formal thinking structures. In other words, in order to use language in an intelligent challenging way and nourish intelligence through the verbal medium, one needs an intelligence that has developed to the stage which Piaget calls formal thinking. These structures begin to develop around twelve to fourteen years of age, certainly not much earlier.

If our educational institutions and rehabilitation efforts misconstrue the role of language and unwisely apply language skills at an early age-level, we are bound to starve the child intellectually, since a child's intelligence is not yet capable of being challenged by language itself. Put differently, a child's intelligence is miles ahead of what he or she can verbalize. It is hard enough for us adults to put into language what we think and expand our thinking through the verbal medium; but we can, at least with assiduous efforts. But the average eight-year-old child does not have this capacity to be challenged by language, and in stressing language and reading, we cannot thereby nourish this child's high-level intelligence.

Qutie frankly, our educational philosophy, with its undue emphasis on reading, writing, and other verbal learning in the primary school, is pathogenic as far as intellectual health is concerned. As long as we continue with this philosophy, we are going to have what has been called "the current epidemic of learning disabilities." This is a cruel misnomer; it should rather be called "schooling disability," that is, the child's school failure is symptomatic of a serious defect in our schools, not in the child. I wish we experts in psychology and education would have the conviction and the courage to tell society that in order to avoid learning failures, we have to change the school system rather than engage in a fruitless effort to prepare and innoculate particular children against a learning system that is basically unhealthy. We need schools that give ample scope for the development of the children's capacities to understand the various facets of reality in which they live. To acquire language, to speak intelligently, to read—all these and other desirable acquisitions have much more to do with developing a certain understanding than with learning and memorizing a certain content or information.

It simply is not true that educational systems have ever given thinking a fair chance. I would not deny that programs exist that foster some aspects conducive to the child's developing intelligence. But what is needed is an all-out effort to provide opportunities for all children in the primary school to engage in challenging intellectual activities appropriate for their ages. This would not mean curricula to teach thinking, since in my perspective, thinking is not something that is taught or learned; it is something the child himself or herself must do and develop. If we had this type of early education, we would find that many so-called learning disabilities or specific reading and language deficiencies would disappear. Such a socially therapeutic outcome would indeed be a most desirable confirmation of a theoretical perspective on language and intellectual development that derives directly from the evidence of psychological studies with profoundly deaf children.

DISCUSSION PAPER:

SOME THEORETICAL AND EMPIRICAL ISSUES THAT ARISE IF WE INSIST ON DISTINGUISHING LANGUAGE AND THOUGHT

Thomas G. Bever

Psycholinguistics Program
Departments of Psychology and Linguistics
Columbia University
New York, New York 10027

INTRODUCTION

When faced with the complexities of the human mind, individual researchers often carve out a piece and ignore the rest. It is hard enough to do research on something called "language" or something called "thought" alone, without worrying about the relations between the two. And then, at conferences like this, these same researchers spend a good deal of verbal energy arguing that there is, after all, a whole mind: that the different abilities are connected in some way, or that they all share some fundamental mental goo.

Language is a manifest skill. The result is that language can be studied in isolation from implicit thought processes. The independent science of linguistics has approached language without concern about its role in thinking, simply viewing it as an isolated capacity. This is an understandable scientific heuristic. It may be, however, that this isolation arises out of the necessity to simplify our scientific lives, rather than out of reality. Accordingly, it would be a mistake to make too much of the distinction between "language" and "thought."

Our options are clear if we insist on distinguishing language from thought. We can say that thought underlies language, that language is the vehicle for thought, or that they both proceed in parallel. Each of the three positions on the relation between "language" and "thought" expressed in this volume represent a different one of these possible positions. All of the authors are concerned with the interrelations of thought and language; so I may be guilty of overcharacterizing each position, simply for clarity's sake. Relatively speaking, however, Dr. Blank's review and discussion emphasizes the role of language as the basis for certain kinds of cognition. Dr. Furth quite unambiguously takes the opposite position, that cognition is the common source from which many skills and capacities spring; language is simply one of those skills. An intermediate position was developed by Dr. Menyuk. We can call it the "who knows?" position, that both language and thought develop together and interact with each other.

A lot of interesting and specific data are presented in the preceding papers; it will require close study to absorb them and to understand their import. So I shall not comment on them specifically.* Rather, I wish to articulate what the common theme is that ramifies the varying viewpoints on the relation of language and thought.

*I should note that I am sympathetic to Dr. Furth's complaints about the possibility that school systems are creating "problem children." I am also sympathetic to the return of "advocacy psychology," in which we should take responsibility for the effects of our science. However, I have little to add to his comments on this issue, other than advancing their direction. The reader will note that the representation and interfaculty translation problems considered in this paper are studied in areas of psychology other than language; e.g., multiple perceptual "codes" (Posner, 1974), "sensory associations" (Hayeck, 1954). The implications of these studies for language are unclear, since they characteristically deal with stimuli more explicit than meaning.

The shared conceptual goal is to specify what property of mind is held in common to all human mental faculties. I shall argue that it is possible that the *only* shared properties are the fundamental units out of which all the varieties of human behavior and knowledge and constructed.

The shared methodology is the concentration on unusual populations having a deficit of some kind. I shall argue that the self-compensating processes of any young damaged organism obscure the interpretation of data from such individuals.

AT WHAT LEVEL IS THE MIND UNIFIED?

A basic conceptual goal in discussions like the present one is that the mind must be *unified* at some level, that there is a common mental capacity that unifies all cognitive faculties such as reasoning (e.g., logic), mental representation (e.g., imagery) and communication (e.g., language). The positions on this differ according to the level at which the unity of mind is posited. The distinguishable mental faculties might express directly a common core; if not, they might communicate with each other in a common language; if not, they still might be constructed out of the same elementary structures.

The different implications of these three positions are clarified if we consider a specific example of behavior in which we relate two faculties. A classic example of such a mapping is the referring relation between words and visual percepts, e.g., "square" refers to "□". Aspects of the referring relation have recently been studied experimentally. Consider the capacity to decide that a particular statement ("that is a square") is true of a particular picture (□ vs. ○). Somehow the linguistic and visual percepts are checked against each other. But how?

The Common Representation Model

The strongest claim is that every faculty that we can isolate close to the mental "surface" is simply an externally differentiated form of the same basic cognitive organization. On this view the ultimate underlying cognitive acts when we understand "that is a square"are literally *identical* to the ultimate acts when we perceive □.† This solves the problem of how we pair the sentence with the visual image by postulating an inner level of mental representation at which the two stimuli *cannot be distinguished*. Such a viewpoint on the psychological nature of stimulus equivalence has a distinguished history. It is, in fact, a structural interpretation of the learning theorist's account of how two stimuli are classified as "identical" (operationally, this means that both stimuli are responded to in the same way; in the sentence-picture matching experimental task the operational test is that a subject responds "same").

This kind of model for cross-faculty equivalences has great intuitive appeal; it provides an understandable mental explanation of equivalence as due to functional identity, just as the "failure-of-discrimination" model provides an understandable explanation of stimulus generalization. However, it is clear that one of the significant difficulties with the functional identity model of generalization is that to be effective and predictive, it requires a definition of the psychophysical dimensions of similarity along which potential discrimination (or lack of it) might occur. For example, it is straightforward to state that an animal will generalize from a 100.0 Hz tone to a 100.1 Hz tone, along the dimension of "tone height." But how do we predict that the animal generalizes to a 200 Hz tone *more* than to a 180 Hz unless we "know"

---

†I am using the term "mental faculty" intentionally, to refer to a mental subsystem organized in aid of a particular kind of behavior. Thus, we have a "faculty of language," a "faculty of imagery," a "faculty of logic," etc. This somewhat awkward terminology is used to avoid confusion with general words like "capacity" and specific ones like "modality."

that 200 Hz is an "octave" above 100 Hz and that octaves can be confused? That is, we need an independent specification of the "generalization space"; or to put it another way, the theory must include an "executive function" that can generate from each stimulus the other stimuli with which it is potentially mentally identical.

The same problem arises for the common-representation theory of sentence-picture matching: there must be an executive function that determines which features of the representation of the stimulus in each faculty can be ignored when matching to the corresponding representation in the other faculty. Consider the four sentences below: each of them *must* have available a different core representation, since they *can* be discriminated (albeit slightly, in certain cases).

> That is a square
>
> It is true that that is a square
>
> You are seeing a square if you are looking at that

(1)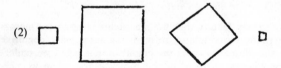

> That geometric figure is the same as that outlined by four lines of equal length joined by right angles.
>
> You are looking at a picture of two right-angle equilateral triangles, each without its hypotenuse, but meeting such that the missing hypotenuse would coincide and the right angles do not.

Similarly each of the figures below *must* have available a different core representation. Yet every sentence in (1) correctly describes every picture

(2)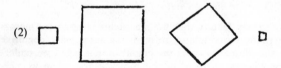

in (2); accordingly, since the available core representations differ, there must be an "executive function" in comparing them that ignores certain differences as irrelevant at certain times. Roughly speaking, it looks as though such a function deletes certain aspects of the core representation of each stimulus modality, and then compares the remaining representations for identity. However, even simple examples show that the "executive function" must be active: mere deletion and identity comparison is not sufficient. Otherwise, how could we decide that the simple sentences below are true of the simple figures on the right?

> That figure is sort of a square
>
> There are two overlapping squares

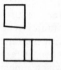

(3)

> It's very hard to tell there's a hidden square

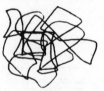

The reader can generate such examples *ad lib.* The point is that the executive function must, in part, actively translate the relevant aspects of the stimulus as represented in one faculty to the other—simple deletion of parts of a core representation is insufficient; what is required is an *active* interpreter between one faculty and another.‡

The Lingua Mentis Model

The notion that there is an active interpreter between mental faculties raises the possibility that the faculties themselves have cognitively distinct forms of representation; that is, they may not assign identical or even partially identical representations to functionally equivalent stimuli. On this view the formal language of visual and linguistic representation differ. Each, however, can be mapped onto the other by a common "language" that assigns identical representations to them whenever cross-faculty matching is required. On this model each cognitive faculty utilizes a potentially distinct set of capacities, but the faculties are coordinated by means of a common *lingua mentis*.

This model has certain virtues: it capitalizes on the fact that even the common core model requires an active "executive function" to match faculties, but leaves open the possibility that each faculty itself involves unique kinds of mechanisms and structures. Accordingly, this model would allow for the notion that distinct linguistic or imagery capacities evolved phylogenetically and emerge ontogenetically separate from other capacities. However, the redundant mystery in this model is how (and why) each faculty is itself couched in distinct terms but is mappable onto a com-com language. Furthermore, there is a direct interpretation of this model on which it is equivalent to the common-core model and also contains the same obscurities. That is, a common language which mediates between formally distinct modalities is the logical equivalent of a common core to which each modality is reduced. This language would require the same mysterious power as the common-core model—the "knowledge" of which features of the representation of the stimulus in each faculty to extract so that the translation would be the same bidirectionally.

The Federated Faculties Model

Suppose, however, that a faculty could be translated into another, and vice versa, by different mapping languages. That is, suppose every sentence describing a geometric figure could be mapped onto a visual representation and conversely, but by different kinds of mapping languages. Functional equivalence between faculties would obtain whenever the two separate unidirectional mappings exist (albeit non-uniquely in each separate case). If each unidirectional mapping could be distinct, then the problems of the previous models do not obtain; in particular, we do not have to find a common representation (be it in the core or in the interfaculty lan-

---

‡Note that the comparison models proposed by Clark and Chase,[1] Trabasso et al.,[2] Olson and Filby,[3] Just,[4] Carpenter and Just,[5] *all* have certain features of such an executive function. They suggest that a set of operations can match a sentence against a picture. These operations route the comparison of the inner representation of the sentence without requiring complete identity for a match. However, they do require that the *language* in which the picture and sentence are represented be of the same form: spoken-language-like propositions. Of course, this too is inappropriate for many pictures, e.g. (3). See Tanenhaus et al.[6] for a general discussion of these models, with particular emphasis on the fact that they are neither models of sentence understanding nor of picture perception, since they presuppose both processes. At best they are protomodels of certain task-specific verification strategies.

guage) to claim cross-faculty equivalence of two stimuli. Rather, we need only claim that cross-faculty equivalence between "square" (linguistic) and □ (visual) exists, if there is some mapping "square →□" *and* some mapping "□→ square"; the mapping languages themselves may be entirely distinct.

The notion that there is neither a common cognitive core *nor* a common language may seem counter-intuitive, at first. The fact that we can talk about our world and the fact that we can match pictures to sentences would seem to prove that there is a common unconscious language in which we represent all these different faculties. But, in fact, it does not prove this.

Consider an analogy that shows how we can transform information in one modality to information in another modality without a common language of representation or of translation. Consider the typewriter.§ The typewriter regularly and reliably translates into letters the kinetic motion of the fingers placed in certain ways. There is no common language into which both finger motions and letters are reduced by the typewriter. Instead the typewriter is a transducer. It is a mechanism that maps one modality—in this case, the modality of finger motions—onto another modality—in this case, the modality of letters. We can equally well envisage a unidirectional mapping from letters to finger motion that would neither use a common language nor even be a typewriter in reverse. Letter recognition is commonplace even in industry today (by identification of visual features). We could easily attach puppet strings to the fingers in such a way that as the printed page is scanned, the fingers would move as though they were typing the corresponding letters. Then we would have a complete bidirectional mapping system from finger motion to letters (via a typewriter) and from letters to finger motion (via puppet strings), made up of two distinct unidirectional subsystems.

It is entirely possible that the mind is made up of distinct subsystems linked together by such unidirectional complementary transducers with no common cognitive core or common intermodal language. I am not claiming that it is true or that it is not true. I want to point out only that the fact that we can talk about our images and recognize pictures of our words does not prove that there *must* be a common cognitive core or a common inner language that underlies our capacity systematically to interrelate such different domains. The examples in (1, 2) show that cross-faculty mappings can be one-many in both directions. Accordingly, a picture and sentence can be said to match if there is a mapping from the picture to the sentence and vice versa. An alternative procedure would be to map one domain into the other (e.g. the visual image □ into the linguistic object "that is a square") and then check if the two representations are synonomous within the latter domain. Since there is an independent need to be able to check whether two objects in a given faculty are functionally equivalent, this procedure would require no extrafaculty "executive comparator."¶

On this view the mind is a federation of distinct subsystems that assign unique representations to mental objects. Each representation can be mapped onto a representation in (some) other subsystem(s) by a unidirectional mapping. The question arises as to what is held in common to the mind if there is neither a common core nor a common language that unites the different faculties. The highest common denominator possible on the federation model is in the elementary mental opera-

---

§I am indebted to M. Friedman for this example, and to J. Hochberg for general discussions.

¶In fact, this procedure is that assumed by many information-processing models of experimentally confined sentence-picture matching. Accordingly, insofar as these models are correct, they would seem to militate against the common core or common language theory of cross-modal matching; after all, if there were a common core or common language representation, why bother to map pictures onto sentences before comparing them?

tions themselves; that is, there is a common unconscious set of formal operation that are organized into different kinds of capacities.** No common language is implied, but rather, a common set of elementary operations that can be assembled in connection with the mouth (or the hands) into something we can call human language, or that can be assembled into the capacity for visual imagery, and so on. What is in common is neither a common language of representation nor of translation, but a common set of operations, a common set of building blocks out of which different kinds of capacities can be constructed. That seems to me to be a possible view, a way of looking at the situation that avoids some unnecessary rigidity on the question about the relationship between one mental faculty we call "language" and another mental faculty we call "thought." What would be at issue on this model is to try by induction and deduction to triangulate on the unconscious to decide on the elementary set of operations and discover how they are organized.

The Limits of Studying Abnormal Populations

The essential problem that the three preceding articles address is this: Human beings appear to assemble distinct faculties to act intelligently; how do they assemble the faculties of "language" and "thought" in particular? I have outlined three possible models of the relationship between differential mental faculties; on the common representation model all faculties derive from the same internal mental states; on the *lingua mentis* model the faculties may use distinct mechanisms, but can be represented in a common language that "translates" from one faculty to another; and on the federation model, the faculties are distinct and are mapped by unidirectional transducers. On this model, only the elementary mental operations are in common.

No doubt, the reader can construct intermediate models between these extremes. The question remains: What kinds of facts should we look for to decide which model is correct? If we focus on the relation between language and thought, our options are limited. It often appears that the conceptually precise experiment would be one in which one faculty is removed and behavioral changes in the other faculty are examined. If the remaining faculty is behaviorally intact, we conclude that it is independent of the one that was removed; if the remaining faculty is impaired, then we would conclude that it depended in part on the one that was removed. Although such experiments are impossible, nature sometimes performs them for us in the form of people whose abilities are selectively impaired. Thus, it is no accident that each of the preceding papers focuses on people who lack the fullest range of "normal" adult capacities, people who are deaf, people who are retarded, people who are still children. The methodology shared by the authors is that examination of people deficient in one faculty may reveal the role of the faculty in the development of the others.

Unfortunately, there is a difficulty with this kind of methodology that makes it nearly impossible to interpret, especially when it is applied to a developing organism. The fact is that developing organisms are *self-compensating*.†† The effects of a deficit in one area may be obscured by a partial take-over by another system which does not ordinarily organize the behavior in question. (For example, the alleged take-over of language by the right hemisphere if there is severe left-hemisphere damage in early childhood.) That is, organisms remain whole organisms, even when they sustain specific deficits; this reduces and distorts the apparent effects of a deficit, especially

** Note that these operations should not be confused with the formal operations in a Piagetian framework. The latter are designed ultimately to represent epistomological structures.
†† Dr. Menyuk's paper is most concerned with this fact.

if the deficit occurs early in the development when the organism's mental organization is relatively malleable. Since human "intelligence" obviously involves both "language" and "thought," it is quite likely that a deficit in one would be masked by compensatory application of the other.

Let me finish with a zoological illustration of this point. Suppose that what is important about kangaroos is that they hop. Ordinarily they do this by application of both legs and the tail. One could argue, however, that the basis for hopping in the kangaroo is "really" its hind legs. To show this, one could perform an ablation experiment, in this case a leg ablation. Remove the legs, and one would find that the kangaroo does a terrible job of hopping. Ergo, one would conclude, it is the legs that are central to hopping.

On the other hand, one might support the theory that it is the tail that is essential. To prove this we would cut off the tail. And now the kangaroo also does a terrible job of hopping. (It falls over backwards every time.) Ergo, one would conclude, it is the tail that is vital to hopping.

Finally, I could maintain a third position which is: It's both. To prove this, all we do is cut off a little bit of both the tail *and* the legs. And we find that indeed the animal still can hop; it doesn't like to and doesn't do as good a job as a normal kangaroo. But it does, in fact, manage to hop, because these different organs have been maintained in balance. The conclusion from all these experiments would be that neither the legs nor the tail is the essential basis for hopping; rather it is a balance between them.‡‡

Suppose we agreed that such ablation experiments are as immoral as they are for the study of cognition and language. Now, we would have to limit our data to observations of hopping-impaired kangaroos (whether due to infantile disease or genetic mutation that damaged the legs or tail). What we would undoubtedly find is that such kangaroos manage to rely relatively more on whatever organs remain intact, leading to aberrant hopping, but hopping, nevertheless. Whatever the clinically observed results, however, we would know little more than before about the organization of hopping in a normal kangaroo. Suppose we found that legless kangaroos compensate by hopping with their front paws, just as the deaf talk with their hands. This would not prove that the legs and tail are irrelevant to hopping in a kangaroo, any more than the ability to sign in the deaf proves that language is not important to thinking.§§

I do not mean that we should not use data from special populations. But I do mean to emphasize how hard it is to understand the implications of those data. This is particularly difficult with respect to language and cognition, insofar as we can separate them. Like everything else about life (that I can understand, at any rate), they seem to be engaged in a dialectic; our whole being is essentially the maintenance of a balance between such faculties. If there is an impairment in one, of course, it will unbalance the system and may result in an apparent impairment of the other. The whole system may ultimately appear impaired, but as long as there is a relative balance between them, some functioning can occur.

Conclusion

I have tried to articulate some conceptual and empirical issues in the study of the artificial separation and reunification of language and thought. My own belief is that

‡‡Lest the reader think this example to be misleadingly fanciful, consider experiments showing that brain lesion-caused behavioral deficits actually can become *less* severe if further complementary lesions are surgically induced.

§§Note that in any case the clear fact that the deaf can think is not relevant to this issue. After all, they can talk too, usually with hands, but sometimes also with their mouths.

since all organisms are self-organizing, the distinction has only heuristic merit. If the distinction causes more intellectual trouble than it is worth, we should drop it. The reason to maintain it is that if we separate the mental faculties for purposes of analysis we may gain initial insight into the mental structures which underlie all the faculties of the mind. That is worth a little intellectual trouble of the type we are having today.

Summary

The distinction between the faculties of language and thought in an intact organism may be arbitrary, but can have heuristic value in isolating the basic organizing functions of the mind.

Three models of the universal mental structures are compared. On the *common representation* model every superficially different mental faculty (e.g. logic, imagery, language) derives from the same common core. On the *common language* model, faculties may arise and function separately, but the representations they assign are intermappable by a common internal language of the mind (*lingua mentis*). On the *federated faculties* model the faculties are separate—they are mapped onto each other by couplementary unidirectional transducers; on this model the basic mental units are the common structures which are assembled differently in the service of different faculties.

These models explain the referring relation of a verbal name and a visual image in different ways. The common representation model explains such interfaculty equivalence in terms of representational identity in the common core. The common language model explains it in terms of identity in the interfaculty language. The federated faculties model explains it in terms of (1) simultaneous mapping between representations (by unique mapping languages) or (2) translation of both stimuli into one of the faculties and equivalence within that faculty.

The obvious data on the role of a faculty in the normal mind derive from comparing the mental functioning of people who lack the faculty with those who have it. However, the developing mind is self-organizing and compensates for specific deficits. This makes congenitally deaf or retarded children difficult to use as sources of data about the relative mental importance of "language" and "thought."

References

1. CLARK, H. H. & W. G. CHASE. 1972. On the process of comparing sentences against pictures. Cognitive Psychol. 3: 472–517.
2. TRABASSO, T., H. ROLLINS & E. SHAUGHNESSY. 1971. Storage and verification stages in processing concepts. Cognitive Psychol. 2: 239–289.
3. OLSON, D. R. & N. FILBY. 1972. On the comprehension of active and passive sentences. Cognitive Psychol. 3: 361–381.
4. JUST, M. A. 1974. Comprehending quantified sentences. Cognitive Psychol. 6: 216–236.
5. CARPENTER, P. & M. A. JUST. 1975. Sentence comprehension: a psycholinguistic model of sentence verification. Psychol. Rev. 82: 45–73.
6. TANENHAUS, M. K., J. M. CARROLL & T. G. BEVER. Information processing models of sentence-picture matching tasks are not theories of sentence comprehension or picture perception: at most they provide isolated examples of verification processes without a theory of verification. In preparation.

DISCUSSION

Lawrence Raphael, *Chairperson*

Department of Speech
Lehman College, City University of New York
The Bronx, New York 10468

DR. RAPHAEL: Before we turn to your questions, I'd like to know if any of the speakers would like to respond to Dr. Bever.

DR. MENYUK: Dr. Blank and I agreed, and perhaps Dr. Furth will, also, that the kangaroo analogy was a very good one.

DR. FURTH: I don't think it's a good analogy at all. If the animal could still hop when you cut off the tail, then you have conclusively shown that the tail is not necessary for hopping. It's not the deficit that tells you anything; it's whether the animal performs. If a deaf child can still perform classificatory behavior without knowing language, that shows that language isn't necessary for classificatory behavior. If he failed, there could be many other reasons why he failed.

DR. JOHN ALBERTINI (*Georgetown University, Washington, D.C.*): I'd like to address my question to Dr. Blank. I wonder if you would please tell us the size of your population and some of the conditions under which the questions were administered.

DR. BLANK: We had eight children in each group, so we had sixteen children at each age. They were matched for all of the usual variables, like sex, age, race, and so on. All told, there would be sixteen times four, sixty-four. But we have really far more extensive data than that. We've limited it because we wanted to have a perfect match, with the only difference being well-functioning and poorly functioning children. But the total sample is based on three hundred children, and it basically bears out the same kind of findings.

DR. ALBERTINI: What about the conditions under which you administered the tests?

DR. BLANK: They were tested in a school setting. It's interesting, although I don't know if this is what you're touching upon—but the whole "difference-deficit idea," that we're putting these children in an alien environment—is that what you're trying to get at?

DR. ALBERTINI: I was wondering if they were tested in play or in isolation.

DR. BLANK: This was done in a classroom, where we took the children out to a small room in the school and worked with them. I don't know if you intended this, but I'll take off from that point. If, in fact, as many people have been claiming, there is a difference in style rather than a deficit in style, then it doesn't explain the fact that these skills do come in. If there was truly a difference, the skills shouldn't come in order. You should maintain a qualitatively different pattern. One of the things I didn't have a chance to stress is that the skills appear in exactly the same way. The patterns of the wrong responses are identical. It's just that the child is now ten years of age instead of five.

There's another interesting idea, and I'll mention it for discussion. It's related to a point that Dr. Furth raised about adolescents. My own hunch—and this is really a hunch—is that there are two enormous bursts of intellectual skill. One is the preschool era, which Piaget has downplayed. I think the conceptual development in the preschool era is remarkable. The second is the early adolescent era. My feeling about the poorly functioning disadvantaged child is that when he has his final intel-

lectual spurt in preadolescence, he is developing the conceptual skills that the preschool child was developing. This leaves him ultimately at a tremendously high disadvantage. At the point when he can really develop the highest level of skills, he has
to exert his energies in developing skills he should have mastered in the preschool
years.

DR. JACK KAPLAN (*Cornell University, Ithaca, N.Y.*): I was curious about one
of Dr. Bever's comments about the possibility of substituting an assemblage of
transducers for a representational format. Have you thought about extending it beyond such a simple example as you've used? A slightly more complicated example
would be the Chase and Clark or Trabaso-type work on matching sentences and
pictures. Can you give a transducer assemblage account of that?

DR. BEVER: Let me amplify your question for people who aren't familiar with
it. There is a sizable line of research devoted to a task in which people compare pictures of simple scenes like a star above a cross, and they read or hear very simple
sentences, like "The star is above the cross," or "The star isn't above the cross." Response times are measured to determine how the people verify that the setence is
true of the picture, or conversely. A basic presumption—there are a lot of presumptions in those models that we believe to be false or trivial—but one basic assumption
is that there is a common language representation into which one can place both
the picture and the linguistic material. That, too, is false, but it requires attention.
So, the answer to the question is yes, we're very much concerned about that particular line of experimentation.

DR. HARWOOD FISHER (*City University of New York, New York, N.Y.*): I have
two questions. They're somewhat related. The first I would like Dr. Bever to respond
to. In any human context, language seems to have some part in the definition of an
object. Any set of elements would have to have been prelabeled, and hence, whoever has to deal with them, in the face of a deficit, must be taking in some kind of
linguistic information. Would not this definition of objects affect one's view of
whether or not language and cognition come together?

DR. BEVER: I believe the question was to the effect that object-recognition involves in humans the recognition of what the object is, in the linguistic domian. The
question is: doesn't this indicate that in fact language is influencing the way we even
perceive our world, never mind higher levels of thought? I think there are two answers, and I'll give them both. One is that I think looking at very simple case studies
in the work of Piaget on object permanence is useful. Let us consider object permanence in the recognition that an object is the same object it was, after it has gone out
of sight. In what seems to be the prelinguistic child, that capacity would indicate
that those human children can recognize that the object is the same, and can therefore recognize what the object is, at least in relation to their domain of experience,
without language. Therefore, I would suggest that naming is not a necessary part of
human perception or cognition of objects.

On the other hand, it also seems clear that both the syntactic rules that are different in different languages and the existence of particular lexical items in one
language and not in another certainly influence heavily what turns out to be easy to
talk about. In particular, it makes it very difficult to translate poetry, because the
syntactic form that has one meaning, literal meaning or logical meaning, in one language may have quite a different affective meaning in relation to the other syntactic
forms in another language. Similarly, the choice of vocabulary would have certain
kinds of connotations in one language that it might not in another. An example regarding the word, "why" was pointed out to me by Dr. Clement. In many languages
the different functions of the word "why" are carried out by different words, for example in German. Presumably, this might have some impact on how children deal

with the concept of "why" as we know it, as they learn German. I'd say it's reasonable to believe that since language is a very frequent activity, it has some influence on how we represent the world to ourselves. But I think the fundamental point is that we represent the world to ourselves without language. We can.

DR. STERN (*College of Physicians and Surgeons, Columbia University, New York, N. Y.*): I don't really want to ferment a fight here between Dr. Blank and Dr. Furth, but I would like some clarifications. This question should be directed to both of you. Dr. Blank, to what extent do you think that the differences you find between the high and low performers is a function of the educational system? Dr. Furth, to what extent do you think that the differences that she is finding are functions of simply individual differences, and are not truly important except as seen in the educational system?

DR. BLANK: The question you asked is central, but an adequate answer would require a great deal of time, for the issues are intimately bound up with the problem of how we evaluate the cognitive behaviors that are possible in the human being. If we are willing to limit our study of cognitive behavior to those skills necessary for "adaptation to the physical world," then by the end of the preschool period, the human being can be considered almost fully competent in "cognition". For example, the five-year-old knows very well how to maneuver in his environment, how to secure the objects he needs and wants. Then, should his own skills fail him, he knows how to turn to others to get their help. In this context, mastery of a term such as "why" is superfluous and may well be, as you termed it, a skill specific to the educational system.

But now for the other side of the coin. I do not believe that the skills and operations useful in the school are just simply those of learning to cope with arbitrary demands in an artificial institution. While such arbitrariness does exist at many points in schools, I believe also that schooling, or rather, success in schooling, is intimately bound up with the mastery of literacy. The demands of written language, however, are very different from those of spoken language. It is for this reason that I believe the mastery of "why" to be so central. The argument is a rather long one and I cannot present it here, but in brief, I believe that the skills typified in the mastery of "why" are similar to the skills needed for the mastery of the written language system. In this sense, the seemingly "unnecessary verbal games" present in many homes can be seen to be essential preparation for later literacy.

So, in summary, my answer is: if you wish to abandon literacy as a goal for the poorly functioning child, then I say the skills I defined are "unnecessary" in that they are relevant only to the school setting. If, on the other hand, you wish to maintain literacy as a goal for these children, then I believe that you must start helping them cope with this type of language production.

DR. FURTH: I believe that these children have been disadvantaged, and there is no question that they are socially disadvantaged in our society as it exists. We cannot change society as such. But I believe that these children would be better off in an educational setting where they would be encouraged to use their general cognitive skills, rather than to experience themselves as failures when stress is on skills like reading and language, in which they are poor. We just make things worse for them. They are even more disadvantaged than they would have to be had they been in a different educational setting. So I'm not denying the disadvantage, but I am thinking that what we are doing educationally for them may be making things worse for them, rather than helping them.

DR. MARY CATHERINE BATESON: I wanted to raise an aspect of Dr. Blank's data which widens the area we're speaking about. I don't think one can examine children's use of "why" without regarding it as related to behavior that Dr. Menyuk called, on her chart, "keeping something interesting going." The fact is that the question "why" works differently on different kinds of parents. I, and probably a great many of us here who are parents, feel it almost immoral not to produce a response to the question "why." We operate with rules of discourse that require an answer. Hence, "why" becomes a very useful term, not only in terms of the cognitive area, as you've been exploring, but also in terms of keeping the interaction going.

Now, what struck me in the comparisons of the errors made by your two groups is that in the error patterns you may have some very good evidence for the fact that your more successful group of children were acknowledging a social necessity to give an answer, even when they could not produce a cognitively appropriate response to the question "why." In other words, the "don't know" and "no answer" categories descended almost to zero, whereas for your less successful group of children, throughout the period, the possibility of just not answering remained much stronger. It seems to me to give some evidence of the kind of thing Basil Bernstein talks about, regarding whether or not they have grasped the cognitive implications of "why." They also are operating with different rules of discourse to say that "why" does not always produce an answer and a sustained interaction.

DR. BLANK: I certainly agree. However, I do not think that the choices you proposed represent "either/or" alternatives. I think both interpretations are valid. They simply focus on different aspects of a complex human behavior. I would like to add, however, that initially the child's production of "why" does not lead to continuation of the dialogue; it almost always disrupts the dialogue. Accordingly, for the child who "believes" in dialogue, the break impels him to "keep going" to find out how he can eventually use the term so as not to disrupt the dialogue. In other words, the problem he confronts is essentially, "What can I finally do to formulate a 'why' that will get me an answer, that will keep the dialogue going?" It is this search that, I believe, ultimately yields a tremendous by-product effect for certain cognitive skills, in that the child has to employ a variety of forms of reasoning so as to finally extract the "why" that he needs to keep the dialogue alive.

DR. REED BATESYOUNG (*Austin, Texas*): This question is for Dr. Blank, but I think she almost answered it. I'm curious, when you say that for six months the child's initial production of "why" seems to be just completely nonsensical. It seems to me, as a linguist, that if there are so many functions for the word "why," and I wish Dan Slobin were here to back me up, maybe the children are trying to elicit one of those responses. Perhaps they've locked onto a meaning for "why," and they want a response to that meaning, but they're just not getting it. Then, after six months, they just get disgusted and give up because they're not ready to answer questions about "why" that are directed to them. The fact that all of these "why's" are connected with negation—and you pointed this out, too, that there's always a negative involved—may mean that they're actually testing a linguistic theory, almost the "mapping derivation problem." They're testing whether they can connect "why" with a negative. I just ask for your response to that.

DR. BLANK: You've raised a valid point, and I'm not sure which view is correct on this. By this, I'm comparing (a) the idea that the children may have a concept which somehow doesn't match the adult concept (b) with the idea that they really don't have the concept. Clearly, if they have a concept, such as pairing "why" with negation, it is a very simple concept. It is much more a form of associational learning, which significantly is not characteristic of their use of other types of words. So, at the very least, it's a low-level concept. Additional data against the idea that they have some concept derives from the fact that all their other question forms are much more advanced than their use of "why." For example, Dusty would use two- and three-word questions with "where," "who," "which," and "what." She never did that with "why." This type of behavior occurs not only in our data; it occurs in all the data that we've been able to find in this area. The children just try the word, but then drop the conversation once the word is out. This suggests that they are not really striving for an answer, probably because they're overwhelmed with the frustration aroused by the adult's response. What's interesting is that the frustration that Dusty showed at twenty months is almost identical to the frustration that Mary Catherine Bateson just pointed out for the five-year-old disadvantaged child who's poorly functioning. Hence, this is a very, very difficult situation for the child. I think what happens is that if he is interested in pursuing it, he has to go on to the next level.

DR. GEORGE ALLEN (*University of North Carolina, Chapel Hill, N.C.*): My question arises out of Dr. Bever's analogy, but I believe it is directed to all the speakers. It is relevant to all their discussions. There is some evidence to suggest that in hard-of-hearing children, the performance—their performance on syntactic function words—is highly correlated with their nonverbal intelligence as measured by any of the lousy nonverbal intelligence tests we have, so long as you correct for the hearing loss. This suggests that the child who cannot hear everything that he is supposed to, can, if he is smart enough, get along and figure out what the system is, anyway. This would suggest that for the disabled child, if not the disordered child, in contrast to the normal child, the name of the game is not balance, but compensation. This suggests that there is quite a strong relationship between cognitive development and linguistic development in the disabled child.

DR. MENYUK: The only comment I have is that there may be aspects of lousy intelligence tests that are germane to particular tasks that are involved in the acquisition of function terms. But there is an interactive thing going on here. In the study of the autistic children that I referred to, there was an overall effect: the measured intelligence could predict the development of these children over a six-year period. However, in the initial evaluation and in the postevaluation, there were particular aspects of task involvement, both in the verbal and in the nonverbal domain, that were differentiated among a population of children of a certain measured I.Q. So you get an overall effect, but it doesn't really tell you anything specific about how the children are functioning and why they are functioning the way they are functioning.

DR. BEVER: There's a point that's interesting in what was asked, which hasn't yet come up. We have naturally assumed that if it makes any sense at all to divide mental faculties and to ask about what causes what, an obvious division is between language as a social instrument and something else called "thought." Maybe that's the wrong way to divide things up in the first place. That bears on the question, because if one finds evidence that two things are not balanced, but rather, that one can take over the function of the other under certain kinds of circumstances, it's possible that this indeed is the true state of affairs. Another possibility is that the internal division of different kinds of mental faculties rather imperfectly mirrors the external division between what we call "language" and what we call "thought." There are certain aspects of language and thought which, in fact, form a coherent mental whole; for example, possibly those involved in analytic kinds of processing activities. Other kinds of mental activities may also be in opposition to analytic activity, but in common to language and thought; for example, gestalt sorts of activities, if such there be. Part of the puzzle, when looking at a child that displays an external sensory deficiency, is to know exactly to what internal deficiency that might speak. It might speak literally to the natural modality—namely, language—or our internal organization of these variable external manifestations may be quite different.

VOCALIZING IN UNISON AND IN ALTERNATION: TWO MODES OF COMMUNICATION WITHIN THE MOTHER-INFANT DYAD*

Daniel N. Stern, Joseph Jaffe, Beatrice Beebe, and Stephen L. Bennett

*New York State Psychiatric Institute and Department of Psychiatry
College of Physicians and Surgeons
Columbia University
New York, New York 10032*

INTRODUCTION

Two laboratories studying dyadic communication have joined in an ongoing research project on the ontogeny of communication. One laboratory has engaged in the study of naturally occurring interactions between mothers and infants, particularly their "nonverbal" communication.[1-6] The other has focused on the rhythm of adult conversation.[7,8] Together, we are examining vocal and kinesic behaviors and their integration during the course of development. This paper presents a part of that ongoing study.

During the first half-year of life the infant communicates effectively through a variety of behaviors: head and body movement and tone, gaze, facial expressions, and vocalizations. By the age of three to four months, all of these behaviors can be integrated to form recognizable complex expressive acts. The distinction between vocal and other motor acts is less compelling at this point in development, and in fact, if made too sharply, may obscure a view of early vocalization. For instance, when watching a film of an infant, with the sound turned off, it is impossible to predict reliably when he is vocalizing. In social situations, there exists a wide range and variety of mouth behaviors, especially mouth-opening with head thrown up, which are extremely expressive and evocative.[4] These may or may not be accompanied by a vocalization. When a vocalization is added to the entire kinesic event, that event becomes importantly different. Nonetheless, infant vocalizations rarely occur (in a social situation) as an isolated motor act such as an adult can perform in speaking; rather, they occur as another element in the constellation of kinesic events that make up a communicative act. Furthermore, they occur within an interpersonal context in which the levels of arousal and affective tone are constantly changing. We thus have examined mother and infant vocalization from the viewpoint that they are sound-producing kinesic events, as well as prelinguistic events which later transform into speech.

This paper was initially prompted by an unexpected finding. During play sessions, mothers and their three- to four-month-old infants vocalize simultaneously to a far greater extent than we had anticipated or than had been commented on in the literature. Early vocalizations appear to have at least one beginning within the mother-infant dyad as a *coaction system* in which each member is performing the same or similar behavior at the same time. This occurrence of behavioral coaction between

*This research was supported by The Grant Foundation and the New York State Department of Mental Hygiene.

mother and infant is common in kinesic communication and several examples were already familiar to us, in particular, mutual gaze and posture-sharing in the form of aligning the head in a parallel spatial plane. Both of these require simultaneous performance of the same behavior. Nevertheless, to the extent that we initially viewed early vocalization as "prespeech," we were unprepared for the considerable occurrence of simultaneous mother and infant vocalization. There were several reasons for this surprise. First, adult verbal conversations served as the model. In this situation maximum communication demands that speaker and listener exchange roles in an alternating fashion.[7,8] The difficulty of processing incoming information while simultaneously sending information requires this alternation. Second, it has been described that as early as the first few months of life, when babbling begins, mothers often create or shape an antiphonal or alternating pattern of vocalizations between themselves and their infants.[9] Similarly, we know that infant vocalizations can be conditioned, using the human voice or other social stimuli as reinforcers.[10-12] When the infant vocalization is viewed and treated as a response in the learning paradigm and the adult vocalization is used as the reinforcer, an alternating dialogic pattern will necessarily emerge. The alternating pattern may, in fact, be conditioned along with the vocalizations.

We present evidence that mothers and infants have two modes of vocalizing with each other that differ structurally and functionally: a coaction mode and an alternating mode. We suggest that coactional vocalizing is not simply an early developmental pattern that later transforms into the alternating pattern of conversational dialogue, but that it is also an enduring mode of human communication that shares much structurally and functionally with the kinesic systems of mutual gaze,[1,3] posture sharing,[13] and rhythm sharing.[14]

METHODOLOGY

Subjects

Eight infants, consisting of four twin sets, were observed from their third to fourth month of life. Two monozygous and two dyzogous sets, five girls and three boys, were represented; individual differences or sex differences will not, however, be discussed. All infants had a normal developmental course. The mothers were primiparous, white, and middle socioeconomic class. For further details regarding the subjects, see Stern.[1]

Data Collection

The methods of data collection have previously been described.[1,6] The essential features involved repeated home visits, at least weekly for a month, during which an entire morning was set aside to videotape the naturally occurring, undirected mother-infant interactions as they normally unfolded: the recording on television tape of the gaze direction of each partner (i.e., whether they are gazing at the other's face), and the presence of vocalizations by mother and/or infant. Periods in which the infant was fussing and/or crying were excluded. This exclusion is very important in that mothers commonly vocalize simultaneously with the crying of their infants in order to soothe them. Also, although all infants were twins, only interactions between the mother and one infant were scored; i.e., all triadic interactions were excluded.

Data Scoring of Dyadic Interactions

Television tapes were replayed in the laboratory and viewed by four trained observers who operated a four-channel magnetic-tape event recorder. One observer scored whether the infant's gaze was "on" or "off" the mother's face, another simultaneously scored whether the mother's gaze was "on" or "off" the infant's face. Interrater agreement as to the presence of a gaze at the other's face was .96 and .93 as to its duration. The third and fourth observers separately scored the presence of maternal and infant vocalization, respectively. Interrater agreement as to the presence of a vocalization was .91, and .86 as to its duration. Accordingly, there are four separate behavioral variables: maternal gaze, infant gaze, maternal vocalization, and infant vocalization. Each of these four variables may occur separately or together in any combination. When each variable can either be "on" or "off," there exist 16 possible combinations of the four variables. Each separate combination is designated as a separate dyadic state. For the purposes of this paper we shall discuss only the two channels consisting of maternal and infant vocalization and the four dyadic states that result from their possible combinations: both silent, mother vocalizing while infant is silent, infant vocalizing while mother is silent, and both vocalizing. The magnetic tape with the channels scored is playing through a punch teletype machine which samples the magnetic tape every 0.1 seconds to determine which channels were "on" and accordingly, which of the possible dyadic states were present.

The punch tape is then fed into a PDP 12 computer programmed to print out how often each dyadic state occurred, its duration, and the percentage of time occupied by each state; in addition, a transition matrix is accumulated that shows the probability (in the next 0.1 second) of any dyadic state proceeding to any other dyadic state or remaining in the same state. When the computer print out is "retranslated," many simple questions can be asked, such as, "Are mother and infant vocalizations more or less likely than chance to occur simultaneously?"

An additional methodology was used to score and analyze portions of the data. This additional strategy was addressed to the question of whether incidences of co-occurring mother and infant vocalization might be related to the infant's level of affective arousal. For one infant only, the video recording of a play session was kinescoped and numbers were placed on each film frame. A frame-by-frame film analysis, without sound, was then performed.[15,6] All infant head, gaze, mouth, and, where possible, eye behaviors were scored on a time-flow record. The mother then looked at the film frame by frame, again without sound, and independently judged the infant's level of affectively positive arousal on a one to four scale. (For further details, see Beebe.[4]) The points in time at which the mother judged changes from one level to the next were then added to the time-flow record. Last, maternal and infant vocalization were then independently scored and superimposed on the time-flow record by frame number. By this procedure it is possible to correlate the different types of vocalizations (alternating, coactional, vocalizations occurring alone) with the maternal judgment of arousal level. The mother's judgments agreed (.85) with the independently arrived at experimental judgments of the infant's level of affectively positive arousal.

RESULTS

The Prevalence of a Coaction Vocalizing Pattern and of an Alternating Vocalizing Pattern

To determine whether a predominantly coactional or alternating dyadic vocalizing pattern was in operation, the odds ratio statistic was used[16] (see FIGURE 1). In an

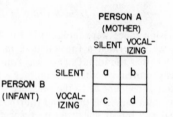

FIGURE 1. Coaction versus alternating vocal dyadic patterns expressed in terms of the odds ratio statistic.

adult verbal conversation in which speaker and listener are exchanging roles, we would expect the greatest frequency to accumulate in cells "b" (when person A is speaking and B is silent) and "c" (where person B is speaking and A is silent). Much lower frequencies would be expected in cells "a" (during joint silence) and "d" (during interruptions where there is simultaneous speech). The odds ratio for such a conversation would be well below 1.0, and indeed, the analysis of 30 polite adult conversations revealed an odds ratio of 0.03.[17] If, on the other hand, persons A and B were engaged in choral speaking, the greatest frequencies would accumulate in cells "d" (when they were speaking together) and in cell "a" (when they were both silent). Lower frequencies would be expected in cells "b" and "c" (during short failures to start and stop speaking together). In such a coaction pattern the odds ratio would exceed 1.0. For analyzing the data, the formula shown in FIGURE 1 was altered to read

$$O.\ R. = \frac{(a + .5) \times (d + .5)}{(b + .5) \times (c + .5)}$$

to account for zero freqencies in one or more cells.

TABLE 1 shows the odds ratio and its level of significance as measured by a chi-square test with a Yates correction[16] for each session of each infant-mother pair. In addition, the mean odds ratio for each infant-mother pair across all their play sessions, and the mean odds ratio across all pairs and all sessions are shown. This analysis revealed that of the 64 separate play sessions, forty showed an odds ratio greater than 1.0 (i.e., a coaction pattern), and fifteen of these reached significance. Twenty-four sessions showed an odds ratio of less than 1.0 (i.e., an alternating pattern), and eight of these reached significance.

When all sessions for each infant-mother pair were pooled, six pairs showed an overall coaction pattern (three reached significance), and two pairs showed an overall alternating pattern (one reached significance). When all sessions for all pairs were pooled the mean odds ratio was 1.20, indicating an overall coaction pattern significant at the .001 level.

It is interesting to note that twins 3A and 3B, who both showed significant patterns but in the opposite direction, are monozygous. This finding will be discussed below.

The Relationship Between the Dyadic Vocalizing Pattern and the Infant's Level of Arousal

In order to test the clinical impression that coactional vocalizing occurs mainly during high levels of infant (and probably maternal) arousal, the frame-by-frame

TABLE 1

THE OCCURRENCE OF COACTIONAL AND ALTERNATING VOCALIZATION PATTERNS BETWEEN MOTHER AND INFANT EXPRESSED AS AN ODDS RATIO (O. R.)*

	Twin Set 1				Twin Set 2				Twin Set 3				Twin Set 4			
	Twin N†	1A O.R.‡	Twin N	1B O.R.	Twin N	2A O.R.	Twin N	2B O.R.	Twin N	3A O.R.	Twin N	3B O.R.	Twin N	4A O.R.	Twin N	4B O.R.
1.	6679	2.48**	8683	1.61	1470	0.19	1098	1.05	4713	2.03*	980	0.68	2061	1.07	2295	1.41
2.	707	1.71	1583	8.07*	2149	1.32	695	3.13***	732	0.29	520	1.94	1424	1.86	4382	0.77
3.	1917	4.65***	11284	3.62***	1006	1.27	854	2.42	1717	5.75***	1122	1.80	2729	0.03***	1451	1.14
4.	3014	0.57			271	0.10	1926	0.50**	1911	1.02	805	1.59	3330	0.78	4643	1.22**
5.	2493	1.26			608	0.85	1102	4.55***	2676	1.19	2538	19.45***	3593	0.81	6501	0.54***
6.					3870	1.87			3317	0.28	2487	0.27***	6646	1.15		
7.					713	0.35			3278	2.53**	1077	0.03***				
8.					502	2.21			1444	0.87	878	13.54				
9.					539	0.41**			1314	1.08	1662	2.23				
10.					790	0.33			3078	1.18	3069	1.74				
11.					1905	1.27			2815	1.28	336	13.76				
12.									4819	0.77	3133	0.62*				
13.											502	0.32				
14.											964	2.13				
15.											2716	0.50***				
16.											2629	0.56				
17.											4313	42.85				
Mean O.R. across all play sessions of each dyad		1.66***		3.32***		1.09		1.35*		1.32**		0.68**		0.96		1.11

*(*p < .05, **p < .01, ***p < .001).

†N = The number of observations taken at a rate of 10/second.

‡Mean O.R. across all sessions and all dyads = 1.20***.

FIGURE 2. The relative occurrence of different types of vocalizations at different levels of affectively positive arousal. (Infant vocalize alone, N = 10; mother vocalize alone, N = 37; infant vocalize in alternation, N = 11; mother vocalize in alternation, N = 15; coaction vocalizations, N = 20.)

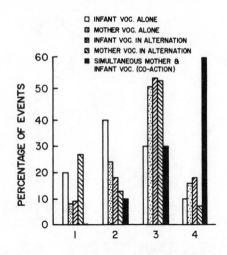

□ INFANT VOC. ALONE
🅑 MOTHER VOC. ALONE
🅩 INFANT VOC. IN ALTERNATION
🅝 MOTHER VOC. IN ALTERNATION
■ SIMULTANEOUS MOTHER & INFANT VOC. (CO-ACTION)

film analysis described above was performed. The five vocalizing categories were: infant vocalize alone; mother vocalize alone; infant vocalize in alternation; mother vocalize in alternation: coactional vocalizations. A vocalization was scored as alternating if it occurred within 1.0 second after the termination of a vocalization of the partner. If more than 1.0 second elapsed the vocalization was designated a vocalization alone.

FIGURE 2 shows the percentage of each type of vocalization that occurred at each level of affectively positive arousal. It can be seen that coactional vocalizations are heavily concentrated (60%) at the highest level of arousal, whereas alternating vocalizations of both mother (53%) and infant (54%) are more manifest at a midlevel of arousal.

The Relative Contribution of Mother and Infant to the Formation of a Coaction Pattern

The following four analyses (A–D) focus on the questions of how and who is mainly "responsible" for creating a coaction pattern.

Operationally, we have asked what the effect is of the presence of infant vocalization on the initiation and on the continuation, or termination, of maternal vocalizations, and vice versa, what the effect is of the presence of maternal vocalizations on the initiation and on the continuation of infant vocalizations.

A. *The Effect of the Presence of Infant Vocalization on the Initiation of Maternal Vocalization.* TABLE 2, Row 1, shows the difference, expressed as $\overline{D}$,[16] between the probability that the mother will initiate a vocalization when the infant is silent, compared to when he is vocalizing. The negative value of $\overline{D}$ in seven of eight dyads indicates that the mother is more likely to start vocalizing during an infant vocalization than when he is silent. This, of course, is contrary to the expected "rules" for adult conversational exchange.

B. *The Effect of the Presence of Infant Vocalization on the Termination of Maternal Vocalization.* TABLE 2, Row II, shows the difference between the probability that the mother will terminate a vocalization when the infant is silent compared to when he is vocalizing. The positive values of $\overline{D}$ in seven of eight dyads indicates that the mother is more likely to stop vocalizing during an infant silence than

TABLE 2

THE EFFECT OF INFANT VOCALIZATION ON MATERNAL VOCALIZATION, AND THE EFFECT OF MATERNAL VOCALIZATION ON INFANT VOCALIZATION*

	$\bar{D}$ Value for Twin-Mother Dyad†							
	1A	1B	2A	2B	3A	3B	4A	4B
The Effect of Infant Vocalization On:								
The initiation of maternal vocalization‡	−.451	−1.393**	−.342**	−.351	−.300	−.369*	−.220	+.096
The termination of maternal vocalization§	+.600	+.525	+.562†	+.032	+.156	−.093	+.518*	+.003
The Effect of Maternal Vocalization On:								
The initiation of infant vocalization¶	−.617*	−1.177***	+.152	−.357	−.261	+.021	−.467*	−.116
The termination of infant vocalization††	−.440	+.121	+.095	−.091	−.014	−.128	−.453	+.093

*(*p < .05, **p < .01, ***p < .001).

†The difference between the two probabilities is expressed as $\bar{D}$ using a chi-square statistic to test the significance of the $\bar{D}$.

‡p (Mother will initiate a vocalization when the infant is silent) minus the p (mother will initiate a vocalization when the infant is vocalizing).

§p (Mother will terminate a vocalization when the infant is silent) minus the p (mother will terminate a vocalization when the infant is vocalizing).

¶p (Infant will initiate a vocalization when the mother is silent) minus the p (infant will initiate a vocalization when the mother is vocalizing).

††p (Infant will terminate a vocalization when the mother is silent) minus the p (infant will terminate a vocalization when the mother is vocalizing).

when he is vocalizing; i.e., she is more likely to continue vocalizing during his vocalization. Again, this is contrary to the expected adult conversational "rules."

C. *The Effect of the Presence of Maternal Vocalization on the Initiation of Infant Vocalization.* TABLE 2, Row III, shows the difference between the probability that the infant will initiate a vocalization when the mother is silent compared to when she is vocalizing. The negative values of $\overline{D}$ in six of eight dyads indicates that the infant tends to start vocalizing during a maternal vocalization.

D. *The Effect of the Presence of Maternal Vocalization on the Termination of Infant Vocalization.* TABLE 2, Row IV, shows the difference between the probability that the infant will terminate a vocalization when the mother is silent compared to when she is vocalizing. No clear trend is evident.

In summary, the mother is more likely to begin vocalizing when the infant is already vocalizing, and she tends to continue vocalizing while the infant is vocalizing. Both effects would tend to increase the likelihood of a coaction pattern. The infant, like the mother, tends to begin a vocalization while the mother is already vocalizing. This also would tend to produce a coaction pattern. However, the infant does not show a tendency to continue vocalizing during a maternal vocalization. This may be simply because his vocalizations are generally much shorter than hers. In any event, the "rules" of adult conversational dialogue are violated by both partners. The mother, however, appears to influence more strongly the production of the coaction pattern, just as it is found that she is more "responsible" for the production of the alternating pattern.

DISCUSSION

The data suggest that we are witnessing the parallel emergence of two separate modes of vocal communication, which differ structurally and functionally. From a larger biological perspective, it is not unusual for different species such as birds to develop both antiphonal and synchronous or coaction communication modes to serve different purposes.[18]

Both dyadic vocal patterns are demonstrable in the interactions of three-to-four-month-old infants and their mothers. The coaction pattern occurs almost twice as frequently as the alternating pattern, but all dyads appear capable of performing in both modes. The majority of individual sessions, however, are not patterned in either direction to an extent that reaches significance. This lack of pattern may prove to be a methodological artifact. Within any single play session the mother and infant may produce several short "runs" of alternating vocalizations, interspersed in the same session with several "runs" of coactional vocalizations. Several switches of pattern within a session may be common, depending on the interpersonal situation and the level of arousal. In fact, it is our clinical impression, although undocumented, that in any session both modes will be employed. However, since the analysis considers one play session as a single event, we can uncover only the predominant pattern for the entire session, thus making the majority of vocal interactions appear less patterned than they actually might be. In any event, at this stage of development most mother-infant dyads will manifest different patterns in different sessions, even though one of the patterns may be significantly more common throughout all their sessions.

At some point in the second year of life when verbal comprehension develops, we would expect the alternating pattern that facilitates this process to be not only well established but also the predominant one. Accordingly, we would expect a developmental shift in predominant pattern from coaction, seen at three to four months, to alternating, seen in adult dyads. (The Odds Ratio would be expected to reflect this shift by gradually falling below the critical value of 1.0 and decreasing further over time until it approximates the value of 0.03 seen in polite adult conversation.) We do not have the developmental data to document this probable course. However, the fact that the alternating pattern must emerge as the dominant one as verbal behavior is acquired does not necessarily argue that the coaction pattern is simply transformed under the influence of maternal shaping into an alternating one, and then disappears from use. The presence of both patterns at the very early developmental stage of three to four months, and the utilization of both patterns throughout life, as described below, suggests a parallel development for each.

A second reason to suggest that these two patterns emerge in parallel as functionally as well as structurally separate communication modes is that each is more likely to occur under different conditions of arousal and affect. FIGURE 2 indicates that the coaction pattern is mainly manifest during the highest levels of arousal, while the alternating pattern is more evident at midrange levels. It is a common experience that at high arousal levels at either the positive or negative end of the affective spectrum, mothers and infants will vocalize simultaneously. While the baby is fretting or crying, the mother most often will simultaneously say something like, "There, there," to sooth him. Similarly, at the far positive end, mothers and infants will laugh in unison. However, even short of this extreme, at moments when the infant (and almost invariably the mother, also) are at a high level of affectively positive arousal, they will vocalize together and appear to derive much enjoyment from it.

A probable explanation of the finding that twin 3A and mother show a predominantly coaction pattern while her monozygous sister, 3B, and mother show an alternating pattern relates to this issue of the influence of arousal level on vocal pattern. At each morning visit, this mother always awakened twin 3A first, fed her, and played with her. The mother then repeated this sequence with twin 3B. By the time mother got around to twin 3B, she was relatively "played out," and instead of pursuing the highly arousing, spontaneously playful behaviors she showed with twin 3A, she interacted with 3B at a relatively lower level of arousal and centered her play more around instructional behaviors. This clinical vignette supports our overall impression that during those parts of a play session when the mother is "teaching" her infant, an alternating pattern is mainly used. However, when the two start to really have fun together, they move into a coaction pattern. Given "identical" constitutions, it is striking that the mother can by three to four months so markedly influence in differential ways the vocal interactions she helps form with each twin. This is consistent with the finding that it is mainly the mothers' influence that determines the dyadic vocal pattern. A possible reason for the generally large amount of coactional vocalizing observed is that these mothers generally sought and achieved highly arousing interactions with their infants.

The existence of coactional vocalizing under conditions of high arousal is not unique to the mother-infant dyad but continues throughout life. It is instructive to consider occurrences of simultaneous vocalization among adults. As the interpersonal situation moves toward intense anger, sadness, joy, or expressions of love, the alternating dialogic pattern "breaks down" and coactional vocalizing again becomes a crucial communicative mode. Mutual declarations of love and vocalizations during love-making are an obvious example. In fact, an operatic love duet can be viewed as an excellent cultural representation of this phenomenon. Arguments provide another example. As an argument gets more "heated," interruptions (which are a form of coactional speaking) become more frequent and longer. At some point, the information in the verbalizations of the antagonists recedes in importance compared to the fight for the "floor"; i.e., the experience of being interrupted and talked at, while talking, becomes the primary communicative event, overshadowing whatever is being said.

Coactional vocalizing is a common occurrence among adults in a related human situation, namely, in defining group membership for a given purpose, or to state or establish group bonds. A variety of examples can serve: choral speaking, as in a pledge of allegience; prayer, in recitative form; work songs or any group singing or chanting; political rallying behavior such as leader, "What do we want?", followers, "FREEDOM," etc.; peer group taunting of another child, "Sally is a yah-yah"; peer group celebrating a member during toasting behavior, "Here, here," etc. The joint vocalizations mentioned above usually carry a symbolic meaning that generally passes for their main purpose. However, they also appear to have a strong group-bonding effect, which, though less obvious, is often more important.

A football game provides several examples of how different subgroups can be defined by who vocalizes together; everyone in the stadium, players and audience, stand and sing together the national anthem. This defines the entire group partici-pating in the sporting event. Then the cheer leaders for one side coordinate the coactional vocalization of one half of the stadium. This defines a rooting or fan group. Then the 36 players and several coaches of one team huddle before the start of the game, some rousing words are said, and the group breaks apart, making some vocalization together. This defines the entire working team. Then eleven members of the team go on the field, huddle to make a play, and break huddle, vocalizing together. This defines the playing unit. It is worth noting that each of these "units" is spatially defined, also. However, it is at moments of heightened arousal that they also "define" themselves by vocalizing together.

Many cross-cultural examples of collective simultaneous vocalizing to express group membership can be found in anthropological studies. Related but dispersed tribes gather together periodically to chant and move in unison as part of the cere-mony that reestablishes group bonds.[14]

Byers describes an unusual form of joint vocalizing among the Yanamamo Indians in South America.[14] When two tribes that are potentially hostile come together for a feast, the two chiefs first engage in a ritual greeting ceremony consisting of what sounds like a "shouting match," during which both chiefs are simultaneously shout-ing at each other, each in synchrony with the other's vocalizations. This presumably serves an aggression-inhibiting function. Coberly[19] examined in ten cultures the process whereby Shamans "cure" a deviant member. In all cultures the Shamann collects a group of normals who are then made to chant, sing, clap, and/or move in unison. The deviant is then brought back into the group by his participating in the collective coactional activity.

In previous work we have found that the gaze behaviors of mother and infant form a "conversational" pattern that constitutes an early dialogic system.[1,3] This dialogic system is heavily coactional in that the response biases of both partners tend to create a preponderance of mutual gaze.[1] The present data indicates that the dyadic coactional vocalizing pattern conforms closely to the dyadic gazing pattern between mother and infant. Furthermore, coactional vocalizing occurs almost invariably during mutual gaze.[22] Accordingly, at given moments, the nature of the interpersonal interaction and its emotional tone are communicated by the mutual and simulta-neous performance of both gaze and vocalization. These appear to be quite special moments for the dyad.

To the extent that vocalizing together, especially in conjunction with mutual gaze, is a form of establishing group membership or bonding, particularly under conditions of heightened arousal, the coactional vocalizations between mother and infant may fruitfully be considered an early attachment behavior that contributes to the formation of the mother-infant tie. Vocalizing in unison as a mutual experience of joy or excited delight in being with someone may be central to the creation of a positive experience of relatedness, and should, in this regard, be added to the growing list of human behaviors that bond a mother and infant together.[20,21]

We have provided evidence that two structurally different patterns of dyadic vocalizations exist between mother and infant by the time the infant is three to four months old. We suggest that both patterns develop as distinct modes serving separate communicative functions. The alternating mode transforms into the conversational dialogic pattern to function later in the exchange of symbolic information. The coaction mode transmits emotional communications expressive of the nature of the ongoing interpersonal relationship, as well as contributing to the formation of the relationship.

ACKNOWLEDGMENT

We gratefully wish to acknowledge the statistical advice given by Dr. Joseph L. Fleiss.

REFERENCES

1. STERN, D. N. 1974. Mother and infant at play: the dyadic interaction involving facial, vocal and gaze behaviors. *In* The Effect of the Infant on its Caregiver. Vol 1: 187–213. The Origin of Behavior Series. Lewis and L. Rosenblum, Eds. John Wiley & Sons Inc. New York, N.Y.
2. STERN, D. N. 1974. The goal and structure of mother-infant play. J. Am. Acad. Child. Psychiat. **13**: 402–421.
3. JAFFE, J., D. N. STERN & J. C. PERRY. 1973. "Conversational" coupling of gaze behavior in prelinguistic human development. J. Psycholinguistic Res. **2**: 321–329.
4. BEEBE, B. 1973. The ontogeny of positive affect in the third and fourth month of the life of one infant. Doctoral dissertation. Columbia University. New York, N.Y.
5. BENNETT, S. L. 1971. Infant-caretaker interactions. J. Am. Acad. Child Psychiat. **10**: 321–335.
6. STERN, D. N. 1971. A micro-analysis of mother-infant interaction. J. Am. Acad. Child. Psychiat. **10**: 501–517.
7. JAFFE, J. & D. A. NORMAN. 1964. A simulation of the time patterns of dialogue. Scientific Report No. C5-4. Center for Cognitive Studies. Harvard University. Cambridge, Mass.
8. JAFFE, J. & S. FELDSTEIN. 1970. Rhythms of Dialogue. Academic Press. New York, N.Y.
9. BATESON, M. C. This annal.
10. RHEINGOLD, H. L., J. L. GEWITZ & H. W. ROSS. 1959. Social conditioning of vocalizations in the infant. J. Comp. Physiol. Psychol. **52**: 68–73.
11. WEISBERG, P. 1963. Social and nonsocial conditioning of infant vocalization. Child Develop. **34**: 377–388.
12. TODD, G. A., A. GIBSON & B. PALMER, 1968. Social reinforcement of infant babbling. Child Develop. **39**: 591–596.
13. SCHEFLEN, A. E. 1964. The significance of posture in communication systems. Psychiatry **27**: 316–331.
14. BYERS, P. 1975. Rhythms, information processing and human relations: toward a typology of communication. *In* Perspectives in Ethology. Vol. II. P. Klopfer and P. Bateson, Eds. Plenum Press. New York, N.Y.
15. CONDON, W. S. & W. D. OGSTON, 1966. Sound film analysis of normal and pathological behavior patterns. J. Nerv. Ment. Dis. **143**: 338–347.
16. FLEISS, J. L. 1973. Statistical methods for rates and proportions. John Wiley & Sons Inc. New York, N.Y.

17. JAFFE, J. 1975. Unpublished.
18. THORPE, W. H. 1961. Bird Song: The Biology of Vocal Communication and Expression in Birds. Cambridge University Press. Cambridge, Mass.
19. COBERLY, L. 1973. An interactional analysis of ten curing ceremonies. M. A. Thesis. Columbia University. New York, N.Y.
20. BOWLBY, J. 1969. Attachment and Loss. Vol. I Basic Books. New York, N.Y.
21. AINSWORTH, M. D. S. 1969. Object relations, dependency and attachment. Child Dev. **40:** 969–1025.
22. STERN, D. N. & J. JAFFE. In preparation.

$57/24$

MOTHER-INFANT EXCHANGES: THE EPIGENESIS OF CONVERSATIONAL INTERACTION*

Mary Catherine Bateson

Northeastern University
Boston, Massachusetts 02115

INTRODUCTION

The present study reports research that brought a variety of approaches to bear on the description and analysis of one kind of joint performance of mother and child, starting in about the second month of life, which, in spite of the difference between the knowledge each brings to the interaction, seems to prefigure the adult interpersonal exchanges we call "conversations." Here we see infants and mothers gazing at each other, as each smiles and vocalizes, apparently with pleasure and a sort of delighted courtesy. As with adult conversation, there is near-constant communication in one modality (visual) and intermittent, alternating communication in another.

This is a description immediately recognizable to many (but not all) American mothers, and so it may cast light upon the potentialities of infancy, if not upon a necessary course of development. Sequences like these can be studied from a number of points of view, and have most frequently been used to extract evidence about mothering or about child development. Work by other researchers has established the importance of eye-to-eye contact in early social development[1] and the possibility of using operant conditioning techniques to increase the frequency of noncry infant vocalization: a mixed social stimulus serves to reinforce vocalization, but the influence of maternal vocalization (as contrasted with touch, visible presence, smiling, and so forth) is preponderant.[2-4] Such research, however, which sums the total number of vocalizations over a period of time and considers the maternal response automatic, ignores the interplay between mother and infant in which each is affected by the behavior of the other and the two are coparticipants in an on-going event. This coparticipation is only part of the general question of mutual regulation of mother and child.[5] One component of this is apparently based on synchrony of movement,[6] probably depending on an orchestration of physiological rhythms,[7] which may provide an essential starting point.

The first section, THE RESEARCH, will be descriptive, with special attention to the development of patterns of conversation-like alternation and the evidence these may provide of the mutuality involved, and to the characteristics of the infant's vocalizations, vocalizations that have not been systematically described, since most investigators do not start from an interest in the interpersonal aspects of communication. In THEORETICAL IMPLICATIONS we will broaden the scope considerably in order to deal with the theoretical justification of the word "conversation" in the title, the needs for further theory and description, and the importance of this area of research for developmental psycholinguistics and the study of the etiology of communication disorders.

*This research was carried on at the Research Laboratory of Electronics at Massachusetts Institute of Technology, Cambridge, Mass., and was supported by the National Institutes of Health (grant 2 ROi NB-04332). Portions of the present paper appeared in the R.L.E. Quarterly Progress Report no. 100 (January, 1971), and were presented at the 1971 Meetings of the Society for Research in Child Development.

Lincoln Christian College

THE RESEARCH

Mother-Infant Joint Performance: The Sequencing and Temporal Structure of Five Interactions (n = 284 vocalizations)

The present study was conducted on data drawn from a longitudinal corpus collected by Margaret Bullowa following the vocal and other development of five children intensively from delivery.[8] (See also Ref.[6].) Bullowa made weekly observations in the home of each child consisting of one half-hour of tape recording, accompanied by filming at two frames per second and a running commentary. During this time, mother and baby followed their normal routines as nearly as possible, and the camera was trained on the infant, recording scenes of sleeping, crying, playing alone, or being attended to by the mother. The present investigator began by surveying these films and tapes of early infancy generally, looking for the earliest development of social interaction between mother and child and for ways in which this might be characterized that would be illuminating for subsequent language development. The work period included the birth and first year of life of the researcher's own first-born. The brief passages in the film data during which mother and child seemed to be conversing with each other occurred like rare gold nuggets between long sections of other types of material, and it is probably only the fact that the mothers were given no instructions except to go on with their routine, and were quietly in their own homes, that made their natural and unsolicited occurrences possible. This kind of richness seemed to outweigh a number of drawbacks in data of this sort.

Social interactions similar to conversation were recognizable for all of the pairs before three months, but due to the deliberately unstructured data collection situation, not all were equally analyzable; one mother's soft murmurs to her infant were practically inaudible, in another case the arrangement of furniture meant that mutual gaze could not be determined, and there were also variations in instrumentation and regularity of data collection. One pair was selected for a detailed study—a middle class family, mother, and firstborn son, "Mackie." The child is a lively and generally active child (his development is now documented well into elementary school). The mother is cheerful but quiet and undemonstrative, so much so that some investigators working on the same data found her cold and taciturn.

Five interactions between this mother and child that occurred between the ages of 49 and 105 days were subjected to statistical analysis of their sequencing and temporal structure. The following criteria were used in selecting the sequences: frequent vocalization by both mother and infant (excluding crying); generally sustained eye contact; and absence of caretaking activities that might have complicated the temporal pattern of vocalization. Sequences selected by these criteria showed several regularities. They tended to follow periods of active caretaking, and typically, mother and infant were less than a yard apart, with the mother's face frequently at the baby's level. On the other hand, there are occasions in the corpus in which the mother apparently tried to start a "conversation," using the same postures and utterances, but without engaging the infant's attention, so that eye contact and responsive vocalization are absent.

Joint Performances: Analysis of Timing and Sequence

That the mother's participation is patterned on conversation and that her participation is constructed around an implied participation on the infant's part can be seen from her text in FIGURE 1, which also shows the recording techniques used in preparing the data for analysis. In order to obtain an accurate record of the vocaliza-

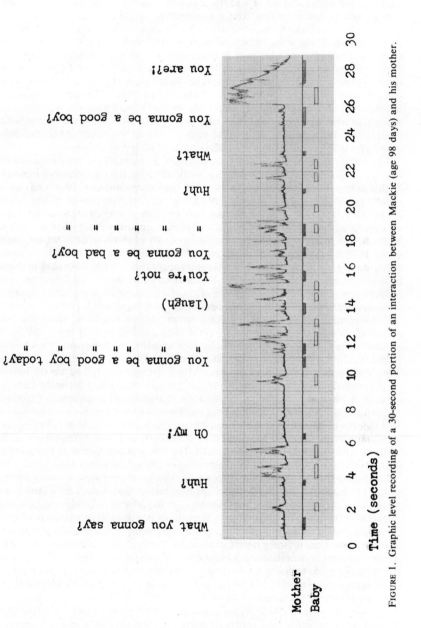

FIGURE 1. Graphic level recording of a 30-second portion of an interaction between Mackie (age 98 days) and his mother.

tions of mother (Mo) and infant (Ba), a number of graphic-level recorder tracings were made of each sequence. These tracings were obtained by prefiltering (to reduce background noise), rectifying, and smoothing the signal. The attribution and sequencing of vocalizations were achieved by focusing on the participants one at a time, marking all the vocalizations of each by hand with a separate stylus and then collating the tracings so obtained. A coded subsonic signal, recorded on a separate channel at the time the data were collected (not shown in FIGURE 1), makes it possible to associate sounds on the tape (and marks from still another stylus on the graphic level recordings) with specific frames in the film. The text represents interpretation, not transcription, since the mother's vocalizations were typically murmured and elliptical. Although the sound was recorded on a single boom-mounted microphone in a naturalistic setting, with considerable extraneous noise, onset figures for vocalizations are estimated as reliable ± 0.2 seconds.

The notion that the participants are alternating is one that can be explored statistically. It is relatively easy to define a vocalization for the mother, since in no case in this sample does the mother speak more than one sentence (with a unifying intonation contour) without a pause. Often her vocalizations consist of single-word sentences. For the infant, a vocalization may be defined in terms of sustained phonation preceded and followed by periods of silence, apparently normally a single exhalation. The infant's vocalizations, while obviously not structured in the same sense as the mother's, are apparently mostly of the type commonly referred to as cooing and grunting, or more generally as "happy vocalizations." For statistical purposes, however, all vocal sounds made by the infant during the analyzed passages were included, including such things as sneezes, and no allowance was made for impressionistic judgments of grouping or communicational significance.

The overall effect of alternating vocalization and the degree to which the alternation of the two parties deviated from the random were computed by pooling the number of runs of particular lengths by each speaker and comparing the observed frequencies of each length with expected frequencies, by chi-square test. The probabilities of particular sequences of either Mo or Ba were computed on the basis of their proportions in the total sample ($p_M = .54$, $p_B = .46$). Thus, the probability of a sequence of only one Mo is $p_M \cdot p_B$, and the probability of a sequence of n Mos is $(p_M)^n p_B$, and similarly for sequences of Ba. Since the total number of runs observed was 183, the probabilities of each length to be expected in a sample of 183 runs, given the constraint that runs by Mo and Ba must alternate and the total number of vocalizations must equal 284, was calculated.† The test was significant at well over the 0.01 level (d.f. = 7) (TABLE 1). In effect, mother and infant vocalize by turns.

The nature of the alternation taking place can be further studied by an analysis of timing, in spite of the occasional rather long pauses that skewed the distributions. Here again, we find evidence that whatever is happening, it is happening in both directions. Thus, when we examine a hypothesis of the mother inserting vocalizations in a stream of random vocalizations by the infant in terms of timing, we find that the mean time between onsets of all infant vocalizations in this sample, regardless of maternal vocalizations, is 3.14 sec ($s = 4.27$); on the other hand, this hypothesis could be reversed, with the infant simply inserting vocalizations. The mean onset to onset time for the mother is 2.96 sec ($s = 2.24$), which is not significantly different from the timing of the infant.

There is also some evidence for a distinction between some utterances as responsive in a sustained sequence, and others as trying to renew the exchange when it lagged.

---

†The method for predicting expected numbers of runs was developed by Prof. D. H. Klatt, of the Research Laboratory of Electronics, MIT.

TABLE 1
OBSERVED AND EXPECTED FREQUENCIES OF RUNS OF UTTERANCES BY ONE SPEAKER

Occurrences of Mo in a Run	Observed Frequencies	p	Expected Frequencies
1	68	.248	33.4
2	10	.134	18.0
3	6	.072	9.7
4	4	.039	5.3
5 or more	4	.047	6.3

Occurrences of Ba in a Run	Observed Frequencies	p	Expected Frequencies
1	62	.248	39.0
2	19	.114	18.0
3	7	.052	8.2
4	3	.024	3.8
5 or more	0	.022	3.5

For both mother and infant, the mean time of utterance onset from onset of previous utterance is longer when the previous utterance was by self than when the previous utterance was by other (TABLE 2). In effect, the time from onset of utterance by other to own onset may be characterized as *response* time, whereas the time from onset of utterance by self to repeated onset by self may be characterized as *elicitation* time; apparently the mother says something (often a question) and waits for a response from the infant before renewing her vocalization. The difference is significant at the 0.01 level for the mother. Although it is not significant for the infant, the tendency is in the same direction, with all interval types somewhat briefer for the infant. It is also notable that mother and child very rarely interrupt one another.

We must assume that some kind of conditioning is occurring for both participants (note that the mother's behavior is also going through rapid modification during these first months) and so it is not possible *per se* to refute the hypothesis that the infant has been conditioned to vocalize in response to the mother, and indeed it has been demonstrated[2] that operant conditioning techniques, with a variety of social rewards, can be used to increase the frequency of infant vocalization substantially. However, a somewhat more complex process is apparently taking place in which *both* mother and child are receiving gratification from the interaction and trying to maintain it. The relationship is a mutual one, and the kind of participation each contributes is symmetrical when seen in relationship to the overall structure of the interaction (but not, of course, the internal structure of the utterances). This fact is obscured by reliance on conditioning theory, which tends to focus on single vocalizations rather than on the structure of an ongoing event.

TABLE 2
ONSET-TO-ONSET SPACING OF VOCALIZATIONS

Preceded by Self	Preceded by Other
Mo $\bar{x}$ = 2.15 sec. s = .96	$\bar{x}$ = 1.43, s = 1.67
Ba $\bar{x}$ = 1.53 s = 1.21	$\bar{x}$ = 1.37, s = 1.26
(Elicitation Time)	(Response Time)

In the statistical analyses described above, we were forced to use simple operational definitions and to treat all of the infant's vocalizations in the same way, but we felt that a much stronger case could be made if they were analyzed in further detail. In particular, we were struck by the number of cases in which the infant vocalized twice in succession, with a second or less from onset to onset. If these doublets (FIGURE 2(a)) were treated as single vocalizations, the statistical evidence would be very much strengthened, since they seemed partly to account for the infant's low elicitation time. In examining suspected doublets, we found that they were generally unexceptional in acoustic form, occurred at the high points of intensity in interaction in the kind of environments where we otherwise found especially long or elaborate vocalizations, and that normally the second was briefer than the first.

Infant Vocalization: Acoustic Study of Two Interactions

Two of the five interactions the sequencing of which is analyzed above were subjected to more intensive study, including acoustic analysis. The idea here was that since this form of interaction depended on the development of patterns of coparticipation in events between mother and child, it might prove a fertile basis for studies of imitation and of the contexts and acoustic and temporal forms of early language behavior *per se*. Therefore, a straight description in acoustic terms of the range of vocalizations represented in the infant's performance seemed worth making. The two latest of the five interactions were chosen for this purpose because these were only a week apart (age 98 and 105 days), and were longer and more varied than others. Furthermore, instrumentation had been improved during the collecting period, and so better acoustic analysis could be done from the later observations.

Narrow-band (45 Hz band width) spectrograms were made (with a Voiceprint Laboratories Spectrograph) of all the infant's vocalizations (n = 75), to be characterized in terms of F_0 (fundamental frequency) and duration. When figures for the two interactions were compared in a Mann-Whitney U-test, it became clear that these could not be treated as two random samples from a single population. They do come, by definition, from the total population of the infant's vocalization during that period, but clearly one or both sequences was not representative, nor do they together represent a definable subset adequately (e.g. total happy vocalizations). In fact, a slightly different mood and structure could be recognized in each interaction.

1. (Age 98 days) This sequence occurred while Mackie was being dressed, having wakened and been bathed and fed. After his clothes were on, his mother paused to chat. Then, when the conversation lagged, she turned to putting on his shoes, at which time he began to whimper and then cry. The analyzed segment lasted four minutes and contained 46 infant vocalizations.
2. (Age 105 days) This sequence occurred at the same time in the caretaking routine, but was generally less intense, with the infant looking away more often. It ended with Mackie burping up some milk and his mother shifting to cleaning him up. It lasted two minutes and contained 29 infant vocalizations, including long crows and chuckles, as his mother tried to keep his attention by tickling him. The running observation mentions several times toward the end that Mackie's attention is wandering, perhaps because of internal events leading to the burp.

In spite of the results of the Mann-Whitney U-test, it was decided to use the available figures for a composite description, since they provide a kind of material not fully described in the literature (see below). Illustrations of typical spectrograms are also included (FIGURE 2).

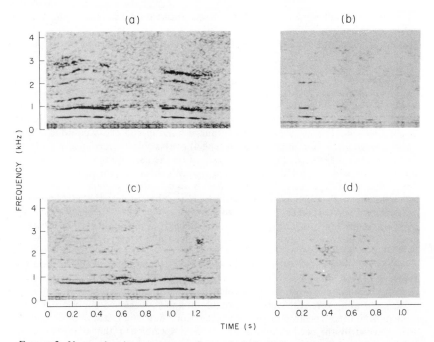

FIGURE 2. Narrow-band spectrograms of several of Mackie's vocalizations showing typical contours. (a): A pair of vocalizations, of the type that seem to function together in the interactions. The first is also a good example of the commonest type of infant vocalization in the sample. (b): The briefest type of vocalization treated. (c): One of the longest vocalizations in the sample, comparable to the pleasure cries described by Wasz-Höckert et al.[11] (d): A whimper.

Duration: range 0.70 to 1.01 sec; $\bar{x}$ = .43 sec (duration was measured from the appearance of clear vocalization, voiced or unvoiced, on the spectrogram to its disappearance). The curve showing the distribution of durations was a very flat one, with no suggestion of multimodality, so that there was no nonarbitrary way of sorting by duration.

Fundamental frequency (F_0): range 260–450 Hz. In general, information on F_0 seems more useful if expressed in terms of position in the vocalization:

> Onset F_0: range 260–440, $\bar{x}$ = 350
> Final F_0: range 310–440, $\bar{x}$ = 370
> Maximum F_0: range 340–460, $\bar{x}$ = 380
> Minimum F_0: range 260–390, $\bar{x}$ = 340

Types of Contours

a) *Convex.* In 34 cases, F_0 rose and then fell, with final F_0 usually slightly higher than initial F_0. Total F_0 changes (increase plus decrease) within these vocalizations had a range of 30–200 Hz, roughly correlated with increasing duration.

b) *Level.* In 12 cases there was no discernible change in F_0. All but three of these vocalizations were less than 0.20 sec in duration, and F_0 was generally high.

c) *Rising.* In 14 cases, F_0 only rose between onset and termination. The range on increase in F_0 was 30–60 Hz.

d) *Falling.* In eight cases, F_0 only fell between onset and termination. The range of decrease in F_0 was 10–80 Hz.

e) *Concave.* In four cases, F_0 fell and then rose. Total F_0 changes (decrease plus increase) within these vocalizations had a range of 30–60 Hz.

Variation in F_0 can be a consequence of adjustment of the tension of the vocal cords or can be a natural result of the variation in subglottal pressure due to the infant's exhalation. It is expected that the subglottal pressure during an exhalation would exhibit an initial rise followed by a fall; hence F_0 variations due to respiratory activity would follow a similar contour, a buildup-and-decay contour. Thus a convex curve of F_0 (the most common type above) would be predicted if no laryngeal control or other special activity is assumed on the part of the infant.[9] Very brief vocalizations with apparently level pitch and vocalizations showing change in a single direction (Types c and d and most of b above) might be regarded as cases in which voicing only coincided with a portion of the exhalation, so that all these vocalizations may be regarded as "neutral," with Type a as the most typical case. However, Type e strongly suggests laryngeal activity on the part of the infant, as do the cases of sustained vocalization without pitch change. Once this is granted, it is apparent that such activity may occur as an additional factor in the other types, especially those in which F_0 shift is greatest or most rapid or highly assymetrical with the vocalization. There is no way, however, to partition the material between vocalizations in which F_0 shift is accounted for by the mechanics of exhalation and those in which it is not.

We are dealing here with only a single infant, and so it seemed important to relate these data to other research on infant vocalization. Acoustic research on infants has been marked by the need to obtain strong, clear specimens rather than by concern for subtle communicational contexts. Furthermore, less has been done to try to describe the happy vocalizations of infancy than cries of distress.[10] Some comparison with the present data, however, is provided by the discussion of "pleasure cries" in Wasz-Höckert et al.[11] By contrast with the presented study, those cries were collected in a controlled environment from 72 different infants and pooled for study. The authors describe a situation comparable to Mackie's: a fed and comfortable baby, gazing into the eyes of an adult (in that case holding the baby) and vocalizing happily. However, although Wasz-Höckert et al. studied vocalizations from birth on, the type of vocalizations they categorize as "pleasure cries" did not appear at all before three months (Ref. 11, p. 7), whereas interactions too brief for statistical study but with vocalizations similar to those described here appeared in our data at just over one month of age. The vocalizations Wasz-Höckert et al. describe are very striking, with an average length of 1.1 sec,[11] whereas only two vocalizations in the whole of the present sample were longer than 1 sec (FIGURE 2 (c)). We suspect that Wasz-Höckert et al., having set the problem in terms of the study of cries, simply ignored the little murmurs and coos that occur in some of the same kinds of contexts, which are more difficult to study and acoustically less striking. Although they should certainly be noted as part of the repertoire, only an interest in their interactional importance in context would have justified focusing on them. The contrast with Wasz-Höckert et al. is shown in TABLE 3. There seems to have been a difference in contour as well, since 46% of the Wasz-Höckert sample is described as "flat," although this term is not quantitatively specified. The two vocalizations in the Mackie sample that were more than one sec in duration have maxima of 450 and 410, in spite of the fact that F_0 in general is lower for older children,[12] so that a drop in F_0 would be expected as a result of growth. The difference might, of course, be due to some exceptional fact about the child Mackie, but that seems unlikely on the basis of comparisons with the other five children considered, all of whom sometimes murmur in situations of happy communion with their mothers. It could also be in some way culturally conditioned, since Wasz-Höckert et al. worked with Swedish and Finnish children, although they suggest that they have some basis for claiming that cultural differences are not to be expected.‡ The difference seems to arise from a difference in sampling technique, where Wasz-Höckert et al. focused on describing an acoustic phenomenon and we are concerned with describing the acoustic aspects of an interpersonal process.

The same bias appears in their disinterest in distress noises preceding full crying, which we investigated briefly to see whether the happy conversational noises of this analysis could be distinguished from whimpers (FIGURE 2(d)). Spectrograms were made of two sequences that were followed by crying in the data. Except perhaps for the very briefest, these were readily distinguishable from conversational vocalization. As the child worked up to true crying, his face beginning to pucker, his vocalizations were also altered, becoming increasingly jerky and tremulous. They tended to be higher in F_0 (range 390–550), with more energy at the harmonics at higher frequency ranges, and to have a glottal onset with irregular glottal pulses producing a "creaky" sound.

In general, the acoustic study did not yield results that seemed to illuminate further the communicational dynamics of the interactions in quantifiable ways. No promising way of partitioning the sample was found that seemed to fit with differences in

TABLE 3
COMPARISON OF VOCALIZATIONS

	Samples	
	Wasz-Höckert et al.	Mackie
Age	3–7 months	1½–3½ months
Sample Size	n = 72 vocalizations (from 72 infants)	n = 75 vocalizations (one infant)
Duration	$\bar{x}$ = 1.1 sec	$\bar{x}$ = .43 sec
Maximum F_0	$\bar{x}$ = 650 Hz	$\bar{x}$ = 380 Hz
Minimum F_0	$\bar{x}$ = 360 Hz	$\bar{x}$ = 340 Hz

context, and all the trends that were observed seemed to have exceptions. At the same time, the very close attention required for these computations strongly increased our impression that each whole interaction had a "plot" with considerable interior diversity of structure, and that within each interaction there were periods of mild crescendo alternating with slight withdrawal on the part of the infant. Thus, seven subsections could be discerned in the interaction at 98 days, and six at 105. The longest fully sustained exchange, 30 seconds, also included the longest and most elaborate vocalizations. A fuller study of conversation at this period of infancy would ideally compare the "plots" of a much larger number of whole episodes, checking the mother's role and striving to correlate position in the plot with acoustic variables.

THEORETICAL IMPLICATIONS

The results of this research seem to confirm the importance of studying infant vocal behavior in interactional context in several ways. The analysis of temporal

‡William Caudill, however, has shown that American mothers "chat" more with their infants and the infants produce more "happy" vocalizations than Japanese infants, who in turn have more direct body contact with the mothers than U.S. babies. See Ref. 13.

structure and sequencing supports the observer's impression that interactions of this type are indeed joint performances, governed by rules of coparticipation between mother and child. Therefore, it seems clear that the attempt to describe the behavior by examining only the infant's performance is unlikely to succeed. Although in this study the data and instrumentation were only adequate for an acoustic analysis of the infant's vocalizations, even here attention to the interactional context produced interesting new results, since it led the investigator to describe a range of vocalizations that had not previously been explicitly recognized as a part of the infant's acoustic repertoire. An interest in natural interaction was an important factor in the original data collection and led to the decision to record routinely in the home. There is a need to overcome the acoustic drawbacks of this approach, but we would urge that such promising areas as detailed "plot" studies of interactions between mother and child (including much more detailed analysis of the mother's own vocalizations and the acoustic properties of all vocalizations by mother and child, in relation to context) can be fruitfully conducted only by investigators for whom the instrumentation and the acoustic analysis are seen as tools of interactional analysis, and not ends in themselves.

Hanging over this discussion from the very beginning—in fact, from the title— has been the impudence of the term *conversation* as applied to interactions in which a one-to-three-month-old infant could participate. It remains necessary to justify the use of this term and suggest the lines of thought that its use opens up.

Adult conversation is familiar to all: often a pleasure, sometimes, we are told, an art, and often a context for learning or change in the participants. Conversation assumes a certain diversity in the participants, but it also assumes a certain similarity. Generally, when we use the term "conversation," we are thinking of situations in which the participants speak the same language, but it is axiomatic that there is at least some degree of difference between their idiolects, which is to say that their linguistic competences are not entirely isomorphic. What is less readily noticed in linguistic approaches, which tend to focus on monologue data (but cf. the increasing attempts in anthropology or sociology to look at interactions[14]), is that coparticipants in a sustained face-to-face interaction like a conversation must possess a second learned system which governs or orchestrates the pattern of interaction. That is, there must be learned regularities governing the *initiation and termination of conversation, alternation and interruption, pacing* and the *interspersing of verbal and nonverbal elements.* When we expand our attention beyond the linguistic line, we notice that communication is normally going on in other modalities, so that there may also be switching between linguistic and other codes (whatever their structure) or indeed switching between several linguistic codes. Thus, we recognize the need to seek another set of rules, rules of *code-switching* in performances. These rules of code switching include switching registers (one type of linguistic code switching, between dialects associated with different degrees of formality). Register switching, (for instance, going from formality to informality and then before termination, back to a greater degree of formality) occurs in most conversation, and much more complex patterns of register switching occur, for example, in religious ritual.[15]

In order to refer to the full range of patterning of this type, we initially used the phrase *performance code.*[16] However, especially in the context of the shifting understanding of the competence-performance distinction in linguistics, the use of the term is likely to cause confusion. In the following, we will refer to performance coding as *praxis.* Since adult systems of praxis are clearly at least partly learned and do vary from place to place, they are cultural and represent a kind of competence. However, when we look at interactions between individuals who bring highly discrepant knowledge to the interaction, we can observe the presence of an *ad hoc* patterning, or, rather, use the concept of praxis to describe the emergent structure of the interaction, the characteristics of the jointly sustained social performance.

The concept of praxis has special importance in our attempt to understand the mechanism by which performances are maintained in spite of code differences, and this problem is heightened in the case of highly discrepant codes: across dialect barriers, between immigrant and native speaker, and, above all, between parent and child. We routinely observe mothers with infants and young children, but rarely do we emphasize that the competences which each brings to the interaction may be more diverse than, say, the codes of a Bengali monolingual and a Texan trying to make friends in a railroad car. The fact that, as one part of the overall mutual regulation that characterizes mother-child relations (a mutual regulation that must adapt to very rapid change in the infant), mother and child are able to engage in joint social performances at all commands respect and investigation. It is necessary only to watch the differences between mothers, or differences in the way the same woman interacts with different infants, to see that there is a real question of the form and development of praxis.

To relate such interactions to conversation may seen to some readers perverse. After all, isn't the whole point of conversation the exchange of information and opinion that closely similar linguistic competences make possible? By contrast with this, our analysis depends on a concept of conversation that focuses primarily on the importance of vocal exchange in affirming and maintaining social contact, rather than on content.[17] This orientation has been followed in a number of studies of adult communication.[14, 18] From this point of view, the vocal exchanges of preverbal infants and their mothers can be treated as "proto-conversations," equivalent at their level to the conversations of adults. They can also be equated because of the similarity in pattern of the praxis of the mother-child pair to types of praxis encountered in adult conversation. Considering these very early conversations from that point of view, and remembering that when "the women come and go, talking of Michelangelo" they may, in a real sense, be said to be using the specific content as a vehicle for a search for relatedness, we may say that mother and child here have achieved a great part of what we value in conversation. Possibly this insight is most readily accessible to those who go through a period of increasing deafness and manage to maintain their interpersonal relationships.

More important, however, for the study of developmental psycholinguistics and communication disorders is the fact that in the development of praxis we can see the progressive construction of contexts of communication, and these are surely also contexts of learning. The development of the capacity for participation in complex sequenced behavior must lay the groundwork for participation in games,[19] and for the development of playful patterns of imitation. An ability to manipulate and recombine sequences within larger frameworks may be significantly related to the development of linguistic competence. An interpersonal failure may underlie a failure in individual development; for instance, in autism. Furthermore, disturbances in areas that have been included above in the concept of praxis have been related to other types of mental disorder. Odd patterns of pausing and interruption are diagnostically useful, and temporal characteristics and hesitations, for instance, which are important for conversation, have been studied intensively by psychologists.[20] The double-bind, which has been put forward as one aspect of the etiology of schizophrenia conceptualized as a communicational disorder,[21] depends on an aberrant pattern of correspondence between codes within larger contexts of relationship (e.g. a contradiction between that which is linguistically encoded and gesture or tone of voice), also an aspect of praxis.

It is clear that language learning must proceed hand in hand with an implicit knowledge of when and how to practice or use language. Here we come to the justification of the term *epigenesis*.[22] The analogy from embryology to behavior is a familiar one; just as types of tissues are progressively differentiated in the development of the embryo, so new behavioral variants are not added on but developed by differentiation from existing patterns. The place filled by speech in the behavior and relationships of an older child is not a new place, but a development of context of previous types of behavior. These earlier patterns of behavior, which will be differentiated into a wide repertoire of interpersonal modes, each governed by learned interpersonal patterns, may be of importance to us precisely because of the differentiation that lies ahead.

Thus, if we consider the interactions of Mackie and his mother described in this paper, treating Mackie's vocalizations, by a convenient fiction, as sentences, we can say that the entire structure of the interactions *above the sentence level* is equivalent to conversation. That is to say, we have identified a structure which, *by progressive differentiation of the component parts*, could become conversation. It seems clear that there is a convergent progress to be accounted for in the development of linguistic competence that is progressively expressed in other interpersonal contexts like those described here, including play and mimicry; that is to say, in successive performances governed by shared rules, rules which are also subject to progressive adjustment. To put the point a little bit differently, we have attempted a partial answer to the question: what part of behavior was conversation before it was linguistically differentiated? What is the *Anlage* of conversation? Probably such a discussion could be expanded to consider all of the functions of communication, but we find the type of communication discussed here, because of its emotional and interpersonal tone, an especially important one. We would hypothesize that to the extent that any disorder in communication involves interpersonal factors, the optimum place to study its etiology would be in conversations between the future patient and caretakers, "conversations" beginning long before the patient knew how to speak.

NOTES AND REFERENCES

1. ROBSON, K. S. 1967. The role of eye-to-eye contact in maternal-infant attachment. J. Child Psychol. Psychiatr. **8:** 13–25.
2. RHEINGOLD, H. L., J. L. GEWIRTZ & H. W. ROSS. 1959. Social conditioning of vocalizations in the infant. J. Comp. Physiol. Psychol. **52:** 68–73.
3. WEISBERG, P. 1963. Social and nonsocial conditioning of infant vocalization. Child Devel. **34:** 377–388.
4. TODD, G. A., A. GIBSON & B. PALMER. 1968. Social reinforcement of infant babbling. Child Devel. **39:** 591–596.
5. SANDER, L. W. 1964. Adaptive relationships in early mother-child interaction. J. Amer. Acad. Child Psych. Vol. 3 (2): 231–264.
6. BULLOWA, M. 1967. The onset of speech. Presented at the Soc. for Res. in Child Devel.
7. CONDON, W. S. & W. D. OGSTON. 1966. Sound film analysis of normal and pathological behavior patterns. J. Nervous Mental Dis. **143:** 338–347.
8. BULLOWA, M., L. G. JONES & T. G. BEVER. 1964. Development from vocal to verbal behavior in children. Monographs of the Soc. for Res. in Child Devel. 29.
9. LIEBERMAN, P. 1967. Intonation, Perception and Language. MIT Research Monograph no. 38. Cambridge, Mass.
10. TRUBY, H. M., J. F. BOSMA & J. LIND. 1965. Newborn Infant Cry. Acta Paediatrica Scandinavica Suppl. 163. Almqvist & Wiksell Boktrycki AB. Uppsala, Sweden.
11. WASZ-HÖCKERT, O., J. LIND, V. VUORENKOSKI, T. PARTANEN & E. VALANNE. 1969. The Infant Cry: A Spectrographic and Auditory Analysis. Clinics in Developmental Medicine.

no. 29. Spastics Inter. Medical Pub. in Association with William Heinemann Medical Books Ltd.

12. WOLFF, P. 1969. The natural history of crying and other vocalization in early infancy. *In* Determinants of Infant Behaviour. Vol. 4. B. M. Foss, Ed. Methuen. London, England.

13. CAUDILL, W. 1973. Tiny dramas: Vocal communication between mother and infant in Japanese and American families. *In* Mental Health Research in Asia and the Pacific. William Lebra, Ed. East-West Center Press, Honolulu, Hawaii.

14. Some scholars have tried to use methods related to linguistics to describe interactions. See for instance, McQUOWN, N., Ed. 1971. Natural History of an Interview. University of Chicago Library Microfilm Collection of Manuscripts in Cultural Anthropology, series 15, nos. 95–98; SCHEFLEN, A. E. 1965. Stream and Structure of Communicational Behavior. Behavioral Studies Monograph No. 1. Eastern Pennsylvania Psychitric Institute. Philadelphia, Pa. BIRDWHISTELL, R. L. 1970. Kinesics and Context. University of Pennsylvania Press. Philadelphia, Pa. See also some of the work now developing around the concept of ethnomethodology, by such researchers as E. SCHLEGOFF. For an assortment of these, see R. TURNER, Ed. 1974. Ethnomethodology. Penguin Books, New York, N.Y., and recent works by HYMES, D., e.g. 1972. Models of the interaction of language and social life. *In* Directions in Sociolinguistics. J. J. Gumper & D. Hymes, Eds. 35–71. Cambridge University Press, London, England.

15. BATESON, M. C. 1975. Ritualization: A study in texture and texture change. *In* Pragmatic Religions: Contemporary Religious Movements in America. I. Zaretzsky & M. Leone, Eds. Princeton Univ. Press. Princeton, N.J.

16. BATESON, M. C. 1976. Linguistic models in the study of joint performances. *In* Festschrift for Carl Voegelin. Ed. D. Kinkade. Peter de Ridder Press, Lisse, The Netherlands. In press.

17. MALINOWSKI, B. 1968. The problem of meaning in primitive languages. *In* The Meaning of Meaning. C. K. Ogden & I. A. Richards. 296–336. Harcourt, Brace & World. New York, N.Y.

18. CHAPPLE, E. D. (with C. M. ARENSBERG). 1940. Measuring Human Relations: An Introduction to the Study of the Interaction of Individuals. Gen. Psych. Monog. **22:** 3–147.

19. CALL, J. D. 1970. Games babies play. *In* Psychol. Today **3:** 8, 34–37, 54.

20. SEBEOK, T. A., A. S. HAYES & M. C. BATESON, Eds. 1964. Approaches to Semiotics. Mouton. The Hague, The Netherlands.

21. BATESON, G. 1972. Steps to An Ecology of Mind. Chandler. San Francisco, Calif.

22. This use of the term *epigenesis* to discuss behavior patterns is derived from ERIKSON, E. H. 1963. Childhood and Society. 2nd edit. W. W. Norton. New York, N.Y.

A DESCRIPTIVE STUDY OF THE EFFECTS OF SELECTED VARIABLES ON THE COMMUNICATIVE SPEECH OF PRESCHOOL CHILDREN*

Suzanne Salzinger, Jeanne W. Patenaude, and Ann Lichtenstein

Biometrics Research Unit
New York State Psychiatric Institute
New York, New York 10032

INTRODUCTION

To whom do very young children talk? Why do they choose to talk to the people they choose to talk to? And why, indeed, do they take the trouble to talk to anyone at all? These three deceptively simple questions are not, as they appear to be, distinct, but rather tend to emphasize different aspects of the same basic question which is the focus of the present investigation.

The question has to do with defining the communicative function of speech, and our attempt to begin to answer it reflects an underlying functional behavioral approach to the problem. It suggests that the basic question can be rephrased as a hypothesis which states that early speech is a function of the extent to which the child's environment "compels" the child to speak. The approach directs us to describe both the immediate and remote stimulus characteristics of the child's social environment in order to locate those aspects of it which exert discriminative control over the child's speech. In other words, we hope to be able to find those stimuli which tend to elicit, or cue, the emission of communicative speech due to the fact that when the child has spoken before in the presence of those classes of stimuli, speech has been positively reinforced.

Egocentric and Communicative Functions of Speech

Speech can be characterized as serving either one of two functions, an egocentric role or a social role. The literature on the function of speech in the very young child has been dominated by discussion of the first, the egocentric role of speech.

Many investigators such as Paiget,[1] Kohlberg et al.,[2] Vygotsky,[3] Luria,[4] and Flavell[5] have been quite explicit in setting aside egocentric speech as a unitary class of behavior which functions systematically with situational demands for cognitive activity, and their work has been concerned with studying its developmental course. Some other investigators, however, have not been explicit in differentiating egocentric from social speech, and when referring to language acquisition, have in fact meant often only its nonsocial, cognitive function. To take just a few examples, all of which represent important areas of work, the studies in mediation by Kendler and Kendler[6] certainly fall within the province of nonsocial egocentric speech. Huttenlocher and her colleagues' work[7] on the situational determinants of the syntactical structure of children's speech exemplifies another area mainly concerned with the nonsocial cognitive function of speech; and Bloom's extensive work[8] on lan-

*This research was supported by NIMH grant MH 21431; GRS Research Foundation for Mental Hygiene, New York State Psychiatric Institute 303 - E 239 G; and The Grant Foundation, Inc., New York, N. Y.

114

guage acquisition, even with its insistence on considering all the contextual determinants of young children's utterances, has not generally made explicit the differentiation between the cognitive, nonsocial aspect of speech and its social or
communicative function.

If one couples both the literature which deals explicitly as well as implicitly with
the cognitive, nonsocial function of early language development, then it is clear
that the bulk of the work in language acquisition has dealt with this function and
not with its communicative function.

This overriding emphasis on egocentric speech is probably due to Piaget's
influence, since having attributed such an important role to self-reference in the
development of cognitive and intellectual functions, many investigators following
him have felt it to be of primary importance in explaining very young children's
overall language development as well. Indeed, although the consensus of the evidence from many sources[2] has supported his idea that the role of egocentric, or private, speech has been critical in cognitive development, it has not been as widely
agreed that egocentric speech necessarily comes prior to social speech in a developmental sequence. In fact, it seems more plausible to consider the fact that since social
forms of speech serve a communicative function, they develop concurrently alongside of private speech forms, and that therefore their development and separate
function can be best examined in the light of other different controlling influences.

Influence of Sociolinguistics on the Study of Communicative Speech

Perhaps the most influential recent factor supplying a new impetus for the study
of social or communicative speech has come from the emergence of the field of sociolinguistics which insists that the characteristics of the social environment systematically determine the forms of speech appropriate for use within various speech
communities. Indeed, it goes further, and insists that speech can not be fully understood unless it is examined with reference to the social context in which it occurs.
Some examples of work already classic in this area can be mentioned.

Labov[9] in his work on Black English in older children has found that certain distinct features of the standard spoken language are either changed or omitted as a
function of the social situation in which they are emitted (e.g., whether it is casual
or formal), or as a function of the norms of the speech community of the speaker
(i.e., children tend to speak like the adult members of their own community), or
according to the speaker's "knowledge" of the prestige forms of the language. In the
latter instance people tend to use the prestige forms or not, depending upon the
person to whom they are speaking. Work on what has been variously described as
speaking code or speech mode or register was originally carried out by Bernstein[10] in
which he characterized middle class and lower class speech as making use of elaborated or restricted codes and claimed that although lower class speakers confine
themselves to the restricted code, middle class speakers use both on occasion. A final
example is a study by Houston,[11] who found that black children in northern Florida
were more or less communicative and more or less fluent depending upon whether
they were speaking in or out of school. She attributed this to a change in what she
called speech register.

Communicative Speech Studies with Young Children

The influence from sociolinguistics has resulted in an increase in the number of
studies of communicative speech with young children, and, hopefully, as this work
continues we will develop a more complete picture of early speech. In a recent reas-

sessment of the importance of social and egocentric speech, Garvey and Hogan[12] suggested on the basis of studying 3½–5-yr-old children's conversations that the children were capable of genuine social behavior, that early forms of social speech entail a surprising level of interpersonal understanding, and that these forms are amenable to systematic study. Schacter[13] found increases in socialized forms of speech in children from age three to five in free play periods in nursery school. Mueller,[14] examining children's conversations, found that a number of variables combined to predict successful communication of an utterance: listener attention; context, i.e., direct reply; form, i.e., command or question; content, i.e., utterances about listener's activity; and attention-getting techniques. In addition, he found that the indicators for failure of communication tended to be lack of clarity, speech fragments, content concerning the speaker's as opposed to the listener's activity, and lack of speaker attention to the listener. Keenan,[15] in observations of twin 2½-yr-olds' conversations, has noted that the children tended to maintain extended sequences of exchanges, certainly reflecting a communicative rather than a nonsocial aspect of speech. Other communicative speech studies have been task-oriented. Alvy[16] found decreases in egocentric communications and increases in verbal exchange as children's ages increased from six to twelve years; and Glucksberg and Krauss[17] have examined the development of success in communicating verbally in some ingenious experimental situations.

Generally speaking then, there appears to be renewed interest in the study of communicative speech and concomitantly, a need for answers to some basic questions of definition as to just what is meant by communicative speech; i.e., what variables function as its determinants.

Between-Subject Paradigm for Studying Communicative Speech

Within the framework of a behavioral discriminative control model, we decided to investigate the problem using two experimental paradigms. The first paradigm involves a between-subject design and consists of tentatively defining communicative speech as a separate class of verbal behavior, then placing children in a setting in which this class of verbal behavior can be emitted, and finally examining its occurrence as a function of a number of independent variables, selected on the basis of both the literature and our own best guesses concerning the relative significance of these variables for controlling the emission of communicative speech in young children.

Our tentative definition of communicative speech, i.e., the major dependent variable of the study, was the proportion of conversational speech that was directed toward another person and that was at the same time articulate and audible (the latter two criteria were taken as a further indication of communicative intent). In addition, we examined two other aspects of the childrens' conversational speech that we felt might be closely related to communicative speech. The first was the total number of words a child emitted during a conversation, and the second was a classification in terms of comprehensibility of all the spoken utterances a child emitted during a conversation. The reason for looking at comprehensibility was that it seemed likely that children who tended to exhibit more communicative speech would be those needing to be more comprehensible to a listener. Judgments of comprehensibility involved not only decisions as to whether utterances were incomprehensible, but also, when comprehensible, whether they could be understood alone, or if not, in what kind of context.

The setting we chose in which to examine the occurrence of communicative speech was a small playroom equipped with toys, in which the children were placed two at a time and tape-recorded. Although two adult experimenters were present they did not initiate speech. The children were free to play and speak as they wished and to whom they wished. The reason for sampling child-child conversations rather than child-adult conversations is that we felt that adults would tend to dominate the conversations and we might therefore find ourselves obtaining a measure of communicative speech reflecting the adult's rather than the child's initiative.

The choice of the independent variables was based partly on a growing literature and partly on our own hunches as to what might make children talk to other people. The variables fall generally into three categories.

The first and, we felt, relatively most important (powerful) predictor in accounting for children's communicative speech is the children's spoken interaction with peers. This is based on the fact that children's playing together is intrinsically positively reinforcing, and that therefore the more a child has spoken to other children in peer play situations, the more such a child will tend to speak communicatively in a setting in which one of the options open to the child is to converse with another child about playing. The literature on this point, admittedly sparse, does not, however, indicate support for this as a strong variable. Rubin et al.[18] found that only-children were less egocentric in their speech, and that there was no difference in egocentric speech for child-child and child-adult conversations. Kohlberg et al.,[2] too, found more egocentric speech indicators in child-child conversations than child-adult conversations.

Nevertheless, based upon the fact that peer play is very reinforcing and that positive reinforcement contingencies operate to produce stimuli that can then exert powerful discriminative control, the selection of this as the major variable seemed more feasible. We felt that the stimulus cues yielded by the presence of other children to whom each child had spoken in varying amounts during free play situations would generalize most readily to our experimental situation and thus provide an immediate source of discriminative stimulus control over the occurrence of communicative speech in conversations.

The second category of independent variables we chose was the effect of the mother's speech on the child's speech. There is currently a growing literature on this which centers mainly on describing how mothers' speech changes as a function of the age and some of the speaking characteristics of the child. Snow,[19] Vorster,[20] and Drach[21] have fairly consistently shown that mothers' speech to children is simpler and shorter than their speech to adults, and Baldwin[22] and Moerk[23] have found that systematic changes in mothers' speech take place with the increasing age of the children. Our own emphasis has been somewhat different, for we were interested in seeing whether selected aspects of mothers' speech could account, at least in part, for children's use of communicative speech. Accordingly, we examined the extent to which each child's mother actively elicited verbal responses from the child during conversations, the extent to which her questions were open-ended, and whether she responded to her child's questions.

The third category of independent variables sampled aspects of the child's social environment that were somewhat more remote. (Unfortunately they were, in addition, somewhat more "remotely" measured, since they were based on interviews with mothers rather than on direct observation.) They had to do with trying to characterize each child's speaking environment at home in terms of how much and to whom it obligated the child to speak.

Deciding to examine the "how much" aspect was the result of our underlying functional behavioral model which would predict that the amount of speech generated, and presumably reinforced, in one situation would determine how likely it would be to generalize to another. To measure this, we simply counted the total number of people with whom each child had regular contact at home. There has been only a beginning made, although an interesting one, in quantifying the verbal home environments of children. Friedlander et al.[24] time-sampled natural language environments in the homes of two infants and found them very different, and Rebelsky and Hanks[25] measured the extent to which fathers spoke to infants and found it to be surprisingly little.

The decision to measure to whom the children spoke was made as a result of studies in the literature suggesting that certain characteristics of the child's social background have differential effects on such aspects of speech as style, concreteness, and abstractness. Williams and Naremore[26] found that social class affected speech mode such that lower-case children's speech was more context-contered and more personally oriented. Jones and McMillan[27] also found differences between lower- and middle-class children in the length of communication units and the amount of contextbound meanings. Baldwin et al.[28] found middle SES children to be more accurate in communicating descriptive information than lower SES children. In view of these findings, which suggested to us that such variables might affect the communicativeness of speech as well as its comprehensibility, we characterized the children's closest and most significant speaking contacts at home in terms of whether they were children or adults or standard english or nonstandard english speakers.

Within-Subject Paradigm for Studying Communicative Speech

The second experimental paradigm makes use of a within-subject design that was yielded by the fact that the study was set up as an investigation of a total social network (Mitchell[29]). It involved sampling a complete matrix of the conversations with each other of all the children in the closed social network of a nursery school class. The design enabled us to investigate the discriminative effect that different children having specific relationships with each speaker exerted on a child's communicative speech during conversations. We had some indication from a study conducted by Salzinger et al.[10] that for adults, social distance determined the communicability of speech within a social network.

In order to measure the characteristics of peer audience that were likely to modify the extent of communicative speech emitted in conversation, the study sampled the complete matrix of spoken interactions among the children in the network in an independent situation. It also measured how often each child in each pair had chosen to sit next to each other in school—hopefully, an indicator of friendship—and whether the conversation involved speaking to a child of the same or different sex. These measures are closely akin to recently reported work by McGrew[31] with young children in the area called *proxemics*.

The decision to examine the discriminative effect of an audience was based on evidence in the literature documenting such an effect. In an interesting study by Shatz and Gelman[32] it was found that children as young as four modify their speech by shortening and simplifying it when they speak to children younger than themselves, much in the same way as do adults. The effect of an audience was also demonstrated by Maratsos,[33] who found that three-to-five-year-olds' speech became more explicit when the listening child could not see what the speaking child was referring to.

In the present study, therefore, we planned to test the hypothesis that the closer the social relationship between two children, as measured by both spoken and nonverbal forms of interaction, the more a child when functioning as a listener in a conversation, will serve to elicit communicative speech from the speaker. Certainly, this relationship holds for adults; the question is whether the social behavior of different children exerts differential stimulus control over communicative speech in three-year-olds.

METHOD

Subjects

Subjects consisted of thirteen children, five boys and eight girls, attending a cooperative nursery school in New York City. The school was staffed by one teacher, assisted in rotation by each of the mothers. The children were tested first in the fall and again in the spring. Nine of the children were present during both sessions. Two were present only in the fall and two others only in the spring. At the beginning of the study the children ranged in age from 33 to 45 months with a mean age of 38 months. The group was heterogeneous with respect to race, socioeconomic status, and ethnic group. Although English was spoken in all the homes, only in seven of them was standard english usage predominant.

Procedure

Data were collected during an initial (fall) and a final (spring) period of the school year, during which time two investigators were present on a daily basis. Variables representing the children's speech and interaction were derived from several sources of data, as follows.

Conversations Between the Children in an Experimental Playroom

Tape recordings of each child's conversation with each other child in the group were made twice, once in the fall and once in the spring. The recording sessions took place in a 10 X 12 foot playroom draped like a circus tent and provided with a standard array of toys.

Recordings were made on a stereo Tandberg tape recorder. Each child wore a microphone around the neck. In order to help distinguish between the two speakers, each of them was assigned either a high or low tone at the beginning of the recording session. Using two hand-manipulated switches, E activated the appropriate identifying tone during the speech of each child, and the signal was fed onto a second track on the tape recorder. At the same time, a second E took running notes on what the children were playing with.

Prior to their first introduction into the tent, all the children were read a story about "Happy-the-Clown" from a specially prepared, colorfully illustrated book. The children were then invited to come into "Happy's tent" in pairs, "to play with Happy's toys." A papier maché puppet clown was present in the room and introduced as "Happy." The Es were seated and their speech was limited to replies to the childrens' questions and occasional guiding comments.

Each session lasted seven minutes, at the end of which the children were allowed to select a few small trinkets and invited to "come back and see Happy again another time."

Transcripts of each of the seven-minute conversations were processed to yield a number of dependent variables.

The first variable was the total number of words each child spoke during any one conversation. (For analysis this variable was transformed to the $\log_{10}$ total number of words.)

The next variable was the proportion of each child's total number of words that was communicative. The coding of the transcripts for communicative speech was based on a content analysis in which communicative speech consisted of words clearly addressed to another person that were sufficiently articulated and audible. How well the speech was understood, or whether it was responded to by the listener, were not used as criteria. Speech reflecting only the child's own play activity was classified as noncommunicative. Both grammatical forms and surrounding context were used to help classify the speech. The transcripts were coded by at least two coders who were trained until reliability was almost perfect.

The third variable was a multicategory classification of the comprehensibility of each child's speech. A two-step procedure was used to so classify the speech. First, the children's speech in each transcript was divided into units, each of which consisted essentially of the specification of a single topic coupled with something said about the topic. Changes in topic, or changes in what was being said about the topic, or changes in the syntactical structure that signalled changes in topic were used to mark the boundaries of each unit. Long pauses and intonation contours were used to help unitize the speech. Second, each unit was then rated for comprehensibility in terms of the following categories: a) the unit was comprehensible on its own (e.g., "I like Happy-the-Clown,"); b) in order for the unit to be comprehended, the immediate physical environmental stimuli had to be taken into account (e.g., "It took off!", where *it* refers to a toy rocket); c) in order for the unit to be comprehended, the speech of another person had to be taken into account (these were primarily answers to questions where the form wouldn't be such as to enable the unit to stand alone); d) in order for the unit to be comprehended, the child's own prior speech had to be taken into account (e.g., "It's under the table. *It really is.*"); and e) and f) incomprehensible units where the meaning of the unit was either ambiguous or entirely incomprehensible, and none of the available context could resolve the classification. The number of units assigned to each category was expressed as a proportion of the total number of units a child used during a conversation. (In the analysis the proportions were transformed to 2 arcsin $\sqrt{\text{proportion}}$.)

Observation of Spoken Interactions Between the Children in the Classroom

During both fall and spring periods, daily two-minute observations were made of each child during free play in the classroom or playground. The observations consisted of recording all the occasions on which a child spoke and who the listeners were for each speech event. The observers were trained until the reliability of the observations was very high.

The main independent variable, the rate of spoken interactions with peers, was derived from these data and expressed as the number of spoken interactions directed toward each other child in the group divided by the number of minutes the speaker was observed when the listener was also present in school. (For the analysis this rate was transformed by means of square root.)

Sociometric Seating Choices in the Classroom

Each day diagrams were made of the children's seating choices during snack, story time, and informal games involving the group. Each child's choice of each other child was expressed as the proportion of opportunities to sit next to another child each child actually availed himself or herself of. Since these proportions were taken to express the measure of friendship between the pairs of children, they were used only for the within-subject analysis.

Conversations Between each Child and His/Her Mother

Following the fall period, tape recordings were made of the conversation of each child with his or her own mother. These were recorded under the same conditions as the children's conversations with each other. The children were instructed to "show mommy Happy's toys."

The transcripts yielded three measures of the mothers' speech: The first was a measure representing the total extent to which the mother tried to elicit a response from her child and consisted of a count of all questions and mands, mands being both the use of the imperative form as well as attention mands; the second was a count of all the mother's open-ended questions; and the third measure was the proportion of her child's questions that she answered. (The latter proportion was transformed by 2 arcsin $\sqrt{\text{proportion}}$.) The three variables representing the effect of mother's speech were used only for the between-subject analysis.

Interviews with Mothers about Home Speech Influences

Each mother was asked to describe the child's living arrangements at home and the resultant opportunities for speech available with parents, caretakers, siblings, friends, and other relatives. Persons within the child's speaking environment were classified both in terms of closeness to the child and in terms of characteristics that might affect their speech, such as class, economic status, ethnic group, and whether they spoke a standard or nonstandard english dialect.

These interviews were coded so as to yield the following variables: The first was the total number of persons each child comes into fairly regular contact with in the household. It included, as well as the immediate family, close friends, caretakers, extended family, and family friends. An additional four variables were based only on the children's significantly close contacts; i.e., primary caretakers and persons with whom the child shared living space. The first indicated on a scale of one to three whether there were more children than adults among the child's significant standard english speaking contacts (A→C SE); the second, whether there were more children than adults for significantly close non-english speakers (A→C NSE); the third, whether there were more standard english speakers than nonstandard english speakers among the child's adult significant contacts (NSE→SE A); and the fourth, whether there were more standard english than nonstandard english speakers among the child's significant child contacts (NSE→SE C).

Sex

The children were classified for the within-subject analysis in terms of whether they were conversing with a child of the same or opposite sex.

RESULTS

The results are presented in terms of three different analyses. The first is a between-subject analysis that examines the relationship between a group of three variables representing measures of conversational speech with three classes of variables representing, respectively, spoken interactions with peers in school, indices of the mothers' speech in conversation with her child, and the spoken contacts characteristic of the children at home.

The second is a multiple regression analysis that measures the relative amount of the effect of three prespecified indices of the three classes of variables; i.e., peer interaction, mother's speech, and spoken contacts at home, on the two conversational speech indices of total speech and communicative speech.

The third analysis is a within-subject analysis that utilizes correlation to investigate whether the social relationship between a listening child and a speaking child modifies the speech of the speaker during conversation.

Between-Subject Analysis

This analysis examines the relationship between the children's conversational speech and a number of different speech-eliciting situations in which the children have been reinforced for speaking to other people.

The means and standard deviations for the three dependent variables representing conversational speech, i.e., the total number of words emitted during conversations, proportion of communicative speech, and proportions of different categories of comprehensibility of the children's speech, are shown in TABLE 1. For the group as a whole, these measures seem to be stable over the course of the year.

Correlations were used to estimate the relationship between the preselected independent variables of spoken interaction with peers, the effects of the mother's speech, and spoken contacts at home with the major dependent speech variables of total speech, communicative speech, and comprehensibility. These data are shown in TABLE 2. They are displayed separately for fall and spring data in order to have some idea of the consistency with which the relationships hold up.

Total Speech

Examination of the correlations in TABLE 2 representing relationships with total speech output show that the most striking relationships are with spoken interactions with peers ($r = .82$ for the conversations in the fall and $r = .54$ for those in the spring); with the measure representing the extent to which the children's mothers elicit responding, i.e., her questions plus mands ($r = .50$ in the fall and .60 in the spring); and with the total number of people having regular contacts with the child at home ($r = .58$ in the fall and .53 in the spring). In addition, the number of open-ended questions the mother uses with her child may have a positive relationship with total speech ($r = .30$ in the fall and .66 in the spring), although because of the difference in effect for fall and spring, it is tenuous.

Communicative Speech

Turning to a consideration of the relationship of communicative speech with total speech, it should first be noted (see TABLE 1) that communicative speech accounts for an average of 66% of the children's total speech in the fall and 70% in the spring. In addition, communicative speech is highly correlated with total speech ($r = .87$ for the fall data and .70 for the spring data). (See TABLE 2.)

Further examination of the determinants of communicative speech in TABLE 2 shows that, like total word output, it is related most to spoken interactions with

TABLE 1

MEANS FOR TOTAL NUMBER OF WORDS, PROPORTION OF COMMUNICATIVE SPEECH, AND PROPORTIONS REPRESENTING DIFFERENT CATEGORIES OF COMPREHENSIBILITY FOR FALL AND SPRING DATA

	Fall			Spring		
	M	SD	Range	M	SD	Range
Total No. Words	106	90	6–252	111	96	8–264
Proportion Communicative Speech	.66	.15	.36–.81	.70	.16	.30–.86
Proportion (a)* units	.22	.10	.10–.35	.19	.08	.07–.33
Proportion (b) units	.22	.08	.06–.38	.23	.08	.05–.34
Proportion (c) units	.09	.05	.03–.20	.13	.05	.05–.23
Proportion (d) units	.04	.03	0–.10	.05	.03	0–.10
Proportion (e + f) units	.40	.16	.24–.73	.32	.12	.14–.60

*(a) = units comprehensible with no additional context; (b) = units comprehensible only with physical context provided; (c) = units comprehensible only in the context of another person's speech; (d) = units comprehensible only in the context of more of the child's own speech; (e + f) = units either ambiguous or totally incomprehensible.

TABLE 2

CORRELATIONS BETWEEN TOTAL NUMBER OF WORDS, PROPORTION OF COMMUNICATIVE
SPEECH, AND PROPORTION OF INCOMPREHENSIBLE SPEECH WITH
SELECTED VARIABLES

	Log Total Words			Communicative Speech			Incomprehensibility		
	Fall	Spring	Both	Fall	Spring	Both	Fall	Spring	Both
Log Total No. Words				.87	.70	.80	−.39	−.04	−.22
Proportion Communicative Speech							−.69	−.61	−.65
Spoken Interactions with Peers	.82	.54	.71	.78	.45	.64	−.34	−.19	−.26
Mother's Questions plus Mands	.50	.60	.55	.49	.31	.41	−.38	.16	−.12
Mother's Open Questions	.30	.66	.50	.15	.17	.16	−.06	.50	.24
Mother's Prop. Questions Answered	.09	.52	.32	.16	.11	.14	−.29	.37	.05
Total Contacts at Home	.58	.53	.56	.34	.49	.42	−.04	−.09	−.06
Significant Contacts A → C SE	.18	.18	.18	.01	.00	.01	.00	−.08	−.04
Significant Contacts A → C NSE	.02	−.20	−.09	.16	−.20	−.02	.21	.10	.16
Significant Contacts NSE → SE A	.08	.28	.18	.29	.31	.30	−.64	−.17	−.32
Significant Contacts NSE → SE C	.28	.29	.29	.65	.33	.51	−.69	−.24	−.50

peers (r = .78 in the fall and .45 in the spring); somewhat less to the extent to which
the mother tries to elicit responses, i.e., her questions plus mands, (r = .49 for the fall
and .31 for the spring); and similarly related to the children's total contacts in the
home (r = .34 in the fall and .49 in the spring). One additional correlation should be
noted. If more of the children among the speaker's most significant home contacts
speak Standard English, rather than Nonstandard English, the speakers show higher
proportions of communicative speech (r = .65 in the fall and .33 in the spring).

Incomprehensibility

The correlations in TABLE 2 with incomprehensibility show its relationship to the
other conversational speech measures as well as its relationship to the three classes
of independent variables of the study. Incomprehensibility does not seem to be a
function of the extent to which the children speak with peers (r = −.34 for the fall
and −.19 for the spring); nor is incomprehensibility related to how much the child's
mother tries to elicit responses during conversations; i.e., her questions plus mands
(r = −.38 for the fall and r = .16 for the spring). Nor is incomprehensibility at all related
to total home contacts (r = −.04 and −.09 for fall and spring, respectively). It is possibly a function of having more standard english-speaking children among the
child's most significant home contacts (r = −.69 for the fall and r = −.24 for the
spring) although the lack of consistency from fall to spring makes the relationship
tenuous.

The interesting finding here is seen in how incomprehensibility relates to the two
other dependent speech variables of total speech and communicative speech. Although there is apparently no relationship between incomprehensibility and total
speech (r = −.39 and −.04 for fall and spring), incomprehensibility does seem to be
a function of communicative speech (r = −.69 and −.61 for fall and spring), implying
that only when the children make an attempt to communicate with each other do
they try to make their speech more comprehensible.

Comprehensibility

Since comprehensibility seems to be characteristic of communicativeness, we
examined the four different types of comprehensible units (i.e., excluding those units

which were incomprehensible) in some detail. Since they do not occur at all equally in the children's speech (see TABLE 1) (the mean proportions for fall and spring, respectively, of (a)-type units are .22 and .19; of (b)-type units are .22 and .23; of (c)-type units are .09 and .13; and of (d)-type units are .04 and .05), the relationships between them and other variables we are reporting cannot be taken to be equally reliable or valid. Results concerning these relationships must therefore be interpreted tentatively. Correlations between categories of comprehensibility with other conversational speech variables and with the independent variables of the study are to be found in TABLE 3.

It is of interest to note that the occurrence of (a)-type units, which need no additional context to be understood, are highly and positively related to communicative speech (r = .81 and .61 for fall and spring data) and total speech, although the latter relationship is not as consistent (r = .79 and .30 for fall and spring). In addition, (a)-type units appear to be a function of both of the independent variables of spoken peer interaction (r = .60 and .36) and to a lesser extent a function of total home contacts (r = .47 and .44). They are not clearly related to the mother's speech. The occurrence of (b)-type units, which require physical context to be clearly understood are also positively related to total words (r = .34 and .61) and communicative speech (r = .58 and .33). In addition, they seem to be positively although not strongly related to the mother's speech (r = .35 and .37), and may be a function of the children's having standard english-speaking children among their most significant home contacts (r = .50 and .28). Both (c)-type units, which require another person's speech as context, and (d)-type units, which require more of the child's own speech to be understood, reverse these relationships and show negative relationships with total speech, communicative speech, peer interactions, mother's speech, and home contacts. Most of these units, although understandable, are fragmentary and relate to the other variables much like incomprehensible speech. However, in interpreting them it should be kept in mind that their incidence is very low in the entire sample of units.

Multiple Regression Analysis

A major hypothesis of the study posits that the extent to which each independent variable accounts for the children's communicative speech depends upon the strength of its discriminative stimulus control, which is determined by how immediately relevant each variable is to the conversational situation in which the children speak to each other. In order of immediacy of discriminative control, we would therefore expect that the spoken interaction with peers would be strongest, the effect of the child's mother's speech during conversations next, and the overall home contacts, least of the three. In addition it seems likely that two of the variables, i.e., the extent to which the mother elicits responding and the total contacts in the child's home, would tend to increase the total output of all kinds of speech, regardless of whether it is communicative or not. Therefore, we might expect these variables to add less to the relationship with communicative speech than with total speech output during the conversations with peers.

To test this we used a multiple regression model to account for both total word output and communicative speech as an increasing function of the three variables. For total word output in the fall, the initial R^2 between total speech and peer interaction was .68. The addition of the partial correlation of total speech with the most remote of the three variables, total contacts, yielded no significant increase in effect. However, the addition of the partial correlation for total speech with the mothers' total effect significantly increased the R^2 to .83. Correcting for chance, using a shrinkage formula, R^2 becomes .76 representing an increase of 8%. For the spring data

TABLE 3

CORRELATIONS BETWEEN FOUR DIFFERENT CATEGORIES OF COMPREHENSIBLE UNITS WITH TOTAL NUMBER OF WORDS, PROPORTION OF COMMUNICATIVE SPEECH, AND SELECTED VARIABLES REPRESENTING SPOKEN INTERACTION WITH PEERS, MOTHERS' EFFECT, AND SOCIAL CONTACTS AT HOME

	(a) Clearly comprehen. units			(b) Units requiring physical context			(c) Units requiring other person's speech			(d) Units requiring more of own speech		
	Fall	Spring	Both	Fall	Spring	Both	Fall	Spring	Both	Fall	Spring	Both
Total No. Words	.79	.30	.60	.34	.61	.48	-.78	-.76	-.77	-.57	-.56	-.57
Communicative Speech	.81	.61	.73	.58	.33	.47	-.61	-.13	-.40	-.52	-.27	-.40
Spoken Peer Interaction	.60	.36	.49	.14	.24	.19	-.56	-.22	-.40	-.75	-.17	-.52
Questions and Mands (Mother)	.39	-.01	.20	.35	.37	.36	-.29	-.49	-.39	-.01	-.64	-.36
Open Questions (Mother)	.00	-.13	-.07	.11	.19	.15	-.19	-.69	-.47	.09	-.54	-.25
Prop. Answers (Mother)	-.18	-.26	-.22	.22	.33	.27	.09	-.62	-.31	.03	-.48	-.24
Total Contacts (Home)	.47	.44	.46	-.13	-.07	-.10	-.40	-.21	-.31	-.23	-.13	-.18
Sig. Cont. A → C SE	.05	.37	.22	.27	.23	.25	-.31	-.27	-.29	.13	.32	.22
Sig. Cont. A → C NSE	-.08	-.55	-.33	.11	-.04	.04	-.27	.17	-.05	-.48	-.41	-.44
Sig. Cont. NSE → SE A	-.08	-.14	-.11	.23	.16	.19	.38	.01	.18	.01	-.28	-.14
Sig. Cont. NSE → SE C	.33	-.08	.13	.50	.28	.39	.02	-.05	-.02	-.24	-.31	-.28

on total speech output, the effect was not as strong, but the addition of the two independent variables changed the initial R^2 in the same way. The initial R^2 between total speech and peer spoken interaction was .29 and when one added the partial correlation with the mother's effect, this significantly increased the relationship to $R^2 = .56$. Again correcting for chance, the shrunken R^2 becomes .37, representing an increase of 8%. The addition of the variable of total contacts in the home was not significant.

Using the same procedure to account for the proportion of communicative speech, we found, for the fall data, that the initial R^2 between communicative speech and peer contacts was .61, which significantly increased to $R^2 = .76$ when the partial correlation with mother's total effect was added. Correcting this R^2 for chance, the shrunken R^2 becomes .66 representing an increase in effect of 5%. Again the addition of total contacts in the home, the most remotely related variable, did not account for any more of the relationship.

Because the spring data showed an initial R^2 between communicative speech and peer interaction that was not significant, the other variables were not added.

In general, then, the results of this analysis indicate that conversational speech is best accounted for by the added contributions, in order, of peer spoken interaction and the effect of the extent to which the mothers elicit verbal responses during conversations. Furthermore, the independent added effect of the mother's speech is somewhat larger for total speech output (8%) than for communicative speech (5%).

Within-Subject Analysis

The question of whether the characteristics of individual children exert discriminative control over (modify) the speech of children who are talking to them is examined in this analysis.

Correlations were computed for each child speaking to each other child for selected pairs of speech variables and social interaction variables.

The speech variables were the same as those used in the between-subject analysis. They consisted of a measure of the total number of words each child spoke in conversation with each other child; the proportion of communicative speech each child spoke in conversation with each other child; and the proportion of incomprehensible utterances each child emitted in conversation with each other child.

The social interaction variables consisted of the proportion of spoken interactions each child directed at each other child during free play, the proportion of occasions each child chose to sit next to each other child in class, and whether the experimental conversation was taking place with a child of the same or opposite sex.

Correlations among the social interaction variables are displayed in TABLE 4 for data representing the fall, spring, and both periods. These show a substantial degree of relationship among all three variables, and most particularly between the spoken

TABLE 4
AVERAGE CORRELATIONS*

	Seating Choice			Same Sex–Diff. Sex		
	Fall	Spring	Both	Fall	Spring	Both
Spoken Interactions	.61	.73	.67	−.40	−.44	−.42
Seating Choice				−.35	−.56	−.46

*Computed within subjects between spoken interactions with peers, seating choices, and same sex-different sex.

TABLE 5

AVERAGE CORRELATIONS COMPUTED WITHIN SUBJECTS* BETWEEN TOTAL WORDS,
PROPORTION OF COMMUNICATIVE SPEECH, AND PROPORTION OF INCOMPREHENSIBLE
SPEECH WITH SELECTED SOCIAL VARIABLES

	Log Total No. Words			Communicative Speech			Incomprehensible Speech		
	Fall	Spring	Both	Fall	Spring	Both	Fall	Spring	Both
Communicative Speech	.34	.00	.28						
Prop. Incomp. Speech	-.40	.26	-.11	-.62	-.25	-.49			
Sp. Int. with Peers	.36	.20	.22	.08	.17	.15	-.18	-.30	-.19
Seating Choices	.20	.32	.27	.10	-.02	.02	-.22	-.13	-.06
Same Sex–Diff. Sex	-.12	-.07	-.06	.16	.06	.13	.13	.04	.03

*Children who did not speak to a number of other children are omitted from this table.

interactions with peers and seating choices (r = .61, .73, .67). This indicates that children who choose to sit next to specific other children also tend to speak to them in free-play situations. The correlations also indicate that it is more likely that children will talk to other children of the same sex rather than of the opposite sex (r = -.40, -.44, -.42), and that they are more likely to choose to sit next to children of the same sex than those of the opposite sex (r = -.35, -.56, -.46).

We then examined the relationship between these social interaction variables and the speech the children emit to each other during the experimental conversations with each other. The correlations among the pairs of conversational speech variables and social interaction variables are to be found in TABLE 5. Although the three social interaction variables were shown to be substantially related, including the verbal interaction variable, there does not seem to be any strong relationship of these variables with the characteristics of the way the children converse with each other.

Specifically, we did not find that the sex of the child who was being spoken to made any difference in the speaker's total conversational speech output, the proportion of speech during a conversation which was communicative, or how incomprehensible it was. Both a given child's spoken interactions with each of his/her peers and a given child's seating choices were unrelated to how much that child spoke to other children during conversations. Finally, neither the child's spoken interactions with peers nor his/her seating choices were at all related to whether the child's speech in conversations was communicative or whether it was incomprehensible.

Among the conversational speech variables themselves, there was no relationship found between the total amount of speech emitted during a conversation and how comprehensible or communicative it was. That is, how much a child chose to talk to another child did not determine how communicative and comprehensible the speech would be.

It was found, however, that if a child talked communicatively to another child during a conversation, the child's speech became proportionately more comprehensible. The correlations between the proportion of speech that was communicative and the proportion of speech that was incomprehensible were r = -.62, -.25, -.49 (see TABLE 5).

In general, then, the within-subject analysis indicated that in conversational speech the children's total speech output, the proportion of communicative speech, and the proportion of incomprehensibility during speech emitted in conversation did not change as a function of each child's social relationship with specific other children.

Only for speech directed at other children in open free-play situations did the social relationship with the listeners have a positive effect.

During conversations it appears that only when a child attempts to communicate to another child, regardless of his/her social relationships with that child, do the characteristics of the child's speech change such that it becomes less incomprehensible.

DISCUSSION

The answers provided by this study to the questions posed initially concerning the function of communicative speech must be taken as suggestive rather than definitive due to the nature of the network design of the study, which prohibits the use of a substantial number of subjects. Nevertheless, a number of relationships appear among the variables measuring conversational speech and the other selected variables of the study that make sense in terms of the discriminative control model which we used to yield a functional account of the emission of communicative speech in very young children.

Essentially, the model predicts that the extent to which any variable will account for the communicative speech of children conversing with their peers has to do with how immediately relevant it is (i.e., how easily it can be generalized) to the situation in which the child is talking.

Before going on to summarize our conclusions, some of the problems with the study must be mentioned, as well as the attempts we made (and did not make) to cope with them. Two characteristics of the study were sources of major methodological difficulty.

The first, as was mentioned, was the network design. Although it has the distinct advantage of sampling an entire matrix and thereby enabling us to analyze the relationships between variables within each of the subjects, a procedure well suited to test the effects of listeners on speakers in conversations, at the same time it produces extreme dependencies between estimates of the variables, since each subject provides a number of correlated rather than independent measurements. The results may therefore be typical only of this particular network of subjects. To cope with this difficulty one would have either to expand the network to include substantially more subjects—a procedure frightening to contemplate—or to replicate the study a few times on new small matrices. We did neither, but instead attempted some replication by sampling the network twice, which in fact merely gave us some notion of how stable our estimates were for this particular network and did not really tackle the problem of generalizing to larger populations.

The other major source of methodological difficulty came from the fact that the study utilized correlational procedures to estimate relationships among many different variables (many more variables, in fact, than subjects), thus increasing the possibility that the relationships were a function of chance. In order to cope with this problem and avoid the all-too-common "fishing expedition," we carefully preselected, by means of literature surveys and our own hunches, those variables which we felt would be predictive of communicative speech, and then instead of searching our resulting correlation matrices for high correlations, we looked only at the relationships we had expected to yield results, and reported only those. In accordance with this approach, the variables used in the multiple regression analysis, as well as predictions of the order in which the variables would contribute to the prediction of speech, were dictated by the discriminative control model before we ran the analysis.

Other problems were problems of measurement of the extremely diverse kinds of variables used in the study. Some of these, like observational procedures and content analyses, were handled by rigorous training of experimenters and coders to achieve reasonably reliable estimates. Others are more difficult to handle and include problems of scaling variables for which the underlying metrical relationships are unknown, such as home contacts. Also, there are special problems with the shape of distributions yielded by data obtained from very young subjects whose developmental levels (e.g., in speech output) differ enormously.

Despite these problems, the study yielded a number of interesting and reasonable findings.

Placed in a situation in which children are able to converse with a peer or not, as they please, three-to-four-year-old children tend on the average to devote a substantial proportion (over 60%) of their speech to communicative speech.

The extent to which children engage in communicative speech during conversations appears primarily to be a function of how much they engage in spoken interactions with peers during free-play situations. In other words, it may well be a function of a social type of play activity.

To a somewhat lesser degree, communicative speech is also a function of the overall extent to which their mothers tend to elicit responses from them during conversations, and is related, although not independently, to the extent of the children's network of speaking contacts at home. In addition, if the child's closest home contacts consist of more standard english-speaking children than nonstandard english-speaking children, this tends to account for an increased proportion of communicative speech in peer conversations.

There is a strong positive relationship between the proportion of communicative speech and the total amount of speech the children emit. Therefore, the somewhat less strong relationship between communicative speech and the more remote (i.e., less immediately relevant than peer interaction) variables of mother's effect and total home speaking contacts may be partly accounted for by their stronger relationship with total speech. In this respect we might also note that the mothers' use of open-ended questions relates a good deal more strongly to total speech output than to communicative speech. The main effect of these variables might be to increase the total amount of children's speech regardless of whether or not it is communicative.

Communicative speech tends to be characterized by less incomprehensibility. Since incomprehensibility is unrelated to total speech output, it would therefore seem to be a function of speech that is emitted only when the children are trying to talk to each other.

The high proportion of clearly comprehensible speech units requiring no additional context to be understood seems to relate mainly to the proportion of communicative speech, and somewhat less to total speech.

The high proportion of speech units requiring the context of another person's speech relates negatively to total speech output, indicating that children who don't converse much confine their speech to answers to questions.

All of the foregoing results describe relationships with variables accounting for the general characteristics of the children's conversational speech, regardless of whom the child is speaking to.

Turning to the discriminative control exerted by peer listeners in the immediate situation, we found some highly suggestive findings which must be viewed carefully, since these data are much less reliable than the between-subject data.

It seems that for children of this age, the characteristics of their conversational speech did not vary as a function of their social relationship with each of the other children to whom they were talking.

Only for speech directed at other childen in open free-play situations did the children's social relationships with the listener have a positive effect.

For conversational speech the listener exerted discriminative control only by virtue of the fact that if the speaker attempted to communicate with him or her, regardless of the listener's social relationship to the speaker, the speaker's speech became proportionately more comprehensible.

ACKNOWLEDGMENTS

The authors wish to thank Richard Sanders for his help in collecting the data, George Fein for his help in analyzing it, and the Lutheran Advent Church on 93rd St. and Broadway, New York City, for their generous cooperation in this study.

REFERENCES

1. PIAGET, J. 1926. The Language and Thought of the Child. Routledge & Keegan Paul. London, England.
2. KOHLBERG, L., J. YAEGER & E. HJERTHOLM. 1968. Private speech: four studies and a review of theories. Child Development 39: 691–736.
3. VYGOTSKY, L. 1962. Thought and Language. M.I.T. Press. Cambridge, Mass.
4. LURIA, A. R. 1961. The Role of Speech in the Regulation of Normal and Abnormal Behavior. Liveright. New York, N.Y.
5. FLAVELL, J. H. 1966. Le langage privé. Bulletin de Psychologie. 1966. 19: 698–701. Presented at meetings of the American Speech and Hearing Assn. San Francisco, Calif. 1964.
6. KENDLER, H. H. & T. S. KENDLER. 1970. Developmental processes in discrimination learning. Human Development 13: 65–89.
7. HUTTENLOCHER, J., K. EISENBERG & S. STRAUSS. 1968. Comprehension: Relation between perceived actor and logical subject. J. Verbal Learning Verbal Behavior 7: 527–530.
8. BLOOM, L. 1970. Language Development: Form and Function in Emerging Grammars. M.I.T. Press. Cambridge, Mass.
9. LABOV, W. 1965. Stages in the acquisition of Standard English. In Social Dialects and Language Learning. R. Shuy, Ed.: 77–103. National Council of Teachers of English. Champaign, Ill.
10. BERNSTEIN, B. 1964. Elaborated and restricted codes: their social origins and some consequences. In The Ethnography of Communication. J. Gumperz & D. Hymes, Eds. Vol. LXVI (Part 2): 55–69.
11. HOUSTON, S. H. 1969. A sociolinguistic consideration of the Black English of children in northern Florida. Language 45: 599–607.
12. GARVEY, C. & R. HOGAN. 1973. Social speech and social interaction: egocentrism revisited. Child Development 44: 562–568.
13. SCHACTER, F. F. 1973. Everyday preschool interpersonal usage: developmental and sociolinguistic studies. Presented at meetings of the Society for Research in Child Development. Philadelphia, Pa.
14. MUELLER, E. 1972. The maintenance of verbal exchanges between young children. Child Development 43: 930–938.
15. KEENAN, E. O. 1974. Conversational competence in children. J. Child Language 1: 163–183.
16. ALVY, K. T. 1968. Relation of age to children's egocentric and cooperative communication. J. Genetic Psychol. 112: 275–286.
17. GLUCKSBERG, S. & R. KRAUSS. 1967. What do people say after they have learned to talk? Studies of the development of referential communication. Merrill-Palmer Quarterly of Behavior and Development 13: 309–316.
18. RUBIN, K. H., D. F. HULTSCH & D. L. PETERS. 1971. Non-social speech in four-year-old children as a function of birth order and interpersonal situation. Merrill-Palmer Quarterly of Behavior and Development 17: 41–50.
19. SNOW, C. E. 1972. Mothers' speech to children learning language. Child Development 43: 549–565.
20. VORSTER, J. 1974. Mothers' speech to children: some methodological considerations. Publikatics van het Instituut voor Algemene Taalwetschap, Univ. Amsterdam. 8: 1–44.

21. DRACH, K. 1969. The language of the parent: A pilot study. *In* Working Paper No. 14: The Structure of Linguistic Input to Children. Language Behavior Res. Lab. Univ. of California. Berkeley, Calif.

22. BALDWIN, C. P. 1973. Comparison of mother-child interactions at different ages and in families of different educational level and ethnic background. Unpublished mimeo.

23. MOERK, E. 1974. Changes in verbal child-mother interactions with increasing language skills of the child. J. Psycholing. Res. **3:** 101–116.

24. FRIEDLANDER, B. Z., A. C. JACOBS, B. B. DAVIS & H. S. WETSTONE. 1972. Time sampling analysis of infants' natural language environments in the home. Child Development **43:** 730–740.

25. REBELSKY, F. & C. HANKS. 1971. Fathers' verbal interaction with infants in the first three months of life. Child Development **42:** 63–68.

26. WILLIAMS, F. & R. C. NAREMORE. 1969. On the functional analysis of social class differences in modes of speech. Speech Monographs **36:** 77–102.

27. JONES, P. A. & W. B. MCMILLAN. 1973. Speech characteristics as a function of social class and situational factors. Child Development **44:** 117–121.

28. BALDWIN, T. L., P. T. MCFARLANE & C. J. GARVEY. 1971. Children's communication accuracy related to race and socioeconomic status. Child Development **42:** 345–357.

29. MITCHELL, J. C. 1969. The concept and use of social networks. *In* Social Networks in Urban Situations. J. C. Mitchell, Ed.: 1–50. Manchester Univ. Press. Manchester, England.

30. SALZINGER, K., M. HAMMER, S. PORTNOY & S. K. POLGAR. 1970. Verbal behavior and social distance. Language and Speech **13:** 25–37.

31. MCGREW, W. C. 1974. Interpersonal spacing of pre-school children. *In* The Growth of Competence. K. J. Connolly & J. S. Bruner, Eds.: 265–281. Academic Press. New York, N.Y.

32. SHATZ, M. & R. GELMAN. 1973. The development of communication skills: modifications in the speech of young children as a function of listener. Monographs of the Society for Research in Child Development. **38** (152).

33. MARATSOS, M. P. 1973. Nonegocentric communication abilities in preschool children. Child Development **44:** 697–700.

INDIVIDUAL DIFFERENCES IN EARLY SEMANTIC AND SYNTACTIC DEVELOPMENT

Katherine Nelson

Department of Psychology
Yale University
New Haven, Connecticut 06510

The question raised for this session of the conference (The Influence of Verbal and Nonverbal Factors in the Acquisition and Development of Language) assumes implicitly that there are important differences among children in some aspects of their language development that are accessible to possible external influences. And indeed, several of the papers given here have presented analyses of differences between normal children and children with deficits of some kind. There still, however, appears to be an underlying assumption that *normal* children follow a universal path of language development. I would like to point out here some ways in which normal children may differ in their acquisition patterns and to suggest what the meanings of these differences might be.

The papers in this annal represent an increasing consensus that language is not a thing apart, that in fact, cognition and language interact in various ways. In addition, as has been emphasized in previous papers, we need to consider the impact of the social context of the child. When we do this, we become concerned with the total communication act: its function, intended meaning, its interpretation by others, as well as its cognitive complexity. It is becoming increasingly clear that these varying components may themselves interact to influence the total course taken by the child in achieving (to put it neutrally) a competent level of language performance. That is, even though all children may rely upon the same underlying systems, structures, or processes of cognition, and may learn the same language, the way in which these are used by the child in the language learning task and in their interaction with environmental conditions may result in very different patterns of both the learning and use of language.

In this light it is not surprising that several investigators have recently found considerable variation in early patterns of language acquisition, not only in terms of the rate of acquisition but also in terms of patterns or strategies reflected in language use. An important question to be considered is whether these differences have any implications either for theory or for predicting other developmental achievements, and if so, what they might be. On the one hand, we might find considerable variation in the strategies used by young children to master the language initially but find that all children emerge with equal communicative competence at a later point in development. In this case, studying individual differences might shed light on the basic processes of language acquisition but would have no policy implications for teaching or treatment of individual children except the negative stricture to leave well enough alone. On the other hand, we might find that early differences were related to other aspects of the child's functioning, concurrent or delayed, linguistic, cognitive or social. In this case, the early differences might be at least diagnostic of future performance, whether good or ill, and might even in some cases indicate the need for particular educational approaches or early intervention of some kind. Dr. Blank's data on *why* questions seem to be a good example of this possibility.

What differences then do exist? Most basically, of course, *rate* of acquisition of linquistic forms and structures varies among children. The age at which normal children begin to say words ranges over as much as a year, and the age range at which they begin to combine words into sentences, although narrower, is still substantial. Children also vary in the age at which they begin to interpret what is said to them, and particularly in their ability to interpret complex inputs. In this area, Huttenlocher[7] has published some preliminary data on the comprehension of early language, and Helen Benedict[1] at Yale has supporting data from a dissertation now under way, which show that the ability to understand increases in a regular manner for most children in terms of both length and complexity of input. However, the age at which the child can process a given level of complexity varies by as much as six months within her small sample of eight children, and its relation to the child's productive language is also highly variable. For both comprehension and production, furthermore, we have to ask the further questions: Rate of what? Vocabulary? Semantic relations? Syntax? Morphology? Phonology? Function? Reference? Predication? Communicative force? The list grows ever longer.

There do appear to be some consistent differences in patterns of acquisition, however. For example, in the sample of 18 children that I studied and reported on previously,[9] I found a striking array of differences in the early stage of vocabulary acquisition, many of which appeared to be related to the child's apparent theory of language function. In many cases, these differences were related also to the mother's style of interaction with the child. Other investigators have reported differences that appear similar to these in many ways, although derived from other analytical systems (e.g. Bloom,[2] Bloom et al.,[3] Bruner,[4] Dore,[6] Limber[8]). I referred to the differences in my sample, which appeared to be related to the style, function, or strategy of speech acquisition as "Referential vs. Expressive," and these are the terms I will use here, although there are other equally valid and probably correlated classifications. In any event, it should not be inferred that these terms refer to a dichotomy but rather a continuum along which different individuals are distributed.

In this sample of 18 children, these terms distinguished a group of ten children whose early vocabulary acquisition was primarily object-oriented (the Referential group) from a group of eight children whose early vocabulary was primarily personal-social in orientation. While this was the primary *identifying* characteristic, it was associated with other aspects of the language-acquisition pattern. Unlike Referential speakers, Expressive speakers acquired vocabulary at a slow and steady pace, with many whole phrases and short sentences interspersed at a time when R children were using only single words. At two years, R children used significantly larger vocabularies, but there was no difference between the two groups in their mean length of utterance (MLU) levels. The difference between the groups thus appeared to be one more of direction, type, or pattern than one of rate, and it seemed to be related to lexical rather than syntactic acquisition.

The meaning and long-term significance of these differences, however, was unclear. By two-and-a-half years there were no longer any significant group differences in the gross measurements of MLU and vocabulary in use. Recent, more detailed analyses of language samples from the same children at 24 and 30 months, however, have revealed speech differences at these ages. Let me summarize briefly two analyses.

Both of the analyses that I want to consider here involve the differential use of parts of speech; one the analysis of nominals—nouns and pronouns—and the other the analysis of nominal modifiers—adjectives and possessives. These were chosen first because they seemed especially relevant to the original distinction that was made between the R and E children, since the R children had learned more lexical items referring to objects, largely nouns, and it seemed likely that adjectives might serve an important role in further distinguishing among classes as the child grew older. In addition, the assumption underlying the study was that the child's language development depended upon the development of a conceptual base prior to language, involving the formation of concepts of objects, actors, and so on, and the ability to relate these to each other in underlying conceptualizations. This assumption made the study of differences in the use of nominals and modifiers seem especially pertinent. It was thought that some children might be able to translate their conceptualizations into language more easily because they had acquired particular forms that made such translation possible. But what of those who had fewer relevant forms available? Did that mean that they would have more difficulty with communication? What would the implications be for further conceptual development?

For the purposes of both analyses, 24 transcripts of 100 utterances each were analyzed, including six each from Referential and Expressive speakers of high or low MLUs. High MLUs ranged from 2.5 to 4.5 morphemes and Low MLUs ranged from 1.0 to 2.5 morphemes. With two exceptions, all high MLU children were 30 months of age and all low MLU children were 24 months of age; thus, age was roughly equivalent to MLU status. There were 10 boys' records and 14 from girls. Sexes were as evenly distributed as possible but not completely balanced across groups, and sex differences were not analyzed.

In the first analysis, the balance of noun and pronoun use was considered by language type and MLU status. Although the substitution of pronouns for nouns might seem, off-hand, to involve more a question of semantics or pragmatics than of syntax, the data show that for two-year-old children, sentences imply pronouns and pronouns imply sentences, whereas nouns are frequently used alone or in disconnected noun phrases. For the purpose of this analysis, sentences were defined in line with Chafe's[5] definition as "either a verb alone, or a verb accompanied by one or more nouns," and for our purposes, also a relational construction involving a noun or pronoun from which the required verb was missing. Thus noun-complement sentences with missing copulas were considered sentences, but single-noun phrases or such common child constructions as negations, attributions, and possessives would not be. In the analysis of noun relations, Chafe's classification system was followed, with minor exceptions.

FIGURE 1 shows the relative use of nouns and pronouns in all utterances and in sentences only for the two language-learning types and for high and low MLU levels. It can be seen here that overall, 72% of the nominals used in sentences were pronouns. Only the Low MLU Referential group used pronouns in sentences less than 70% of the time, and for this group the percentage was 63.8%. Two contrasting effects can be seen in this figure. First, the Expressive children were quite uniform in their proportional use of pronouns at both MLU levels and in sentences as well as out. However, they increased dramatically in the number of *nouns* that they used from age two to age two and a half. As shown in TABLE 1, it could not properly be said that they were actually shifting from pronoun to noun use, however, because their noun-pronoun ratios stayed more or less the same at both periods: 1.2 to 1.1. The Referential children, however, did show a marked shift, both in their overall noun-pronoun ratios and in the noun-pronoun ratio in sentences. In fact, the mean number of nouns used by these children per 100 utterances showed an absolute drop, whereas the mean number of nouns used by Expressive children rose significantly.

Thus a striking relationship emerges. Sentences imply pronouns and pronouns

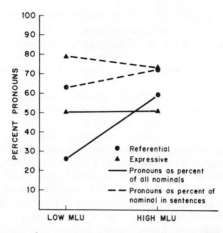

FIGURE 1. Relative use of nouns and pronouns in all utterances and in sentences only for the two language-learning types and for high and low MLU levels. (By permission of the publisher of Cog. Psychol.[11])

imply sentences, and Expressive children show a more mature—that is, more sentential and more pronominal—pattern at the Lower MLU level than do Referential children. But remember that these children also had smaller vocabularies and used both fewer nouns and fewer noun types at the Low MLU level.

Were these differences related to the particular semantic relations into which the nominals enter in the children's sentences? Overall, there was a general uniformity of pronoun use for the various roles such as agent, patient, and experiencer, and of the percentage of sentences using one of these relations across MLU levels and

TABLE 1
NOUN-PRONOUN USE BY LANGUAGE GROUP

Nominal Variable	Referential		Expressive		Correlation with MLU
	Low	High	Low	High	
Mean Number Nominals	89.0	126.2	75.2	130.5	.884*
Mean Number Nouns	63.3	51.5	36.8	62.5	.281
Percent Nouns used in Sentences	14.8	52.1	17.1	39.9	.749*
Mean Number Pronouns	25.7	74.7	38.3	68.0	.790*
Percent Pronouns used in Sentences	63.2	91.0	85.0	94.0	.588†
Noun-Pronoun Ratio	5.50	.783	1.23	1.12	−.424‡
Noun-Pronoun Ratio/Sentences	.682	.393	.287	.383	−.074
Pronouns as Percent of Nominals/Sentences	63.8	72.7	79.6	73.1	−.056
Personal–Impersonal Pronoun Ratio	.301	.648	.557	.824	.628†

*p < .001.
†p < .01.
‡p < .05.

language types. The correlation of MLU with the percentages of use of a given semantic relationship was significant in only one case. That is, the semantic relations expressed were on the whole increasing in proportional numbers as the total number of utterances rose with development. Again, it was true that pronouns were used primarily to express each of these relations at both MLU levels and for both language types.

The only difference between language types in regard to semantic roles is in the comparison of use of agents and experiencers, where the Referential children showed greater use of agents and the Expressive greater use of experiencers, although this difference did not reach statistical significance. These relations are, of course, entailed by the verbs used, agents being appropriate to action verbs and experiencers to mental states such as wanting, knowing, seeing. There is a suggestion here that the Expressive children are more oriented to the personal-social and the Referential to the action of things, which is, of course, consonant with the original basis of their selection. Although both agents and experiencers are animate in child speech, the fact that experiencers are more likely to be "I" or "You" may account for another difference between these groups, namely, that the ratio of personal to impersonal pronouns is higher for the E group than for the R group. Again, this ratio rises for both groups with development, but it is higher by about 20 points for the E group at both MLU levels.

The analysis thus far is in striking agreement with a report by Bloom[3] and her colleagues on contrasting trends for the four children she has studied intensively. She has reported that two of these children used pronouns for the agent relation in the early stages while two used nouns, and that the two tended to converge at a 2.5 MLU level. She reported also that object affected was always expressed most frequently as a noun, while the present data show that pronouns were most frequent in all roles (except complements) for all speakers at both levels, and that the convergence of noun-pronoun use takes place primarily through the elimination of nonsentential uses where nouns predominate.

We have seen, then, that the E children used sentence patterns that were more mature at the early stage, whereas R children seemed to concentrate on lexical knowledge—for example, labeling. The use of adjectives in adjective-noun constructions seems obviously related to this distinction, since adjectives can be used to extend the lexicon productively and to name concepts or distinguish among concepts in a more complex way than simple labeling can do. Thus, it was supposed that the children who were ahead in lexical information (the R children) would also be advanced in terms of the adjective uses to be found in their speech at this age.

Again, it was found that modifiers served the same functions in speech for both groups of speakers; that is, they were used for commenting on the states of things, and for classifying or distinguishing among a group of things with advancing MLU and increasing age. There was an indication, however, that the E speakers used more possessives, and more possessives in proportion to adjectives, for the purpose of distinguishing among objects, as shown in TABLE 2. This was primarily true at the higher MLU level. As can be seen here, there was also a significant interaction between language group and MLU level in regard to the ratio of adjectives to nouns. This interaction was the result of the fact that the R speakers used twice as many nouns at the Lower MLU level (as noted earlier), but the two groups were approximately equal in noun use at the higher level. At the latter point, however, the Referential speakers were using adjectives far more frequently than the Expressive group, thus producing the higher adjective-noun ratio.

The use of adjectives, while not importantly related to syntactic development, is related to semantic or conceptual development. Their use enables the child to expand his lexicon productively and to refer to concepts that cannot be expressed in a single, already-known term. There are, of course, many charming examples of child speech that illustrate the child's use of this strategy.

We have seen then that Expressive and Referential speakers originally identified at an average age of 19 months still show some continuing differences in language at 30 months, approximately a year later, and that these differences are of a semantic rather than a syntactic type. That is, R speakers have higher adjective-noun ratios and lower adjective-possessive ratios. They seem to use more agents and fewer experiencers in sentences, and they have higher proportions of impersonal to personal pronouns. Both of the latter factors appear to be related to a continuing preoccupation with things and actions on things by R speakers in contrast to the continuing preoccupation with people and their relationships by the E speakers. It should be emphasized, however, that on most of the language measures there are no longer any significant differences between the groups. The same basic types of semantic relationships are being expressed and the same kinds of forms tend to be used; for example, most children use pronouns in preference to nouns in conversation most of the time at 30 months. Are the remaining differences important to either

TABLE 2

POSSESSIVE-ADJECTIVE RELATIONS
BY LANGUAGE GROUP

	Referential		Expressive	
	Low MLU	High MLU	Low MLU	High MLU
Mean Number of Adjectives	6.17	13.33	6.33	7.50
Mean Number of Possessives	4.50	2.83	4.17	7.33
Possessive–Adjective Ratio	.786	.209	.753	1.052
Adjective–Noun Ratio	.117	.297	.148	.116

language or cognition, and are they likely to persist, or are they vestigal remnants of early learning styles?

Of course, there is no firm answer to this question, because there are no relevant follow-up data available for these or a similar sample of children. Let me, however, suggest some hypotheses as to the meaning of the data we do have. First, let me note that the finding of significant differences on any dimension between these two groups at 30 months is notable in that they were divided into two somewhat arbitrary dichotomous groups on the basis of vocabulary data gathered before they had begun to form two-word utterances, on the average 11 months prior to the 30-month measure. It was clear, too, by 24 months that many of these children had shifted gears, so to speak, and had balanced their Expressive style with a Referential style, or vice versa. Eventually, of course, all children must learn to communicate in both modes. Thus the most reasonable expectation might be that the differences discovered in the course of language learning would disappear as the child discovered and began to use language for all kinds of his communication needs.

That some differences do remain and that these tend to be lexical or vocabulary differences is noteworthy. I have previously suggested that R and E styles or strategies were partially related to the mother's speech to the child, particularly to speech that was object- or child-related, respectively. Thus, it could be that mothers who were inclined to focus on objects and their relationships early in the language-learning process, who taught the child names of things, for example, would continue to do so as the child advanced in speech function and ability. Those mothers who focused more on the child's activities and were more directive would tend to continue that style. These emphases, in turn, would probably continue to be reflected in the child's speech.

An alternative or additional possibility is that some characteristic of the child continues to be reflected in his speech and that external verbal and nonverbal factors play little part. For example, it might be that, although both R and E children express the same basic semantic relations, the R children have actually a larger store of "thing" concepts which they translate first into larger object-word vocabularies and then proceed to differentiate through the increasing use of adjectives. This possibility gains plausibility from consideration of the E children's dependence upon pronominal use early in the game. That is, for example, "it" is used to stand for many objects without regard to their particular definitions or features. At this point, however, we know too little about the relation between the child's use of the names of things to his formation of concepts about those things, and to his ability to formulate propositions about those concepts, relating them to self and others, to draw any firm conclusions. In fact, some recent data reported by Keith Nelson and J. D. Bonvillian[10] seem to indicate that naming and action schemes may be alternative approaches to objects for very young children.

An alternative interpretation consistent with these data is that the E and R speech styles were both generated from a similar conceptual base but that different aspects of that conceptual base became translated into the speech code initially. In one case, the child begins by learning specific lexical terms for specific concepts and must thereafter learn the sentential rules for combining these relationally in the language. In the other case, the child begins by learning more general (pronominal) terms tobether with some relational structures and must learn thereafter the specific lexical terms that enter into them. This, in fact, appears to be the most plausible interpretation of the present data, and it seems to reflect more an effect of cognitive style than of either basic cognitive or linguistic abilities. This is not to say that environmental factors would not affect this development; surely they would. What is important is that some internal factor—affective, social, cognitive—might direct the child to emphasize one aspect of the language more than another.

It would be premature to conclude that the spech differences analyzed here have *any* continuing effects beyond 30 months of age. However, on the basis of present evidence, it does not seem premature to conclude that *if* there are enduring effects, the place to look for them would be in the realm of the variety, differentiation, and use of the child's concepts, rather than in the area of language skills per se.

This discussion has not, unfortunately, answered the questions with which it began. It is becoming clearer, however, that there is a wide variety of strategies or styles with which children approach the language-learning task and a variety of ways by which they translate their meanings into forms that have meaning in the parent language. Even if there is only one language to be learned, there is more than one way to learn it. At the least, this should cause us to ask, "What are the possible ways of learning language?" in order both to build better theories and to understand better the developing child.

REFERENCES

1. BENEDICT, H. The development of language comprehension in 9–16 month old infants. In preparation. Doctoral dissertation.

2. BLOOM, L. 1970. Language Development: Form and Function in Emerging Grammars. M.I.T. Press. Cambridge, Mass.
3. BLOOM, L., P. LIGHTBOWN & L. HOOD. 1975. Structure and variation in child language. SRCD monographs. In press.
4. BRUNER, J. 1973. The ontogenesis of speech acts. Mimeo.
5. CHAFE, W. L. 1970. Meaning and the Structure of Language. Univ. of Chicago Press. Chicago, Ill.
6. DORE, J. The Development of Speech Acts. Mouton. The Hague, The Netherlands. In press.
7. HUTTENLOCHER, J. 1974. The origins of language comprehension. In Theories in Cognitive Psychology: The Loyola Symposium. R. L. Solso, Ed. Erlbaum Assoc. Potomac, Md.
8. LIMBER, J. 1971. The genesis of complex sentences. Presented at the NSF Conf. Developmental Psycholinguistics. State Univ. of Buffalo, N.Y.
9. NELSON, K. 1973. Structure and strategy in learning to talk. Monograph of the Society for Research in Child Development. 38 (1-2, Serial No. 149).
10. NELSON, K. E. & J. D. BONVILLIAN. 1973. Concepts and words in the 18-month-old: Acquiring concept names under controlled conditions. Cognition 2: 435-450.
11. NELSON, K. 1975. The nominal shift in semantic syntactic development. Cog. Psychol. In press.

PSYCHOPATHOLOGY AND ATYPICAL LANGUAGE DEVELOPMENT

Harold J. Vetter

Criminal Justice Program
University of South Florida
Tampa, Florida 33620

Certain patterns of unusual or deviant language and communication occur with sufficient frequency in particular personality disorders to constitute an essential part of the process by which such disorders are diagnosed. The disorders of affect and cognition known in the aggregate as schizophrenia, for example, are identified clinically by peculiarities of language usage, ranging from the intrusion of idiosyncratic meanings into approximately normal speech to incoherent "word salads" and gibberish. Other configurations of psychotic and neurotic behavior are also identified diagnostically by atypical language and communication.

It should be made clear that we are not dealing here with such primary patterns of language disturbance as aphasia and stuttering. This is not to deny the relevance of psychopathological considerations in such disorders. The importance of emotional conflict in the pathogenesis of stuttering is amply documented, and there is abundant clinical evidence that the aphasic patient may respond adversely to his lowered or altered capacities for symbolizing and communicating, even to the extent of exhibiting what Goldstein[1] called a "catastrophic reaction." However, regardless of whatever psychopathological factors may be present in aphasia or stuttering, both are essentially *linguistic* disorders. Their principal manifestations are present in vocal speech and their treatment requires some or a great deal of speech therapy and retraining. On the other hand, the linguistic phenomena to which I shall refer in this discussion occur as concomitants to conventional psychopathological syndromes.

The objectives sought in research on psychotic and neurotic language have been numerous and varied, but most of the studies reported in the professional literature have reflected a common orientation toward the nature of language behavior and communication in relation to psychopathology. According to this orientation, linguistic phenomena are of concern to the psychopathologist primarily as *symptoms of an underlying pathological condition.* Viewed in this light, language behavior presents a number of undeniably attractive possibilties. Since speech and language behavior are among the more ubiquitous aspects of human functioning, the task of the psychopathologist in gathering appropriate samples of behavior is greatly facilitated in comparison with other types of behavior that are less accessible to observation.

Another beckoning prospect is the possibility that a detailed analysis of language will eventually result in an instrument with diagnostic value for distinguishing the language behavior of patients in various nosological categories. Still further possibilities with regard to prognosis and treatment have not been ignored: it is felt that a closer understanding of language behavior will afford a sound basis for valid and reliable clinical prediction, as well as contribute to the aims of psychotherapy, by clarifying the communication process that takes place between the patient and therapist. These objections have been expressed succinctly by Forrest[2] with regard to schizophrenia:

> Little description is needed with which to recognize the utterances of schizophrenics as such; and were its recognition the only interest in such speech, much of the extensive description that has been attempted would be useless. But psychiatry, having as its concern a system of response whose circuits are beyond tracing and probably beyond chemistry in their ordering, has had little from these circuits by way of data, and is consequently based on the study of communication. If the study of schizophrenic communication is the principal means by which the disease may be understood, its course known, and also its causes discovered, then precise description of schizophrenic language is valuable. (p. 1)

Clinicians who are in daily contact with patients and who are obliged to cope with the problems of communication and interaction posed by psychotic language behavior as part of their ordinary round of activities can scarcely be criticized for setting such pragmatic goals. Unfortunately, this symptom-oriented, functional approach to psychopathological language research has produced rather disappointing results. Although we have amassed a wealth of information about some aspects of psychotic and neurotic performance on tasks requiring "verbal responses" and a large body of observations on the gross characteristics of language usage among several categories of patient, preoccupation with the "semantics of psychopathology" has served mainly to demonstrate the obvious fact that neurotic and psychotic individuals often differ from normal persons in what they choose to talk about and how they choose to talk about it. Much less obvious is the fact that neither the *what* nor the *now* of psychotic and neurotic language usage are related in any simple or straightforward way to the underlying pathology of such conditions.

Only within recent years has the expertise of the language specialist been brought to bear upon problems of psychopathological language. Studies conducted by linguistic and psycholinguistic investigators are beginning to find their way into the professional literature, and the results of such investigations have already aided in the clarification of some basic issues in psychopathological language development. This research, moreover, is informed by a point of view that assigns legitimacy of interest to psychopathological language phenomena *per se* as objects of scrutiny, quite apart from their purely clinical significance as symptoms of an underlying pathological conditions.

Most of my observations will be confined to language behavior in schizophrenia and autism. The reasons for this selectivity are not entirely arbitrary and capricious. Schizophrenia is the psychotic syndrome with the highest incidence rate. In addition, it presents the most complex, challenging, and extensively investigated range of psychopathological language phenomena. By contrast, it seems reasonably clear from the few studies available on language behavior in the affective disorders that there is little evidence of gross pathology or disorganization in cognitive processes. Most of the phenomena in these patients can be accounted for in terms of psychomotor acceleration or retardation.

CHARACTERISTICS OF "SCHIZOPHRENIC LANGUAGE"

Maria Lorenz[3] cautioned against the tendency to generalize from limited samples of language behavior observed in schizophrenic individuals to the assumption of *a* schizophrenic language: "When we have a name for something, we tend automatically to assume the existence of a corresponding reality. Language, as used by schizophrenic patients, becomes identified by the term 'schizophrenic language.' This term suggests an entity with distinct features, a language differing from ordinary language." (p. 95) Says Forrest,[2] with regard to the failure of investigators to establish a "schizophrenic dictionary" for use by the friends and relatives of patients, "Their question—Is there a schizophrenic language?—is as fruitless as the older quest for a poetic language. If one may search in vain for *a* schizophrenic language, one may on the other hand easily find schizophrenic language." (p. 1)

In his presidential address to the Eastern Psychological Association in 1973, Roger Brown[4] reminisced about a period of three weeks of "total immersion in schizophrenia" he had spent at several hospitals in the Harvard locality and at least one meeting of the Cambridge Chapter of Schizophrenics Anonymous. He stated that he found "plenty of schizophrenic thought" but nothing that qualified as "schizophrenic speech." From this he was led to conclude that there is no such critter. If this conclusion raises the eyebrows of those who have spent a good deal longer than three weeks observing and studying persons diagnostically labeled schizophrenic, the exlanation might lie in Brown's definition of schizophrenic speech. Brown equates schizophrenic speech with *regressed* speech, which suggests childlike speech, and tells us:

> While I fairly often heard patients spoken to with what I call nursery school intonation, a kind of exaggerated prosody that most adults use with children, I have to report that in my three weeks I never heard anything childlike from a patient nor indeed anything I would want to set apart as schizophrenic speech. (p. 397)

More specifically, "childlike" refers to several characteristics of speech development in preschool children, which Brown has designated as Stage I:

1. Sentences start short and only very gradually get longer.
2. Consonant clusters, an aspect of phonotactics, are reduced or simplified in various ways.
3. Functional morphemes, like inflections for person and number, case endings, articles, prepositions, and so forth, are almost always omitted, even in contexts in which they are obligatory in the adult language.
4. Semantically, Stage I speech is limited almost entirely to the sensorimotor world; it concerns objects, actors, actions, locations, nominations, recurrence, disappearance, attribution, and a few other things. Notably lacking is talk about emotions, personalities, personal relationships, religion, and all of the things schizophrenics talk about. (p. 398)

His failure to find any of these characteristics in the speech of the schizophrenic persons he met convinced Brown that "schizophrenic speech" is a myth.

The concept of schizophrenia as a "regression psychosis" has been popular with theorists of a psychoanalytic persuasion. Among psychopathologists whose orientation is behavioral rather than psychodynamic, the concept has largely been discredited. As Maher[5] has noted, the mere demonstration of a superficial resemblance between some feature of schizophrenic behavior and that of child behavior does not bring us appreciably closer to an understanding of the psychotic behavior. He concludes that the concept of schizophrenia as a psychosis of regression has not been demonstrated with respect to language, and expresses doubt as to the potential usefulness of such demonstrations in psychopathological investigations.

If schizophrenic speech is not childlike or regressed, what are its salient characteristics?

Just as there is no single, clearly defined entity that answers to the name "schizophrenia," the verbalizations of those who are diagnosed as schizophrenic vary widely, as we have already noted, from approximately normal speech to evident gibberish. Among most authorities in speech pathology, it is generally assumed that the speaker desires to communicate in normal terms and that the cognitive processes are essentially intact. Thus, when an aphasic finds it impossible to dredge up a specific lexical item, the implication is that there is a disturbance in the neurological processes, but his motivation for speaking is not at issue. In the case of schizophrenics, on the other hand, there is usually no assumption of tissue insult, but cognitive processes frequently appear to be disrupted and there is some reason to doubt that the patient desires to communicate in a normal sense. Richman[6] cites an example of the schizophrenic who denied knowing the meaning of the word *intercourse*, then added, "If I don't know [there is] nothing to be afraid of, is there?" (p. 56)

Many clinicians would probably subscribe to Ferreira's[7] notion that the schizophrenic:

> ... develops a language (or reshuffles his former one) so as to hide and conceal all of those statements (verbal and nonverbal) about himself, mother and the relationship, known to be dangerous and forbidden. In "schizophrenese" the schizophrenic finds the only possible compromise: an idiom that not only conceals all that must be concealed but even allows, at a different level, a modest measure of unsuspected satisfaction. For in the privacy of his language, the schizophrenic finds the much looked-after opportunity to say a piece of *his* mind about a relationship the nature of which he could not state publicly. (p. 129)

Schizophrenic speech, then, seems to reflect very general communication problems and simultaneous communication at more than a single level. Indeed, Bateson and his associates[8] have advanced the theory that schizophrenia has its origin in the "double bind" that a youngster finds himself in when a parent consistently conveys simultaneous but incongruent messages. That is, the mother utters words to the effect of "Come here, I love you," but at the same time communicates rejection by tone of voice, gesture, and other subtle cues.

The presentation of these incongruent messages poses a difficult problem for the child. Since the mother is the primary love object, the child needs to be able to discriminate accurately among the messages he receives from her. If he does this, however, he will be punished by the realization that his mother really does not love him. On the other hand, if he does not discriminate accurately between the messages and accepts his mother's simulated loving behavior as real, he will then approach his mother. When he does this, she will become hostile toward him, causing him to withdraw. After he withdraws, she will punish him verbally for withdrawing from her because it indicated to her that she was not a loving mother. Consequently, the child is punished if he accurately discriminates between the messages or if he inaccurately discriminates between the messages. Hence, he finds himself in a double bind.

The only real escape for the child from this situation is to communicate with his mother about the situation in which she has placed him. However, if he does this, she will probably take his comment as an accusation that she is not a loving mother and will punish him for saying it. In other words, the child is not permitted to talk about the situation in an effort to resolve it.

Because this situation and sequence of events occur repeatedly in the child's home life, his ability to communicate with others about their communications with him is greatly impaired. As a result, he is incompetent in determining what other people really mean when they communicate with him and also incompetent in expressing what he really means when he communicates with others.

Due to this impairment of his ability to relate to others effectively, the child may begin to respond defensively to others with incongruent responses when confronted by this double-bind situation. In addition, he may manifest withdrawal and other mechanisms of defense that are viewed as part of the psychopathology of schizophrenia.

Thus, schizophrenic speech is rather like a distorted mirror image of the kinds of communication the patient was exposed to at home, if Bateson and his colleagues are correct in their analysis. Incongruent messages constitute ambiguous communication that is difficult or impossible to interpret—and difficult messages are what the schizophrenic so frequently offers to those with whom he *appears* to be trying to communicate.

Brown[4] questions the validity of the double-bind hypotheses as a potential explanation for the pathogenesis of schizophrenia: "To make the etiological role of the double bind at all plausible . . . one has to explain why some people cannot react in . . . ordinary ways but must feel both sides of the bind intensely, be unable to respond in kind, or leave the field." (p. 402) Perhaps an answer to sorts can be given by citing an illustration of the kind of mother who creates a double-bind learning situation. Searles,[9] in discussing ways in which "one human drives another crazy," quotes an extract from a discussion he held with the mother of a schizophrenic boy:

> He was very happy. I don't and can't imagine this thing coming over him. He never was down, ever. He loved his radio repair work at Mr. Mitchell's shop in Lewiston. Mr. Mitchell is a perfectionistic person. I don't think any of the men at his shop before Edward lasted more than a few months. But Edward got along with him beautifully. He used to come home and say (here the mother imitates an exhausted sign), "I can't stand it another minute!" (Quoted in Vetter,[35] p. 320)

If one imagines the kind of homelife and loving relationship this intriguing anecdote suggests, it is not difficult at all to accept its implications with respect to social learning for the schizophrenic son.

The apparent flatness of affect or the inappropriate expression of affect and withdrawal or loss of interest in the social and physical environment are probably the most widely cited characteristics of schizophrenia. It is withdrawal which seems to be expressed typically in schizophrenic speech. Tangential responses or the pursuing of irrelevant details are easily interpreted as an avoidance of direct communication. The omission of transitional expressions to join disparate ideas (scattering) is less readily interpreted in the same manner, though the effect is poor communication at best. The following written example of scattering from Maher[5] seems almost like a third or fourth approximation to English:

> If things turn by rotation of agriculture or levels in regards and "timed" to everything; I am re-ferring to a previous document when I made some remarks that were facts also tested and there is another that concerns my daughter she has a *lobed* bottom right ear, her name being Mary Lou . . . Much of abstraction has been left unsaid and undone in this product/milk syrup, and others due to economics, differentials, subsidies, bankruptcy, tools, buildings, bonds, national stocks, foundation craps, weather, trades, government in levels of breakages and fuses in electronic too all formerly "state" not necessarily *factuated*. (Quoted in Vetter,[10] p. 5; the underlined words are considered to be neologisms.)

The idea that the schizophrenic employs language in order to *not* communicate is an interesting one and we shall return to the notion shortly in a rather different context. However, there is a contrary school of thought which also claims considerable support. Ullmann and Krasner,[11] for example, argue: "*Much of schizophrenic ideation is not a deficit in the patient but a deficit in the listener.* If the listener were capable of filling in the gaps, he would 'understand' the patient." (p. 359) In other words, where a sufficient context is provided, it is often the case that what appears to be unintelligible makes some sort of sense. There is no denying that the patient and the normal listener are not observing the same interactional rules, but the desire to communicate in normal terms may be present, somewhat in the way that Bleuler[24] considered "disturbances of association" to be a primary difficulty in schizophrenia. Cameron and Magaret[12] report that:

> Schizophrenic patients themselves often complain about the confusion in their talk and thinking, saying that everything seems mixed up, the words do not come as they once did, thoughts rush in and are jumbled ... "There are a million words," one patient said, "I can't make sentences; everything is disconnected." Another patient made several attempts to speak and then gave up; the next day she complained that her thoughts had been rushing through her mind so that she could say nothing. (p. 511)

In some cases, then, it would appear that schizophrenics would like to communicate normally, yet are unable to do so. Robertson and Shamsie[13] have reported a case that casts doubt on the "secret language" hypothesis from a linguistically more technical standpoint. A native of India whose mother tongue was Gujarati and who had an excellent spoken and written command of Hindi and English, as well as a smattering of German and Norwegian, was subjected to a variety of tests and tasks to see if his neologisms were gibberish or whether they were more properly to be considered manifestations of a secret language. If the latter were the case, the neologisms should reappear with some consistency of meaning. This, however appears not to have been the case. The neologisms appear to have been *ad hoc* productions which effectively obscured communication, but which lacked the sort of consistency that would seem to be necessary for so systematic a phenomenon as an actual language. Thus, the communication in this case is "secret" but is not language. Attempts to discuss the Indian's "gibberish" with him proved unsuccessful. As Robertson and Shamsie remarked, "He was prepared to utter unlimited amounts of it, as it were in playful mood, but not to tolerate a direct inquiry into it nor to work elements into it on the explicit instructions of the examiner." (p. 147) In this case it seems that the patient has no objection to communication as such, yet he maintains the privacy of his communication.

In brief, then, the utterances of the schizophrenic cover a spectrum from more or less normal speech with the blocking or disguising of painful or unacceptable notions, to a rather thoroughgoing disruption of normal speech. In the absence of adequate samples of "word salads" or what is loosely called "gibberish" (Robertson and Shamsie seem to feel that merely interspersing neologisms among meaningful strings of familiar words is sufficient to warrant the label of gibberish), it is difficult to suggest how thorough the disruption may be. Thus, the use of expressions such as "hately" is rather minor, intelligible, and probably not uncommon. On the other hand, a rearrangement of the morphemes, such as *ly-hate, or reversal of the order of phonemes, as /*ly yil-tyeh/ for "hately," would be quite extreme. Until we have adequate samples of so-called gibberish, preferably in phonetic transcription, we simply cannot be sure what we are talking about. The same difficulty is found in discussions of glossolalia, of course, and it would be extremely interesting to compare "speaking in tongues" with the Babel of schizophrenia. Presumably there are rules of some sort that underlie both kinds of production, no matter how unintelligible they are. A young man who was active in the Charismatic

Revival Movement in New Orleans once told me that when he spoke in tongues at religious services, he had no idea of the meaning of his utterances at the time. It may very well be that the same would apply to some schizophrenic productions, although it would be hard to be sure, no matter what kind of statement the patient would be willing to make about it.

The bulk of the literature on schizophrenic speech seems to be devoted to oppositions of the sort: literal/metaphorical; concrete/abstract; particular/contextual. In general, such discussions are rather difficult and not terribly persuasive. Similar arguments are raised, again with dubious success, in relation to children, preliterate peoples, and the deaf. In all of these cases, Roger Brown's[14] injunction seems appropriate:

> It is the general rule with these studies [of the difficulties that schizophrenics encounter in dealing with abstractions] to find a statistically significant group difference but also to find that the two distributions (for schizophrenics and normals) have a large area of overlap. This means that these characteristics are not reliably diagnostic. Some of the performances of the schizophrenic clearly involve a preference for narrow categories (e.g., a failure to define a term by its superordinate), but many do not and it is often difficult to figure out the general definition of concreteness under which the performance is subsumed. Furthermore, there are some schizophrenic performances which must be judged abstract by our definition. (pp. 294–295)

As an example of the latter, Brown refers to a study in which the investigator found that schizophrenics would accept an unusually large number of synonyms for words. Not only is it clear that giving a large range of meanings to words is an exercise in abstraction, but in more or less typical examples of what is described as a penchant for dealing concretely with questions, there may be a clear awareness of conceptual categories of kind and type, as Maria Lorenz[3] observed after citing the following example:

> A patient is asked to define certain terms:
> Q. Book
> A. It depends what book you are referring to.
> Q. Table
> A. What kind of table? A wooden table, a porcelain table, a surgical table, or a table you want to have a meal on?
> Q. House
> A. There are all kinds of houses, nice houses, nice private houses.
> Q. Life
> A. I have to know what life you happen to be referring to. *Life Magazine* or to the sweetheart who can make another individual happy. (p. 36)

Linguistically, of course, there is no difficulty. The problem is, in part, one of differing assumptions about the nature or purpose of the communicative act. The questioner expects an abstract, dictionary-type definition to cover the general case, while the subject rejects that expectation. Compare the apparent perversity of the schizophrenic in the above exchange with one of the examples reported by Garfinkel:[15]

> The victim waved his hand cheerily.
> (S) How are you?
> (E) How am I in regard to what? My health, my finances, my school work, my peace of mind, my . . .?
> (S) (Red in the face and suddenly out of control.) Look! I was just trying to be polite. Frankly, I don't give a damn how you are. (p. 44)

Garfinkel's experimenter (E) was not schizophrenic: he was dramatizing the fact that assumptions or common understanding that underlie interaction lack properties of strict rational discourse as these are idealized in rules that define an adequate logical proof:

> For the purposes of *conducting their everyday affairs* persons refuse to permit each other to understand "what they are really talking about" in this way. The anticipation that persons *will* understand, the occasionality of expressions, the specific vagueness of references, the retrospective-prospective sense of a present occurrence, waiting for something later in order to see what was meant before, are sanctioned properties of common discourse. (p. 41)

If Garfinkel is correct, a good deal of our daily interaction depends upon ambiguous or vague communication that seems designed to bind two parties while actually insuring their separation. The particular example quoted from Garfinkel illustrates what Malinowski called *phatic communion*, in which it is the mere fact of exchanging utterances which is important and the content of the utterances is virtually irrelevant. By insisting on a literal interpretation of the greeting, the experimenter was behaving in a way that was perceived as hostile. In other examples, the experimenters were seen as ill or in "a bad mood."

The ethnomethodology studies of Garfinkel and his associates open interesting possibilities for comparing the unspoken rules of normal communication with those which guide the verbalizations of the schizophrenic. In some cases, it would seem, the principal difference between the normal and the schizophrenic is that the latter makes explicit the vagueness which is left in the background in ordinary interaction.

POIESIS AND SCHIZOPHRENIC LANGUAGE

Schizophrenic speech may reflect forbidden thoughts in some cases; it may reflect a general antipathy toward interaction in other cases. Sometimes it appears that the patient wants to communicate in the normal sense but cannot because of severe cognitive disturbances. The evident perversity of the sort illustrated above in Lorenz's example seems to reflect a rejection of the unspoken assumptions of normal routine interaction. Still further in the same direction, perhaps, is what Forrest[2] calls the *poiesis* of schizophrenic productions. Forrest cites one of Kraepelin's cases where, in response to the word "Bett," a patient replied, "Bett, Bett, Bett, dett, dett, dett, ditt, dutt, dutt, daut, daut, daut, dint, dint, dutt, dett, datt. Wenn ich angefangen habe, fahre ich fort bis zu Ende." (pp. 156–157) Says Forrest:

> With his increased preoccupation with the form of words, the schizophrenic, like the poet, finds it more difficult to speak his mind, and may sometimes use his words to fill out a form at the expense of not having them express his thoughts. In other words sometimes the meter displaces the argument. At this point the poet may revise his poem, or else be satisfied with the thought it says, although he did not intend to say it. He may even convince himself that the thought the words say was what he had in mind all along.... (p. 157)

Forrest argues persuasively for the creativity of schizophrenic productions. Neologisms, "involving as they do distortions and condensations, may be of the intensity and vividness of good poetry which has always coined and rejuvenated words" (p. 167) One of Bleuler's patients had been tormented by "elbow-people," which Forrest appreciates from his own experiences on the New York subway. Bleuler himself had commented on the similarity of schizophrenic and artistic productions, citing the "subordination of all thought-associations to one complex, the inclination to

novel, unusual range of ideas, the indifference to tradition, the lack of restraints."
(Quoted by Forrest, p. 187.)

David Forrest's insightful analysis of poiesis in schizophrenic language provided welcome support for a number of conclusions I had reached in a much more plodding fashion concerning similarities between poetic and schizophrenic verbal productions. A study of neologisms is psychopathological language[16] produced no convincing evidence that new word coinage in schizophrenia involved any fundamental distortion at the morphologcal or morphophonemic level. Hundreds of samples of schizophrenic neologisms in several languages provided support for Roger Brown's[14] contention that most, if not all, neologisms conform to the phonological and morphological rules of the patient's native language:

> The disease (schizophrenia) does not seem to disrupt that fundamental pattern. In addition most neologisms are constructed according to some standard morphological pattern. Their meanings can often be guessed from the constituent morphemes. This would simply be linguistic invention were it not for the fact that the patient seems to think his neologisms are conventional forms requiring no explanation. (pp. 292–293)

With regard to more extended schizophrenic verbal productions, in all of the "word salads" I had been served by schizophrenic patients (usually those who would have been labeled "hebephrenic" by the older nosological terminology) in a variety of institutional settings, I had never encountered any instances of the "severe agrammatism" to which older psychiatrists referred. Indeed, I had never encountered *any* schizophrenic who took the kind of liberties with grammar that E. E. Cummings[17] allowed himself when writing passages such as:

> *anyone lived in a pretty how town*
> *(with up so floating many bells down)*
> *spring summer autumn winter*
> *he sang his didn't he danced his did*
>
> (p. 370)

Nor had I ever met a schizophrenic patient who could supply an example of what Schneider[18] called *Abwandlung* (switching grammatical functions of parts of speech) that compared with Cummings' haunting line: "but if a lark should april me."

Several studies (e.g., by Cohen,[19] Hunt et al.,[20] Jones,[21] and Maher et al.[22]) have elicited judgments from experienced clinicians of "schizophrenicity" in brief samples (50 words or so) of schizophrenic spoken or written language. Typically, these are supplied to the judges without identifying information of any kind, and often a control group of "normals" (i.e., college students) is included in the research design. Consistently, such studies have shown high interjudge reliabilities in both experienced clinicians and nonclinicians; and just as consistently they have shown that the formal cues of grammar and prosody are of little or no significance in the judgmental schema of either group. Judgments are guided by the meaning or content of the verbal productions.

Modern deviance theory affirms that a good deal of psychopathology is in the eye of the clinician-beholder. I have often wondered what might happen if, instead of schizophrenic verbal production, an investigator were to use samples of writings by authors like Gertrude Stein, Gerard Manley Hopkins, E. E. Cummings, and James Joyce, who are famous for their linguistic inventiveness and originality. What kind of ranking on a 5-point or 7-point scale of "schizophrenicity," for example, would a clinician give such a selection by Gertrude Stein as:

> Cut a gas jet uglier and the pierce pierce in between the next and negligent. Choose the rate to pay and pet pet very much. A collection of all around, a single person, a lack of languor and more hurt at ease.

Or James Joyce's:

> Dark ages clasp the daisy roots. Stop if you are a sally of the allies. Please stop if you are a B.C. minding missy, please do. But should you prefer A.D. stepplease. And if you miss with a venture it serves you girly well glad.

I suspect that there would be a significant level of agreement among judges that the above samples ranked high in schizophrenicity.

Cummings[23] gave the following advice to students:

> The key seems . . . to be a rejection of ordinary rules. As for expressing nobody-but-yourself in words, that means working just a little harder than anyone who isn't a poet can possibly imagine. Why? Because nothing is quite so easy as using words like somebody else. We all of us do exactly this nearly all of the time—and whenever we do it, we're not poets. (Quoted in Forrest, p. 173)

From this point of view, some schizophrenics would seem to be full-time poets, and perhaps in most cases schizophrenics seek new means of communication, even if through mutism.

Language Behavior in Autism and Childhood Schizophrenia

Autism is a psychotic disorder of childhood and forms part of the psychopathology of schizophrenia. Berkowitz[24] designated two categories of childhood schizophrenia: autism and pathological symbiosis. The latter form of emotional disturbance is characterized by an intense pattern of dependency on the part of the child toward the mother. This relationship is disrupted as the child develops psychosexually and the intimacy with the mother provokes a break that leaves the child on his own for the first time. The child has not developed the ability to become independent and build up defenses for selfprotection because everything has been done for him by the mother. The child cannot cope with the situation and reacts violently in one of two ways: (1) he panics and goes into periods of self-inflicted injury, or (2) there is a revulsion toward the mother and accompanying hostility which the mother is unable to overcome. If she attempts to reestablish the relationship, the child become panicky; but if she does not try to reestablish the relationship, the child withdraws even more. Both of these reactions are accompanied by elective mutism. The play behavior of such children reveals an inability to alter the dependence on the mother: they imitate almost everything the mother does. Speech and communication may have undergone an initial period of normal-appearing development. Following the period of mutism, speech may reappear at a later period either gradually, when the child goes through the whole developmental sequence, or when he resumes speaking at the level of development he had attained prior to the onset of mutism.

The autistic child is unable to establish contact with, and relate to, people. He is capable of understanding and using language, but often employs language for purposes of concealment rather than communication. For example, he may possess a vocabulary that is advanced in comparison with that of a normal child. He may use this development, however, to produce bizarre noises, talk in a repetitive fashion to himself, and speak to an inanimate object such as a television set or to a nonexistent person. In addition to language abnormalities, the autistic child often shows an obsessional preference for relationships with objects and fragments of things he has destroyed. He seems unable to endure change in his environment and becomes extremely difficult to manage if sameness is not maintained.

Kanner[25] first described the syndrome which he called *early infantile autism*. He applied this term originally to children who exhibit "an inability to relate themselves to people and to situations from the beginning of life" (p. 217). Later he extended the concept of autism to include children who seem to have experienced normal development for the first year and a half of life, only to undergo at this point a waning of interest in normal activities, severe withdrawal of affect, arrested social development, and marked disturbances of language and communication. Among the criteria which Kanner considered most significant for autism were: (1) "An extreme self-isolation, or an inability to relate themselves in the ordinary way to people or situations from early in life" and (2) "An obsessive insistence on the maintenance of sameness." Failure to react to the sound of the human voice, as well as to other familiar sounds in his environment, may create an erroneous impression of mental retardation or severe impairment of hearing. Eisenson reports that many autistic children have a history of being quiet from birth and that parents often report little crying and an almost complete absence of sound play.

Cunningham and Dixon[26] have described some of the characteristics of language behavior in autistic children:

> There may be no speech at all. In those who do speak, there is often a failure to use language to convey meaning to others. There is a tendency to repeat the same phrases, rather than to construct original remarks. Immediate echolalia may be present, or delayed echolalia. Affirmation is indicated by the repetition of a question. It takes many years before such a child can use the word "yes." Reversal of pronouns occurs. Kanner's explanation of this phenomenon is worth quoting: "The absence of spontaneous sentence formation and the echolalia type of reproduction give rise to a peculiar grammatical phenomenon. Personal pronouns are repeated just as heard, with no change to suit the altered situation. The child, once told by his mother: 'Now I will give you your milk,' expresses the desire for milk in exactly the same words. Consequently he comes to speak of himself always as 'you,' and of the person addressed as 'I'." (pp. 193–194)

The autistic child may invent his own words for various objects and situations, or he may use conventional words in such an idiosyncratic fashion that he is unintelligible to others. A parent may acquire a limited capacity for "understanding" some of the autistic child's verbal responses by carefully noting the recurrent situations in which his "words" are used.

More than three decades after Kanner's introduction of the term *early infantile autism*, mutism, echolalia, and pronomial reversal are among the traditional clinical signs by which autism is identified diagnostically. The extent of mutism reported by investigators ranges from 28% in the group described by Wolff and Chess,[27] to 61% in a sample studied by Fish and his associates;[28] other studies place the incidence somewhere between these two figures. Mutism typically involves both defective comprehension and a failure to develop nonverbal means of communication; and either the failure to develop speech or loss of speech habits previously acquired appears to be related to various abnormalities of behavior and perception. Rutter[29] has reported a 75% incidence of echolalia and a 25% incidence of difficulties in pronomial usage.

Bartolucci and Albers[30] have noted that syntactic structures in autism have received little attention. Hermelin and O'Connor[31] have reported that autistic children do not appear to make the same use of syntactic and semantic structures in the recall of series of words as normal and mentally retarded children. Other investigators (e.g., Frith[32] and Tubbs[33]) have reported similar findings, suggesting that the autistic child may suffer from a general inability to interpret meaningful structures at the auditory-verbal input level.

Bartolucci and Albers point out that pronominal difficulties and echolalia are both indications of a possible deficit in comprehension. In the absence of any evidence that "pronouns are a self-sufficient syntactic system which can be affected in an isolated fashion,"they hypothesized that autistic problems in pronominal mastery "is only the most obvious aspect of a more general problem, namely, the development of deictic syntactic categories":

> All language typically occurs in a certain space, at a certain time, and between a speaker and a hearer; each of these parameters frequently shifts in the stream of utterances. These orientational features of language are handled at the morphological level primarily by the personal pronouns, the adverbials of place and time (e.g., here, there; now, then), and the verb inflections. Together these are called the *deictic system* of language . . . It was our hypothesis that the deviance in the language of autistic children would be particularly manifest in these deictic categories. (p. 133)

Using drawings and toys, Bartolucci and Albers compared three groups of autistic, mentally retarded, and normal children on their mastery of the tense markers and inflections for the present and past tenses. Significant differences were found in the production of the past tense: while the normal children produced correct responses to 80% of the test items, the percent of correct responses for the autistic subjects was only 8%. The mentally retarded children scored in between with 60% correct responses. Three types of errors were noted: (1) omission of the inflection; (2) use of an inappropriate marker; and (3) other atypical constructions.

In interpreting their results, Bartolucci and Albers exclude the possibility that the inability of the autistic children to produce the regular past-tense inflection is due to some global deficit in linguistic or cognitive development. They also eliminate the possibility of nonspecific inattention or a phonetic inability to perceive the relevant stimuli. That is, the children were able to repeat complex utterances which included the past tense that they had heard over TV or in other contexts. Also, they did about as well as the mentally retarded children in the production of the present tense. The authors conclude that the autistic children in their study:

> . . . seemed to be unable to consistently make a connection between the semantic, deictic, time-related aspects of sentences and the deictic, time-related, morphological function of the inflection or other markers in the past tense of the verb. One corollary of this assumption is that the more adequate use of the present regular third-person inflection and of the progressive present form are probably not due to a good grasp of the time-related deictic aspects of these markers, but to a form of rote-learning which is relatively more successful, possibly because of the higher frequency with which the present tense is used in the linguistic environment of the child. (p. 140)

This would help explain why the older autistic child in the group did better with the present tense than the younger subjects, while being unable to produce an appreciably higher number of correct responses to the past tense.

The Bartolucci and Albers study is a valuable addition to the small but growing body of psycholinguistic research on autistic language behavior. Their research provides an excellent illustration of how testable hypotheses can be derived from areas of linguistic theory and meaningfully applied to traditional clinical problems. Hopefully, their work will encourage other investigators to devote attention to further aspects of atypical language development in childhood schizophrenia.

CONCLUSION: A THEORETICAL PERSPECTIVE

Attempts to interpret schizophrenic language and communication are part of a much larger effort to account for the full range of schizophrenic behavior on a systematic, coherent theoretical basis. Behavior geneticists like David Rosenthal[36] have marshalled an impressive array of evidence for the existence of a genetic predisposition toward schizophrenia. Learning theories, on the other hand, have approached schizophrenic behavior as a problem in stimulus control. They seek to identify those stimulus elements and response contingencies which affect the rate at which a given behavior is emitted. Whether the behavior is produced originally by organic or psychogenic factors is of no particular consequence, provided that stimulus control over the behavior can be achieved by controlling the appropriate reinforcement consequences of the behavior.

Ferster[37] has provided a functional analysis of autistic behavior. He suggests that the autistic child suffers from a deficit of environmental control over behavior, in general, and speech, in particular. The major difference between the behaviors of the autistic and the normal child is not the range of behaviors but rather their relative frequencies. Performances that have only simple and slight effects on the environment occur frequently and make up a large percentage of the behavioral repertoire of the autistic child, while major deficits occur in the area of more complicated social behavior. Much of the child's atavistic and aversive social behavior is reinforced by its consequences; the reinforcement that sustains the primitive self-stimulatory behavior is a result of the small changes in the environment produced by such actions. The child responds with a behavior repertoire that has been shaped in the past by intermittent reinforcement and extinction practices on the part of the parents. The child has found that the physical environment always reinforces behavior by various tactual and postural sensations, while people do not.

The parents of autistic children, because of their own difficulties and interests, have supplied reinforcement in such a way that desired social behaviors have gone unreinforced, while aversive tantrum behaviors have received attention. For example, mothers of autistic children are often described as intelligent, cultivated individuals with manifold personal interests that no doubt preempt paying attention to the child on a significant number of occasions in daily life. As the child prevents the mother from responding to her interests, he becomes a conditioned stimulus for avoidance except in cases where the stimulation he provides becomes so strong as to be aversive. The parents' attention, then, as a generalized reinforcer, has not operated in such a way as to develop the long chains of behavior that are maintained in the normal child by the mother's praise. Without generalized reinforcers, parental stimulus control of the educational process and its consequent reinforcement are all but impossible. In any new situations outside the home, the child is lacking in appropriate behavior and is deprived of further reinforcement by adults and peers because he fails to behave as expected.

Research conducted within the operant paradigm does not distinguish between "etiology" and "treatment." Ferster and DeMyer[38] conducted a germinal investigation in which an attempt was made to alter the behavior of autistic children using both tangible and generalized reinforcers (tokens that could be redeemed for tangible rewards). Their aim was to create an environment that was particularly supportive of the child's strongest behaviors, from which complex forms of responding could be approximated. With the use of games, music, and trinkets, they found that they could sustain complex responding for up to ninety minutes. As this behavior increased, tantrum behavior decreased. The children—in contradiction to the researchers' original expectations—were unusually slow to condition; it was a painstaking effort to expand their limited behavioral repertoires. The very slow development of stimulus control and transfer of training outside the experimental situation indicated an inherent perceptual limitation. Ferster and DeMyer were forced to conclude that a desired behavior must be trained in the exact situation using tangible reinforcers. This is essentially the approach that has been employed in a large number of studies involving the instatement and shaping of verbal behavior in autistic subjects.

Kurt Salzinger[39] has provided an interpretation of schizophrenia which recognizes, in his words, a "restriction which must be imposed on anyone evolving a theoretical description of schizophrenic behavior," i.e., that "it must make reference to the known genetic component of the illness (its physiologic basis) at the same time as it pays tribute to the fact that the behavior of organisms is modified throughout their lifetime as described by the principles of behavior theory." (p. 601) Salzinger's *immediacy hypothesis* states:

> ... that the behavior of schizophrenic patients is more often controlled by stimuli which are immediate in their spatial and temporal environment than is that of normals. It is the compelling control of the immediate stimuli over the behavior of schizophrenics which represents the physiologic basis of schizophrenia. The fact that stimuli which impinge on organisms leave them in a different state from the way they were before represents the environmental basis of schizophrenia. Individuals whose behavior is modified primarily by immediate aspects of the environment would be expected to behave differently from individuals (presumably normals) whose behavior is controlled and modified by both immediate and remote stimuli. Finally, the theoretical system suggested here requires one other assumption ... that whatever the schizophrenic defect is, it fluctuates over time, thus giving rise to the apparently "normal" periods and also providing the periods during which new (different) behavior can be acquired by a patient, one of whose major problems is the fact that the effect of stimuli, and therefore their power of acquiring control over behavior, is not lasting during his abnormal periods. (pp. 601–602)

"Immediate," as Salzinger uses the term, refers to temporal contiguity. If two stimuli are presented in succession, the one closest in time or currently present is prepotent.

The immediacy hypothesis provides an explanation for findings in several types of experimental investigation: (1) the more rapid extinction of verbal conditioned responses in schizophrenics than normals; (2) the tendency for schizophrenics to give a significantly higher number of repetitions on most verbal tasks; and (3) consistent findings of slower reaction times among schizophrenics on a variety of tasks of a sensorimotor type. In addition, the immediacy hypothesis offers a parsimonious interpretation of some widely reported clinical features of schizophrenic behavior.

Problems of communicability in at least one aspect of schizophrenic speech are readily accounted for in terms of the hypothesized prepotency of immediate stimuli. Using the cloze procedure (originally developed by Taylor[40]) in the analysis of typed transcripts of schizophrenic speech samples, Salzinger has demonstrated that a significantly greater number of intrusions attributable to the effects of immediate stimulation are a major source of lowered communicability in schizophrenic verbal productions.

The immediacy hypothesis also helps explain the frequently reported tendency of schizophrenics to show greater responses to private versus public stimuli, particularly in situations in which the resulting behavior is made to appear inappropriate and even bizarre. In episodes ranging from seconds to hours, schizophrenics exhibit what are often referred to as "lapses of attention," during which their behavior appears to be controlled by private stimuli (e.g., hallucinations) rather than public stimuli (e.g., the behavior of an interviewer). In order to account for such phenomena, Salzinger suggests, we have to take into consideration the circumstances of preschizophrenic development:

> The immediacy hypothesis suggests that a person likely to become schizophrenic is also one who has a tendency to respond preponderantly to immediate stimuli. Such a response tendency is quite prevalent in young normal children and given the assumption that it occurs only part of the time in the preschizophrenic, it might take quite a while before it

results in recognizably "strange" behavior. As people surrounding such an individual recognize the strange behavior they begin to ridicule the preschizophrenic, which may result in his avoiding people, or they begin to stay away from him because of his strange behavior. It is the resultant isolation which will promote the importance of the private stimuli (which also act through their immediate stimuli primarily) during the isolation and which make more important the immediate public stimuli after periods of isolation. The importance of immediate private stimuli would then be expected to be greater in those patients who went through periods of isolation than in those who did not. (p. 606)

Much of the eccentric behavior of the schizophrenic would thus result from misunderstandings and faulty interpretations of his social environment. Statements made by other people would be taken out of context, possibly resulting in paranoid delusions of persecution or grandeur. In other cases, contradictions evoked by prepotent immediate stimuli would produce a state of confusion.

Empirical investigation of the immediacy hypothesis by Dr. Salzinger and his associates has already produced a series of important research reports, and the heuristic value of the hypothesis has been demonstrated in a number of areas of inquiry. The immediacy hypothesis represents one of the few attempts to provide conceptual linkage between behavior genetics and behavior theory that has resulted in the derivation of testable hypotheses. It might also be noted, by way of conclusion, that the immediacy hypothesis offers full scope for the contributions and potential contributions of the linguistic and psycholinguistic investigator.

ACKNOWLEDGMENT

I should like to express my indebtedness to my friend and colleague, Dr. Richard W. Howell of the Department of Anthropology, University of Hawaii, in Hilo. I have greatly profited from his expertise in linguistics and ethnolinguistics, as well as his broad experience in all aspects of language analysis. Most of the ideas incorporated in this paper were worked out in a continuing dialogue with Dr. Howell that has spanned nearly twenty years and several continents.

REFERENCES

1. GOLDSTEIN, K. 1942. Aftereffects of Brain Injuries in War. Grune and Stratton. New York, N.Y.
2. FORREST, D. V. 1968. Poiesis and the language of schizophrenia. In Language Behavior in Schizophrenia. H. J. Vetter, Ed. Charles C Thomas. Springfield, Ill.
3. LORENZ, M. 1968. Problems posed by schizophrenic language. In Language Behavior in Schizophrenia. H. J. Vetter, Ed. Charles C Thomas. Springfield, Ill.
4. BROWN, R. 1973. Schizophrenia, language, and reality. Amer. Psychol. 28: 395-403.
5. MAHER, B. A. 1966. Principles of Psychopathology. McGraw-Hill Inc. New York, N.Y.
6. RICHMAN, J. 1968. Symbolic distortion in the vocabulary definitions of schizophrenics. In Language Behavior in Schizophrenia. H. J. Vetter, Ed. Charles C Thomas. Springfield, Ill.
7. FERREIRA, A. J. 1960. The semantics and the context of the schizophrenic's language. Arch. Gen. Psychiat. 3: 128-138.
8. BATESON, G., D. JACKSON, J. HALEY & J. WEAKLAND. 1956. Toward a theory of schizophrenia. Behav. Sci. 1: 251-264.
9. SEARLES, H. 1959. The effort to drive the other person crazy—an element in the etiology and psychotherapy of schizophrenia. Br. J. Med. Psychol. 32: 1-18.
10. VETTER, H. J. 1969. Language Behavior and Psychopathology. Rand McNally & Co. Chicago, Ill.

11. ULLMANN, L. P. & L. KRASNER. 1969. A Psychological Approach to Abnormal Behavior. Prentice-Hall Inc. Englewood Cliffs, N.J.
12. CAMERON, N. & A. MAGARET. 1951. Behavior Pathology. Houghton Mifflin Co. Boston, Mass.
13. ROBERTSON, J. P. S. & S. J. SHAMSIE. 1968. A systematic examination of gibberish in a multilingual schizophrenic patient. In Language Behavior in Schizophrenia. H. J. Vetter, Ed. Charles C Thomas. Springfield, Ill.
14. BROWN, R. 1958. Words and Things. The Free Press. New York, N.Y.
15. GARFINKEL, H. 1967. Studies in Ethnomethodology. Prentice-Hall Inc. Englewood Cliffs, N.J.
16. VETTER, H. J. 1968. New word coinage in the psychopathological context. Psychiat. Quart. 42: 298–312.
17. CUMMINGS, E. E. 1959. Poems 1923-1954. Harcourt. New York, N.Y.
18. SCHNEIDER, C. 1930. Die Psychologie der Schizophrenen. Georg Thieme. Leipzig, Germany.
19. COHEN, A. J. 1961. Estimating the degree of schizophrenic pathology from recorded interview samples. J. Clin. Psych. 17: 403–406.
20. HUNT, W. A., N. F. JONES & E. B. HUNT. 1957. Reliability of clinical judgment as a function of clinical experience. J. Clin. Psych. 13: 377–378.
21. JONES, N. F. Jr. 1959. The validity of clinical judgments of schizophrenic pathology based on verbal responses to intelligence test items. J. Clin. Psych. 15: 396–400.
22. MAHER, B. A., K. O. MCKEAN & B. MCLAUGHLIN. 1966. Studies in psychotic language. In The General Inquirer: A Computer Approach to Content Analysis. P. J. Stone, D. C. Dunphy, M. S. Smith & D. M. Ogilvie, Eds. M.I.T. Press. Cambridge, Mass.
23. CUMMINGS, E. E. 1958. A poet's advice to students. In E. E. Cummings: A Miscellany. G. J. Firmage, Ed. Argophile. New York, N.Y.
24. BERKOWITZ, R. 1960. The Disturbed Child. New York University Press. New York, N.Y.
25. KANNER, L. 1943. Autistic disturbances of affective contact. Nerv. Child. 2: 217–250.
26. CUNNINGHAM, M. A. & C. DIXON. 1961. A study of the language of an autistic child. J. Child Psych. Psychiat. 2: 193–202.
27. WOLFF, S. & S. CHESS. 1965. An analysis of the language of fourteen schizophrenic children. J. Child Psych. Psychiat. 6: 29–41.
28. FISH, B., T. SHAPIRO & M. CAMPBELL. 1966. Long term program and the response of schizophrenic children to drug therapy: A controlled study of trifluoperazine. Amer. J. Psychiat. 123: 32–39.
29. RUTTER, M. 1965. The influence of organic and emotional factors on the origins, nature, and outcome of childhood psychosis. Dev. Med. & Child Neurol. 7: 518–528.
30. BARTOLUCCI, G. & R. J. ALBERS. 1974. Deictic categories in the language of autistc children. J. Aut. Child. Schiz. 4: 131–141.
31. HERMELIN, B. & N. O'CONNOR. 1967. Remembering of words by psychotic and subnormal children. Br. J. Psychol. 58: 213–218.
32. FRITH, U. 1969. Emphasis and meaning in normal and autistic children. Lang. Speech. 12: 29–38.
33. TUBBS, V. 1966. Types of linguistic disability in psychotic children.' J. Ment. Defic. Res. 10: 230–240.
34. BLEULER, E. 1950. Dementia Praecox or the Group of Schizophrenias. International Universities Press. New York, N.Y.
35. VETTER, H. J. 1972. Psycholoy of Abnormal Behavior. Ronald Press. New York, N.Y.
36. ROSENTHAL, D. 1970. Genetic Theory and Abnormal Behavior. McGraw-Hill Inc. New York, N.Y.
37. FERSTER, C. B. 1961. Positive reinforcement and behavioral deficits of autistic children. Child Dev. 32: 437–456.
38. FERSTER, C. B. & M. DEMYER. 1962. A method for the experimetal analysis of the behavior of autistic children. Amer. J. Orthopsychiat. 32: 89–98.
39. SALZINGER, K. 1971. An hypothesis about schizophrenic behavior. Amer. J. Psychother. 25: 601–614.
40. TAYLOR, W. L. 1953. Cloze procedure: a new tool for measuring readability. Journalism Quart. 30: 415–420.

DISCUSSION

Robert W. Rieber, *Chairperson*

Department of Psychology
John Jay College of Criminal Justice
The City University of New York
New York, New York 10019

DR. M. C. BATESON: Before we go on to the discussion, I would like to say a few words about the relationship between my paper and that of Dr. Stern and his group, a relationship that prompted our putting them next to each other. The infants I described are slightly younger than the ones he has described, but the film that he showed is extraordinarily evocative of the area I am talking about. To build a bridge in the other direction, you can take the spectrograms I have presented as illustrations of the kind of vocalization he is dealing with. The first of the doublets in FIGURE 2(a) is representative of the infant vocalizations he described, except that as the coaction pattern develops and rises toward a crescendo, the infant's vocalizations get longer and more like FIGURE 2(c) and like the "pleasure cries" Wasz-Höckert and his group describe.

In the film Dr. Stern showed of an infant-father interaction, we had a very strong sense of the father's leadership in establishing the joint performance. I must say that it delights me to have Dr. Stern showing infants interacting with their fathers alongside my discussion of infants with their mothers, and I wish we knew something about how to relate the differences to biological and cultural differences in sex roles. By contrast with his material, in the dialogues I've been working on, taking the statistical analyses of timing and time lapses, it is not clear who has the leadership. Mother and child are coparticipants in a joint social performance very similar, at a certain level of structure, to conversation. This is essentially symmetrical and contrasts with our tendency to look at interactions between parent and child as profoundly asymmetrical, where, for instance, the infant is seen as being conditioned and the mother is conditioning him.

This is especially true when we consider what I call "elicitation time." That is, just as in conversation, they are taking turns. But in conversation it sometimes happens that you may not answer in the space I leave you for answering, and then I try again, and I say, "Well, what do you think about that?" or "Well?" or "Um?" in order to set up a new context for your expected response. Of course, there is massive assymmetry between mother and child in linguistic competence, but we need to think of language as a social skill as well as a cognitive skill. Thus (as I remarked this morning), it's interesting that "why" questions, as single-word questions, work well for some children in keeping an interaction going, even though a study of their use of *why* in sentences later shows that they have not mastered the cognitive side of it, and indeed that their mastery of the cognitive side will involve a certain loss of social efficacy. Nonetheless, the early mastering of patterns of coparticipation gives them contexts for later linguistic development.

DR. KURT SALZINGER: I'd just like to make one observation, and that is: it seems to me that both Dr. Stern and Dr. Bateson have shown the reinforcement-theory model at work, and that's not surprising at all. That is, the infant is reinforcing the parent; the parent is reinforcing the infant. Here we have a very beautiful picture of it quite early in the game.

DR. STERN: I agree. However, what is more striking to me is that during short "runs" of the interaction, the mother and infant can perform their behaviors almost synchronously with one another, or at least so closely together that there is insufficient reaction time to assign one behavior as a stimulus and another as a response. During such stretches of the interaction, the S-R model appears to be less useful than the notion that each partner is sharing the same program or rhythm. Of course, both partners in the dyad have to be resynchronized frequently, and at such points the S-R model again becomes essential for the understanding of the cuing process. Both viewpoints are needed: an S-R model and a shared program. I suspect that Cathy agrees, and I would like to hear what she thinks about this from her experience.

DR. BATESON: I don't think either Dan or I are wearing any buttons today. I've no objection to noticing that this is a context for learning and that they're clearly having a marvelous time; these two facts are related. I'll go that far. The difficulty with an S-R model, I think, is that you break up the ongoing event. Now, if we can keep from being distracted from the ongoing pattern, in which we get mother and child or father and child doing something together, then I think yours is an enrichng additional point of view.

DR. SUZANNE SALZINGER: Now a comment from the other half of the family. I just wanted to bring up a talk that Dan and I had the other day, when I told him about a recording that we had once made of a three-month-old. I had deliberately reinforced the child's speech and worked on the pattern. The way I did that was to let the child finish vocalizing, and whenever there was a pause I imitated what the child had just done before that. So, in a sense, I was creating an alternation pattern, but the interesting thing was that we got a very high level of arousal, just the way yours did. So, I think that it may not be the natural pattern that's giving you the arousal level. It may be that any pattern can produce that with satisfaction.

DR. STERN: I partially disagree. What you have observed certainly occurs. Arousal may increase progressivey in the course of an alternating exchange. However, as the level gets higher you generally, but not necessarily, start to see a breakdown in a purely alternating pattern, with progressively more vocal overlap and, accordingly, a trend toward a coaction pattern. Then, after some period, the interaction may have moved to a different arousal level and affective tone, and a more purely alternating pattern can again be resumed. My sense of it is that at the higher levels of arousal you generally see more coactional patterning.

DR. BATESON: I think mother and infant learn to manage the arousal level, and this is especially important as an aspect of gaze. What the particular mother and infant that I focused on tended to do was this: there would be an escalation, and a withdrawal, then an escalation and a withdrawal, so that in interactions of four minutes there was a definite plot. There probably were points where they could have gone off in the direction of coaction, and they controlled that, sustaining the dialogue pattern. Dialogue seemed to be a preferred pattern for this pair, whereas the father in Dan's film seems to elicit coaction deliberately.

DR. KURT SALZINGER: Just one more brief remark. I think there is a subtle change in the reinforcement contingency in these interactions. At first, each member of the dyad reinforces the other. Then this changes into a cooperative game. Here the reinforcement is contingent on the relationship of the responses of parent and child, on their cooperating. There is enough experimental data to show that one can reinforce two people for doing things in sequence, in chorus, or in whatever pattern is desirable. I find this to be a more acceptable explanation that the concept of arousal, with its vagueness.

DR. OSGOOD: Kurt, just what kind of a response is "cooperating"?

DR. KURT SALZINGER: Cooperating responses are those in which the reinforcement is contingent on the relationship between the responses of two organisms. In this case, cooperating consists of having two responses follow one another; in another case it might be two responses occurring at the same time; in a third case it might be I say, "Da, da, da," and the other person says, "Da." The definition is entirely functional.

DR. KEN KATOFSKY (*Pittsburgh, Pa.*): I'd like to ask both panelists whether they've thought of looking at the behavior in perhaps a slightly different way. Have you thought of it as imitative behavior on the part of the child? I've been struck in observing this in two-month-old infants. It seemed to me that when the infant would start, the parent could join in, and there would be mutual arousal. But in addition to that, the parent would be talking, and the infant would catch a view of the parent's mouth and start making mouthing motions with or without vocalizations. The infant is trying to imitate some aspects of the mother's or father's behavior by mouth movement, if not by vocalization.

DR. BATESON: I'd be tempted to turn that upside down and say that as the infant is learning to engage in complex sequences involving both himself and the mother, he is also learning contexts for imitation. In other words, you can look at it both ways. It's clearly a closely related phenomenon.

DR. RIEBER: Apparently, anyone can look at things both ways, and that makes a difference.

DR. STERN: I want to respond to something Kurt said before, with regard to arousal. It is almost impossible to understand infant behavior unless you take into account the variable of arousal, however you may wish to measure it. This is extremely important, because if we consider the onset or emergence of vocalizations as having something to do with expressive acts related to emotional state, then very clearly the level of arousal at which vocalizations occur, and at which the dyadic mode of vocalizing occurs, becomes relevant. I agree with you completely that arousal is hard to pin down, even with the help of physiological measures, but I do not agree that we can talk only about different reinforcement contingencies and forget about the level of arousal. The consideration of at least both is required.

DR. MARJORIE ARNOLD (*Rutgers University, New Brunswick, N.J.*): I'm interested in knowing if either of you have found any consistent differences in which member initiates the dialogues, and whether a check was made on the birth order of the child. I'm raising this point because there is a student at Rutgers whose dissertation concerns mothers and infants in interaction at fourteen weeks. The infants were all firstborns. She was very surprised to find that overwhelmingly, the infants initiated interactions. Even though these were the first children of these mothers, it was almost always the infants initiating what then was a dialogue.

DR. BATESON: I've worked only on firstborns. The intensive study was of a firstborn. My problem would be defining a clear point at which initiation takes place, because I recognize the phenomenon at the point where a degree of mutuality is being established. The interactions that I studied tended to come immediately after caretaking episodes. In other words, the mother has fed, bathed, and dressed the baby, and is holding it, so the caretaking has involved a sustained contact and interaction between them. And then there's a sort of pause, and this kind of thing develops.

DR. FURTH: I would just like to comment that deaf children, profoundly deaf children, behave exactly like these children you have seen here, so that there is no way to distinguish the deaf from the hearing child in these communications; so, it's quite clear that whatever interaction takes place, it's not just acoustic, and the deaf child gets enough cues from the kinesthetic behavior itself to behave like a normal child.

DR. DAVID RIGLER (*Children's Hospital, Los Angeles, Calif.*): I think that Dr. Furth anticipated some of my comment. The film was fascinating, partly because it was more than acoustic, because we did in fact see the bodily interaction, the motor movements, the bouncing of the child, the mute facial expressions of the father, the eye contact, and, of course, the smile of the baby. I think all these things have to be taken into account before one constructs an S-R model.

DR. STERN: It is certainly true that vocalizations do not occur alone, i.e., without the concommitant performance of many expressive motor acts. In fact, whenever a mother says something like, "Hi, honey," she doesn't simply say "Hi honey" with a neutral face; she says (with raised inflection), "Hi, Honey," and at the same time performs an exaggerated facial expression that is generally exaggerated in spatial and temporal performance, which we have come to call an infant-elicited variation of behavior. One of the striking things about these unusual or infant-elicited variations in vocalization (baby talk) and facial expression and movement is that they all go together, and it is difficult for a mother, when faced with a real baby, to split them apart. So your point is quite well taken.

DR. RACHEL FALMAGNE (*Clark University, Worcester, Mass.*): I would like to ask Dr. Nelson a question concerning the theoretical implications of these results. You've offered two hypotheses, one of which you favor: the difference in cognitive style, so to speak, and the alternative hypothesis, that the consistency between the children's behavior at an early age and their vocabulary later on is provided by the fact that the mother's speech is oriented toward objects, rather than affects. There seems to be, though, a third possibility, which is a different version of the second one, especially in the light of papers we heard this afternoon emphasizing the interaction in the dialogue between mother and child. The third hypothesis is that the child's early utterances serve as a stimulus for the mother to paraphrase and elaborate on. Either because of cognitive style or the mother's bias, when the young child in your group meets primarily object-words, the mother paraphrases and elaborates with sentences containing adjectives and actions. In other words, the process builds cumulatively from that initial point. I was wondering what comments you might have about that, and also what data might speak to this.

DR. NELSON: Unfortunately, my data don't speak to it. However, from the analyses of the data I have been able to provide, I would certainly agree with you that it's a cumulative interacting process. Some mothers appear to be better at building on what their children are doing than others. But for some mothers who were using object-words with their children, the children themselves were not responding at all, because the mothers were trying to engage the child in a teaching mode rather than in picking up what the child was talking about and building on that. So you have an almost indefinitely large range of interaction patterns that can occur. Certainly, what looks like one of the most efficacious patterns is the case in which the child does produce words referring to objects or events that he's interested in, and the mother builds on those to enable him to go on from there; but it can have a detrimental effect as well.

UNIDENTIFIED SPEAKER: In the Dr. Suzanne Salzinger study, I'm especially interested in Group E, "Incomprehensible Speech Pattern," and the ways that the mother, and perhaps the elementary school teacher, squelches this capacity in the young child in trying to form a rigid, rational, logical mind, as opposed to a creative, looser mind. Perhaps this is asking for a value judgment on Dr. Salzinger's part. If it's shown that the mother is not reinforcing this so-called "incomprehensible category," which could be correlated to the imagination quality, the young child is forced into a rational, logical approach, as opposed to a creative approach.

DR. S. SALZINGER: I'm afraid I can't answer a lot of that. All I can say about the effect of the mother on the variables we did study was that the mother's speech, i.e., the way in which she spoke to the child, did affect how much these children tended to converse with each other, as measured by the total amount of speech they emitted in a conversation with peers in a completely different situation. That effect seemed to depend on her total "push," as we've called it. However, we found that the mother's speech *style* is exemplified by open-ended questions, which many teachers think is the way to teach. We found that although the open-ended questions correlated very highly with *how much* speech the children would give forth, they did not correlate with *communicative* speech. In other words, this speech style did not seem to guide the children toward wanting to speak with each other. I must say that was a surprise to us, but it was in fact quite clear in our data.

DR. REED BATES YOUNG (*Austin, Texas*): I have a complaint about language studies, I don't have the solution. A problem has shown up in several of these papers, and it will probably show up in several others. For at least the last ten years, researchers have analyzed word-counts, and holophastic phrases, and whether an utterance is a noun, an adjective, or a verb. But it's the adults, it's the parents, who define what they think the child is intending: Is it a noun? Is it a verb? Is it "milk," "mommy," and "mine"? It just seems to me that you get into a circular situation I would like to see a way out of. I don't know the way out myself, but I'm saying that this whole thing disturbs me because it has a circular aspect to it.

DR. NELSON: I think the point is very well taken. I think most people who have been doing analyses have tried to classify the speech in terms of what the child intended the word to be. To the extent that that's possible, this is the approach I've taken. I agree with your point from the outset, in that nouns and adjectives and so on don't make that much sense in the early vocabularies. At the same time, they're a convenient way of classifying the language in a way that relates it to later speech. It may be circular, but the better way isn't readily apparent.

DR. SALZINGER: I just want to go further, along with Katherine Nelson's answer. It seems to me that it's not as terrible a situation as the questioner made it appear. In a sense, it's a straw man, because, in fact, the way you define your responses and the things you're going to look at does indeed have to do with your theoretical approach to the field. I really don't think that's such a bad thing, as long as you make quite explicit what you're doing.

DR. MENYUK: Dr. Nelson, in your concluding remarks, if I'm correct, you maintained that there are differences in patterns of language development. I wonder if you are separating or are putting together language development and development of language use. In the categories that you did provide, you very carefully stated that there were no distinctions between the groups. You were suggesting that proportionality might have something to do with cognitive style. Would you comment on language development versus development of language use?

DR. NELSON: I'm not sure I understand the question. The conclusion was that in terms of patterns of language use at thirty months, there were in fact no specific linguistic differences. There were still some differences in terms of the uses of classes of words such as adjectives by the referential children. I was distinguishing that from a specific linguistic performance factor. That is, it's a language-in-use factor. Is that what you're referring to?

DR. MENYUK: Yes, because when you use the term "language development," it is not clear what you are referring to.

DR. NELSON: However, earlier—prior to thirty months—there did seem to be differences. The expressive children, for example, were using more complete sentences at the lower MLU level than were the referential children. Presumably, that is a factor of linguistic form or structure, so that would actually be a difference in their developing linguistic pattern, which had disappeared by the later age.

DR. HARRIET WHITESTONE: (*University of Hartford, Hartford, Conn.*): I wanted to ask Dr. Nelson if she mentioned that expressive children had more mature utterances. Could this possibly have reflected their learning more social idioms or socially enforced routines?

DR. NELSON: Yes, it certainly could have, and it possibly did. I think many of the complete forms that they used were learned as complete forms. However, there is recent evidence that many children learn complete forms which they then analyze and reformulate.

DR. JAFFE: Before I ask my question, from some of the remarks made during the coffee break, I think I'd better reiterate the point that Dr. Stern was making, just to make sure that everyone was really clear about the point of the paper. Though coaction is more frequent in the interaction we examined than antiphony (alternation), both are present at the age of three to four months, and both are present in adult conversations. The only difference is in the ratio, the preponderance being in favor of coaction early; in adult conversations, the preponderance is in favor of antiphony.

Now, the fact that these are twin pairs bears importantly on individual differences. There must be a few people here who are not from the New York State Psychiatric Institute. For those of you who are not, you should know that it has traditionally been twin country, because the genetics of mental illness are being carefully worked out in a population where we can know for sure that people have the same or different heredity, namely, one-egg and two-egg twin pairs. The incidence of mental illness is then studied in these types of siblings.

It is of some importance that one of these twin pairs from a single egg, monozygous, was a pair studied in this paper. A very important part, for which we simply didn't have time, bears on this question of individual differences. Here we have a crystal-clear case in which we know that these two babies have exactly the same genetic make-up, and we can see what effect the environment, which we can observe, has on these types of interaction patterns.

Now I'll give the floor to Dr. Stern to present the piece of the paper that we didn't have time for this morning.

DR. STERN: That was a plant, and I'll make it brief. One twin baby (3a) and her mother showed an overall pattern that was coactional, whereas her *monozygous* twin sister (3b) and mother showed an overall pattern that was alternating (see TABLE 1 in our paper). Both patterns were highly significant but in opposite directions. When we went back to the tapes there turned out to be a potentially simple explanation, which has a good deal to do with some of the subtle ways individual differences can come about, given the same genetic makeup. Every morning and every afternoon momma always woke up twin 3a first, fed her, played with her, and put her to bed. She then woke up 3b, fed her, etc. She was one of the mothers who generally interacted with her twins serially, rather than together. Mothers of twins have this choice, up to a certain age. What this amounted to, then, was that by the time she got to twin 3b, she was pretty played out and she did not utilize the same highly arousing spontaneous behaviors that she engaged in with twin 3a. With twin b, she utilized more instructional-type behaviors which tend to lead to less exciting interactions and which are best carried out with the alternating pattern. She "trained" the twins so that their waking patterns were generally an hour or so apart. She found this easiest. In any event, entirely diverse patterns of interaction resulted for the very probable and simple reason that she kept on waking one up before the other.

DR. BATESON: Dan, could you say a little bit more about the set of families that you were using, and about how you tried to sample them, and so on. You refer to "every morning and every afternoon the mother would pick up the same twin," and so on. What was the socioeconomic background of the families? Were they all first-born twins?

DR. STERN: The mothers were all primiparous, middle socioeconomic class, white, suburban women. We visited the homes at least once a week, often twice. We set aside an entire morning for the observations and called the mother the night before to ask when the babies would probably get up in the morning. We arrived about one half-hour before the expected waking time to set up the cameras, and so on. We visited at least once prior to filming or taping, so that they would begin to get used to us.

DR. BATESON: And how long were you there?

DR. STERN: You mean on each visit?

DR. BATESON: Yes.

DR. STERN: A minimum of three hours, pretty much all morning. We'd usually come at 8:30 or 9, and often stay for lunch, as it turned out.

DR. BATESON: Did you observe individual differences between dizygotic twins?

DR. STERN: Oh, yes. But there were even immense differences between the monozygous twins. The more you look at twins, the more you appreciate the distinction between genetically identical and constitutionally identical infants. Also, each twin is born into a different psychological environment. For instance, the twin who comes out first generally has every advantage in the world, from the Apgar score on up. Second, if they are the same sex, which they will be if they are monozygous, the first twin always get *the* name. There is only one name, you know, the favorite name, which embodies many important fantasies. It is very important. The child with the name will probably become the main carrier of much of the familial and personal legacy and hopes. These are not small issues. In fact, twin A in this set was the first who got *the* name; the other one got a second-rate name that they had to come up with. So whoever comes out first is already a different person in the eyes of its environment.

DR. S. SALZINGER: This is also addressed to Dan Stern. You seem to keep flirting with a functional approach. The answer to the planted question implies that you have some notion of what the functional relationship is between these two patterns and the way that mothers handle babies. I say "flirting" because you really haven't come out with it yet. But it strikes me that if that is, in fact, the case, and you have looked at a lot of twins, you may have some hypotheses which you might want to look at, and that there may be ways of independently, blindly rating mothers' behavior to predict the two patterns in babies. Have you ever thought of doing anything like that? Do you see what I'm getting at?

DR. STERN: I'm afraid so.

DR. S. SALZINGER: You've thought of it.

DR. STERN: I'm not exactly clear about what you mean by "flirting" with a functional definition. Would you define it a little more closely?

DR. S. SALZINGER: Well, you explained the difference in the patterns of the two—of these twins in terms of the fact that the mother woke up one child first and handled her first or him first, as the case may be. Later on, that mother was played out, and therefore the other pattern emerged. There must have been innumerable cases where you observed, or after the fact said, "Oh, yes, well, the mother does such and such, and this is why we get this pattern." The question is: could you prerig your system so that you can predict some of the patterns? It seems to me that might be very interesting.

DR. STERN: Oh, I don't think I flirted with that. I would predict that you will get a coaction pattern, or at least more of one, whenever there is a high level of arousal and a lot of affect, be it positive or negative. Period. The dyadic pattern is not a function of individual differences *per se*, or rather, it is, but only to the extent that those individual differences in baby and mother allow them to get to levels of high arousal and affect. So I would predict that if we could agree on an acceptable measure of arousal and affect, we would find coactional vocalizing to occur more frequently at the higher levels. There will, of course, be individual differences in the infants' arousability and ability to hold the state, as well as in the match between the two of them, which also determines their ability to move from one state to another or to stay in one state. I don't feel I've equivocated on that point.

DR. S. SALZINGER: What I'm really getting at is that it's too bad that you look at it in retrospect and say that this is the way it's happening. I'd like to see you set the stage and predict it, and then see if it does happen.

DR. STERN: I agree with you. We are in the middle of planning studies that are prospective with regard to this kind of issue.

DR. NELSON: Did you ever observe any infant-infant interaction?

DR. STERN: Yes. They don't do an awful lot with each other at this stage, i.e., three to four months of age. An infant cannot provide for another infant the necessary stimulus array (vocalizations, expressions, movement, etc.) with the requisite contingencies that an adult can. Accordingly, they are poor at holding one another's attention.

DR. MENYUK: This is rather related to what Dr. Salzinger asked, and also responds to your descsription of the twins, one of whom was awakened first and the second afterward. Is it not the case that what happens in terms of these interaction patterns is not simply a function of the mother and her view of the situation, but also a function of the baby, and the fact that the babies also have varying thresholds of arousal? Under those circumstances, one would have to set up fairly complex predictive models in terms of mother and child. What would be the possible outcome?

DR. STERN: Your point leads to a larger discussion, which includes considerations of the level of arousal in both the infant and the mother. There is no question about there being individual differences on both sides of the fence. A large part of the problem resides in how to measure and then evaluate arousal. Even if we had EEG, EKG, respiratory rates, etc., the matter would not be easily resolved, since the interpretation of the various combinations of change in physiological and behavioral variables is not agreed upon, or at least not sufficiently understood in this setting.

Alertness, consisting of visual attention with cardiac deceleration, is probably constantly alternating with motor expressivity; that is, activity with cardiac acceleration. Both these "types" of arousal will certainly be operating in this situation, and there are probably several other important combinations of changes. I believe we need a larger body of naturalistic physiological and behavioral data of this nature even to begin to plan the kind of experiment you mentioned. We are currently tackling that task.

DR. GEORGE WELLER (*Montefiore Speech and Hearing Clinic, Bronx, N.Y.*): Could I say something to that point? I'm a little bothered about the use of the term "arousal," as though it's one-dimensional. There are at least two dimensions of arousal, perhaps three. Arousal can be the energy dimension that underlies activity level, and it can be the intensity dimension that underlies emotions. Those two are very similar, and those two you can measure by activity measures. The third kind of arousal may be the most important for our purposes of studying communication development, particularly communication disorders, and that's the alertness factor that underlies intelligence. It's this particular factor which involves attentional focus that is almost impossible to measure by a purely behavioral measure, unless you're very astute, because, as a matter of fact, it tends to be negatively correlative with most measures of activity. In other words, when the child focuses his attention, his motor activity usually stills, and he concentrates. For those of us who work with children with communication problems, say around two and three years of age, this is always one of the great difficulties, separating their ability to communicate from their obvious disability in paying attention; so that kind of arousal is very important. I think you should always make the distinction when you talk about arousal as to what kind of arousal you're talking about.

Let me make one or two other points. Your comment about twins being discordant in terms of constitution is very well made. I'd like to emphasize that this is particularly strong where you have monozygous twins, because they share the same chorion and you get more inequities of blood flow, more inequities of maternal nutrients, and so you get a much higher incidence of death and you get a much higher incidence of brain damage, and, we would presume, on up the continuum, you get a much higher incidence of behavioral differences caused by this fact, that they were monozygous twins. So instead of being unusually similar, they may be unusually different.

UNIDENTIFIED SPEAKER: The comment on twins has aroused my attention, since I am a twin myself. As far as the remarks that have been made, I have no doubt that they are sound as generalizations. I think that I can say rather objectively that they didn't work out in this particular instance. As I reflect on it, I see that I'm putting myself first in relation to my brother, but that's the way I always have done, except at the moment of birth. He did arrive first. I'm not sure why he got the name that he did, but I appear to have gotten what the family considered the choice name, and I appear to have managed to get the greater amount of education and the greater relationship to intellectuals such as yourselves.

DR. RIEBER: Could you give your name, please, and affiliation.

Since, it comes that way, I have to tell you the whole name, because that's part of the story of the name. The name is Wesley Constantine Appenunzio. And that, as my father used to say, is a strangely contrastive blend of conflicting influences.

DR. RIEBER: Anything added to that would be an anticlimax.

DR. AARON CARTON (State University of New York at Stony Brook, Stony Brook, N.Y.): I'm interested in the Jaffe, Stern, and Bateson research and the problems that it raises in respect to modality of communication. It's noontime. I wanted to talk to my friend who is at the other end of the room, and the noise level being what it was, the channel was preempted. At about that moment, I noticed that our deaf colleagues had the advantage over us; they were able to communicate across a large expanse very successfully, very efficiently, at a time when that was closed to us who rely only on a hearing mode.

In the research of Jaffe and Stern, they've been isolating their modalities. Sometimes they work in a visual modality; sometimes they work in the auditory modality. Apparently, to date they haven't reported research where the work is across modalities, where, perhaps, one parent sends a message in the visual or tactile modality and the child responds vocally, or vice versa. When we got into the debate about whether these are stimulus-response and reinforcing relationships, we saw that a tremendous amount of complexity must come to bear in locating them. I wonder if you have any thoughts about research that could tease out a variety of levels of stimulation and the uses of modality.

DR. JAFFE: Believe me, we have rooms full of data, all cranked out by computers, on precisely these four channels; but not from manipulating them. They're naturalistic observations. Today, Dan was concentrating on the vocal channels, since this was a linguistic conference, and mutual gazing would be of less interest here. As he said, most of his work has been on gazing. We also have another paper on the fire, with concommitant timing of both people's gaze and both people's vocalization; in other words, a four-channel system instead of a two-channel system. I think he would have a lot to say about that if you would like to listen. It was the paper we were originally going to give.

DR. BATESON: Perhaps one thing that should be said at this point, if we're discussing modalities, is that when you open it up to all the modalities, you virtually have to say that in most of these interactions there's coaction throughout. The real question is: do we sometimes take turns in one or more modalities as an ongoing interaction?

DR. STERN: That is very well put and changes, in part, the ball park in which we talk about interactions. We frequently see the kind of interaction where the mother may voke and the baby responds by turning away or by turning away with a smile, whereupon the mother says something else, and the baby then may toss his head up and open his mouth, or voke, and then the mother says something again and the baby this time responds by returning his gaze to her, and so on. She reacts to each infant behavior as if it were a verbal response following the adult discoursive model. Similarly, you see many mothers who are terrific with their tactile behavior (I'm sure you've seen this), so that they can keep the ball going, so to speak, by putting the touching or jiggling in at the right places. I quite agree with you; it requires a reconceptualization of what we are talking about.

Changing the subject a bit: to what extent are some of these behaviors evoked in the ethological sense, rather than being responses to a stimulus in a learning paradigm? This is not, of course, a small issue, but it is very germane at this stage of development, when we are talking about the origins of interactive behaviors.

DR. CARTON: I'd like another crack at it, if I may. There seem to be some hints as to what may emerge while one looks at this. You argue, Dr. Stern, that the coactional events take place under a high state of arousal. That makes sense. When the channel is preempted, one can't put the kind of material that Dr. Nelson called "referential" into the channel. One can put only expressional kinds of material into it. One might be interested to see what will happen over the years as you follow your subjects up, regarding whether those subjects who are engaged frequently in coactional patterns don't become the expressional speakers of Dr. Nelson's research.

The one problem with this is, and the thing I find annoying, Dr. Bateson, is that your kids were younger, and you would have thought they would know less about modality than Stern's kids. It's rather too bad, I think, that it came out that they knew so much about alternation.

DR. M. C. BATESON: Yes, but our sampling of situations was very different. I selected the pieces I looked at out of the data because I was interested in alternation, and I was working with one mother-child pair; so there's nothing in my data that says anything about the frequency of coaction. But, I'd like to raise an information point, and ask Dr. Furth this. You mentioned the advantages that the deaf have when we're all making a rumpus. I have the impression that conversation among the deaf—and this is a field that I know nothing about—allows a great deal more coaction without disrupting the referential affect than does vocal conversation. I wondered if a study has been done of coaction versus alternation in signing, and how this falls out in behavior.

DR. FURTH: I don't think a study has been done, but if you observe deaf people together in a group, you will see that that is precisely the case. I attended an international meeting in Rome where there were deaf people. Everybody was talking with everybody else at the same time. It would have been impossible with any other communication channel.

DR. BATESON: You see, vocal communication is additive. If we all talk at once—well, if two people talk at once—it's twice as noisy. This relates to the crescendo effect, where you have a curve of arousal. When two or three people are signing at once, you're not overloading the system in quite the same way, so it's a very different structure. It would affect arousal differently.

DR. FURTH: I wonder whether you could address yourself to this question of gesture language: hand, visual language versus vocal language. Certainly, one reason why deaf people have difficulty learning to speak is that they find gesture language so congenial and so natural, and spoken language so unnatural. Now, probably for hearing children, this spoken language develops in conjunction with gesture language, as you point out. Eventually the spoken language dominates, and the hearing child, the hearing person, feels comfortable in using a spoken language. Don't you think that there is a certain priority in a gesture language that deaf children cannot overcome? Obviously, it's a speculation on my part, but it may explain why they have such difficulty learning speech.

DR. BATESON: It seems to me that there is a very important distinction to be made here that is often confused when we speak of modalities. We're switching back and forth between talking about what sense we're perceiving with, by looking or by listening. And I'm talking about what kinds of things are being encoded in body motion versus vocalization. I think part of the ambiguity that you're raising comes from not making this distinction clearly. There obviously are very great differences between the kinds of things that hearing people encode kinesically and the kinds of things that must be received visually if one is depending on gesture as a substitute for vocalization. This comes out so very different structurally that I don't think one is more natural than the other.

DR. RIEBER: I'm somewhat puzzled by your question about why the deaf have such a difficult time learning speech. Certainly we're not forgetting the fact that they can't hear. It is a fact that the auditory monitoring system is part of that problem. Perhaps you were addressing yourself to why the deaf have such a reluctance to give up signs, which, of course, is another question. I gather you were talking about the latter. Fine!

DR. STERN: Perhaps some light can be shed on this point by considering which expressive behaviors emerge first. Discrete, recognizable vocalizations appear to emerge earlier than well-articulated hand gestures. The child has relatively poor control over his arms and hands until at least the fourth month of life. On the other hand, his control of gaze and head movements is well advanced by three months. From the developmental point of view, then, I would say that facial expressions, head movements, gaze, and vocalizations would be there before hand gesturing.

DR. FURTH: That sounds quite unbelievable. The reason is that the vocalizations that children use at six months of age are not specific in terms of referential meaning. These are very general vocalizations, vocalizations that are manifest by just being in contact with somebody.

DR. STERN: Let me put it this way, then. You can condition vocalizations, sucking, head movements, and gaze, certainly by three months. I have never seen anybody successfully condition any hand movement at that point. So there may be a more mature relationship between cognition and these behaviors than there is between cognition and hand behaviors. That's the point I'm trying to make.

DR. FURTH: Yes, but it still remains that we are talking about a level of symbolization that is one step below language, really. We are talking about signal behavior; yet you condition a particular signal, but this is a hardly human language.

DR. LISA MENN (*Universty of Illinois, Urbana, Ill., and MIT, Cambridge, Mass.*): I'm not speaking now from my own work, but from that of Lonnie Wilbur. She has done some work on children who are simultaneously acquiring signs because they are the children of deaf, signing parents, and they are acquiring speech because they are hearing children. They acquire these things pretty much in parallel. Finger babbling is observed to appear; that is, gestures in the signing area that one naturally wants to call finger babbling, because they seem to have a distinct resemblance to intentions to sign and to communicate. Vocabulary emerges more or less in parallel. Signs, at least over a period of several months for which she did a video-tape study of these children, tended to emerge slightly earlier than words for the corresponding objects. It's a bilingual study, really, in the classic fashion of the Hungarian therpacroatian study that's so well-known. I think she might be a source of further data on that.

DR. STERN: I think that's fascinating, and I stand corrected. I would love to see that work.

DR. NELSON: Did the children have as much exposure to vocal language as they had to the finger language if their parents were deaf?

DR. MENN: I think that point's well taken. They did have less exposure to spoken language, but their parents were very concerned that they should learn to speak, and they were taken care of, I believe daily, by a speaking baby sitter, in order to help them acquire spoken English as normally as possible.

DR. BARBARA HUDSON (*State University of New York at Albany, Albany, N. Y.*): In deciding which of the systems is most effective, I think you might have to consider both which is easiest for self-expression and which is easiest for comprehension. In the situation described, the meeting of deaf people in Rome, it might very well be that these people are fluently expressing themselves at the same time. But unless you have some measure of how they're understanding each other at the same time, whether they're able to divide their attention visually and effectively encode the messages of each other, I think you won't really be able to make any kind of statement. You must know both how effectively you can simultaneously express yourself and simultaneously understand other people. I think that with the auditory system, we can do that more effectively than with the visual system. But I have no more data than any of these other people on that point.

DR. BARBARA PERMAN (*University of Edinburgh, Edinburgh, Scotland*): I wanted to ask Dr. Stern to elaborate further on this gentleman's point about the interaction between the visual and the auditory modalities in your study. I gather, and I'm not familiar with your work, that you haven't at this point in time, put together the interactions between the modalities. Is that correct, or is it not?

DR. STERN: That's mainly correct.

DR. PERMAN: I wondered if you have any impressions on how the vocal interaction and the visual intereaction play each other out, and whether you have gained any insights as to what specific roles each might play? What kind of a design would you use to look at the interactions, in fact? Is this the stage that you're just at now?

DR. STERN: Yes.

DR. PERMAN: Do you have any ideas of how this might proceed, so that we can more precisely, in the next conference, discuss the issue, which is the difference in the modalities and the effectiveness of them, and so on?

DR. STERN: I think that one of the fantasies we had was that the mother would teach the baby the adult (or at least the American English) pattern of coordinating gaze and speech, as described by Kendon and by Argyle, which goes something like this: Let's say I'm talking to this gentleman; if I say a one-to-ten sentence as a speaker, I will say—my finger is now copying what my eyes are going to do—I will say "one, two, three, four, five, six, seven, eight, nine, ten." My return of gaze is a signal that I have finished voking, and he will then look at me and go "one, two, three, etc., nine, ten." So the signal to stop the vocalization is coordinated with the content of the verbalization, as well as the paralinguistics, as well as the gazing system, so that you end up with a really very coordinated pattern of two people getting together. We've tried to see if anything like this exists between the mother and the baby. I can tell you the answer is no. It is a lot more complicated, the major problem being that mothers, when they are with their infants, violate every "rule" I can think of for adult-adult dialogic exchange, be it with their gaze, be it with their face, be it with their voke. For instance, when a mother is playing with her infant, she will gaze at him almost all of the time, because that's the way she knows where he is as far as arousal and affect are concerned, and so, the rules of gazing get very complicated; gaze does not interact with vocalization the way it would when she's talking to an adult.

In general, we have limited ourselves by coding each behavior as only "on" or "off." The interesting patterns of gaze-voke interactions are more complicated. For instance, when the baby wants to put mother in a hold pattern and say: "I've had enough for now, but I don't want you to go away," he will avert gaze, frequently with a smile, so they show propitiatory smiles even by the age of four months. You know, this kind of thing. They will also sometimes voke at the moment of gaze aversion. They'll go, "ah," like this. Sometimes they will voke when they come back. Now, the method of analysis that Joe and I have worked out cannot capture the subtlety of such signals, of which there appear to be many. I must say, the more we see of the actual momentary events and what effect they've got on the mother, the more I feel like throwing out all the print-out and studying in detail these kinds of communicative events. Another example of such an event was found by Dr. Beatrice Beebe, who is working in the lab and who is also a contributor to the work. A behavior that a baby can perform at this age that will most turn on a mother and get her to talk, and to light up the mother's face, is not smiling, as most people would say, and not voking, but one in which the baby opens its its mouth wide and throws its head back. Like this. If, then, you throw a voke on top of it, it adds just a tiny bit more from the point of view of making it evocative. But there are very few mothers that we've seen who don't automatically respond to that with a flurry of behaviors including vocalizations plus the immediate riveting of their gaze, plus the lighting up of their faces, the raising of their eyebrows, the lowering of their jaws, and throwing back their heads. Now, if you want to call that a response to a stimulus, O.K., you can call it that. I'm not sure. I think it's probably much more ingrained in human biology.

So the answer to the question of what about the integration of all these behaviors is this: It's such a rich set of data that I want to run in a lot of directions with it all at the same time.

DR. RIEBER: Your example intrigues me because it is the exact same movement that one does when one says, "Hi." The mouth opens, the head moves up and back, and then comes down.

DR. STERN: Exactly. It's a form of greeting behavior.

DR. S. SALZINGER: I would just like to plead with you not to throw out all the print-outs, because it seems to me that it's a far cry from Joe's adult speaker-speaker interactions and the baby-mother interactions that you're dealing with. I know it sounds terrible to say that you should continue it for year after year after year as your children get older and older, but somewhere along the way some of those print-outs are going to yield statistical (you'll excuse the expression) relationships that are going to be very interesting and will, I hope, approach the adult models.

DR. STERN: I agree with you, Suzy, I really do. And we're going to go ahead with it but, the pull to explore other avenues is strong.

DR. JAFFE: There are some real predictions that could be made. Suzy's question, from before, has been bothering me, and Dr. Furth clearly reminded us that we are not studying speech; we are studying vocal signaling here. But we do know what the childhood pattern is: more coaction, both in vocalization and in looking. Also, there's joint gaze. The adult pattern is more alternation in both vocalization and visual fixation. The listener looks at the speaker, but the speaker doesn't fix continuously on the listener. In fact, a speaker fixing on a listener is actually used in psychophysiological experiments as a stress situation. It's a weird experience to have someone talking to you who never takes his eyes off yours. So we have an adult pattern and we have a childhood pattern, and both adults and children use both. But there's a ratio change. When would we expect an abrupt shift in this ratio? Presumably, that will be when this vocal signaling begins to be processed linguistically. So there is a very definite prediction, which will correlate with everything everyone else is measuring, as to when this ratio will shift rather abruptly.

DR. RIEBER: How abruptly?

DR. JAFFE: This is just speculation. It could turn out to be a very delicate index of when those noises begin to grab the kid as symbolic patterns. This may show up as a discontinuity of rate of change.

DR. STERN: To follow up on that, remember that what we've got is an overall odds ratio of 1:2 in the mother-infant dyads, and when Joe ran through thirty adult conversations, .03. Now, there's a long way from 1:2 to 0.03. I would, in fact, make a delightful developmental study to watch it shift and to see whether it was gradual, whether there were sudden shifts, and at what month.

DR. RIEBER: The reason I reacted to "abruptness" was that I suspect that term has just as much ambiguity as the term "competence." It has many meanings, and we must specify which one we mean.

DR. LISA MENN: This is close to my own present area of research, where I'm working with a single child who is in the process of going through a transition from babbling to speech and doing some things that are rather in-between. One of the things that he learned very specifically, I think, during the first month I was observing him is how long a gap is permissible befre you should answer somebody else vocally. You know that this may be culturally determined, like the gap between speakers, the tone of your voice, and a lot of other things. I don't know whether it's a universal or a language-specific thing, but I do know that after a certain point, lags in conversational interaction, even though his contributions were all babbles of intonation contour, became to seem extremely normal. I would say something, and I would get a response. There were no more of these dead lags. Now, it was pretty sharp. I think it happened within the space of a month. It should be very easy to verify it, and I would suggest that this might be the right spot for the shift you're looking for. It could be earlier, because he already knew a great deal about speech. He was twelve months old at this point. But I would also guess that the shift you're looking for is probably complete shortly after this time. Again, this is subjective. I've got some video tape and tons of audio tape. Anyone is welcome to take them.

DR. KURT SALZINGER: I just wanted to make a comment on whether we're dealing with something that's ethologically an orienting response. I think obviously, there are many such things. But I think that before you jump into that pond, it's very important to establish it quite clearly. For example, consider the notion that the change of speaker is indicated by gazing back at the person that you've spoken to. I happen to have read a dissertation by Mary Ann LaFranz, and if she's here, I hope she'll help me. She had two Black speakers, middle-class Black speakers, and her point was that their signaling of the changing of the speaker was quite different, that they didn't even look at one another. She then went on and said that this is true of Blacks, to which I also object. The point is that you need much more data before you say it's an orienting response, before you say it's an ethnic response. It's too big a jump to say the kid is preparing for a later adult communication: i.e., to look back like this when you say "hello" to somebody.

DR. STERN: I disagree completely. First of all, with regard to whether you look at somebody at the end of a sentence or not, I grant you that's subject to cultural variation. However, the maternal response to the baby throwing his head up and gaping, plus vocalizing, may be a different matter. The reason that I think there's sufficient evidence to speculate about released behaviors is that Eiblsfeldt and Kendon have done cross-cultural studies showing that greeting behavior consisting of mouth opening, eyebrows up, and head back with or without vocalization is one of the most universal gestures among man in all the cultures they've looked at; so that when we see it as one of the most consistent things that mothers do in response to their infant's orientation and especially in response to a highly arousing set of facial behaviors that the infant throws at them, I think that we're on much safer ground and we're not just jumping into the pond.

DR. BATESON: Look, could I throw in one clarification here? We seem to be drifting into the same kind of problem that people who simply focus on language sometimes get into, where when silence occurs, it doesn't count. When gaze is broken, that doesn't mean that communication in that channel has stopped. It may be that the infant has a much, much smaller repertory of communicative gaze patterns than the adult, so that it is more important to focus on the sustained gaze. But when I am speaking to someone and going through this pattern that you describe, they can check throughout that pattern that I'm still handling my eyes in a way appropriate to continued speech. It's part of holding the floor; it isn't just part of not giving up the floor.

DR. RIEBER: We've come to the end of our time period. I do have an announcement or two, but perhaps we might end with an aphorism that summarizes our conversation here this afternoon. The aphorism is as follows: "Speak that I may see thee, but don't look at me in that tone of voice."

THE PLACE OF GRAMMAR IN A THEORY OF PERFORMANCE

David McNeill*

Institute for Advanced Study
Princeton, New Jersey 08540

My point will be that grammar and performance must be sharply distinguished. Indeed, they are so distinct that it is useless to seek relationships between them. They reflect distinct levels of analysis, each associated with a different range of questions about language. There is no a priori relationship between these different levels. In fact, it seems implausible to expect there to be psychologically interpretable connections of any kind between grammar and performance.

My point thus flies in the face of an opinion that has prevailed in psycholinguistics for the past 15 years, a view I will call the Miller-Chomsky requirement, after its first authors. However, the entire history of psycholinguistics, not only the parts of it contributed by Miller and Chomsky, has been dominated by this same view.

The Miller-Chomsky requirement states that performance is related to grammar in the following way: the device for performance generates the same structural description for sentences as the grammar generates. This requirement has been expressed repeatedly, although, in a curious failure of scholarship, successive writers seem to have been unaware that other writers have said the same thing and each thinks he has arrived at an original formulation. But it was expressed most clearly and succinctly the first time by Miller and Chomsky,[1] who put the requirement this way:

> We require . . . that M [the finite performance device] assign a structural description $F_i(x)$ to x only if the generative grammar G stored in the memory of M assigns $F_i(x)$ to x as a possible structural description. (p. 466)

The procedures M employs for computing this structural description are not specified. In particular, Miller and Chomsky do not assert that the rules of the generative grammar provide these procedures (this is contrary to a widespread belief); in fact, Miller and Chomsky barely consider this question at all.

Essentially the same requirement was described by Watt,[2] who, in addition, distinguishes between a formal linguistic grammar, prepared by linguists, and the mental grammar actually corresponding to a speaker's linguistic competence. The performance mechanism, again not discussed in any detail, provides structural descriptions that agree with those in the mental grammar:

> . . . between our MG [mental grammar] and what we say must be interposed a performance mechanism. . . . This performance mechanism composes sentences whose analyses accord with those given them by the MG, and imposes on input sentences the analyses they would have had if generated by the MG. (p. 140)

*On leave from the Committee on Cognition and Communication at The University of Chicago, Chicago, Ill.

A still more recent incarnation is in Fodor et al.:[3]

> There are thus intimate logical relations between an optimal grammar and a model of an ideal sentence recognizer for the language the grammar describes. Since the latter device assigns each utterance one of the structural descriptions that the former device generates, the output of the optimal grammar constrains the output of the ideal sentence recognizer. It should be recognized, however, that the grammar does *not*, in that sense, constrain the operations that the recognizer employs in *computing* its output (p. 277, italics in the original).

The ideal sentence recognizer mentioned here differs from a "real" recognizer in the addition of various psychological limitations, but there is no further discussion of this question.

As these quotes are meant to suggest, the development of psycholinguistics has been continuously under the guidance of the Miller-Chomsky requirement, as if no other conception of the problem were possible. As far as I can tell, there has been no deviation at all, for 15 years or so, from the view that the performance device, whatever it is, will employ operations that, while they do not have analogues in the rules of the grammar, will produce an output whose structure will be the same as the structure generated by the grammar. My view, in contrast, will be that there is no a priori reason to expect the Miller-Chomsky requirement to hold, that it is not even plausible to expect it to hold, and in fact, trying to apply it leads to absurdities.

The reason that it is not plausible for the Miller-Chomsky requirement to hold is that grammatical descriptions and performance descriptions relate to distinct levels of analysis.

The goals of a theory of linguistic performance I will take to include representing and, if possible, explaining the mental processes that listeners and speakers engage in during actual acts of recognizing and producing speech; for example, to describe the way in which speakers assemble utterances on the basis of the conceptual structures that are formed as the speaking process goes on, or the development of semantic images as sentence input takes place. These questions, of course, can be approached on many levels and in a variety of ways. I am not pleading for any special one of these, but only illustrating the goals of performance theory in what I trust is a noncontroversial form.

Why should the mental operations of performance not produce the structures that are generated by a grammar of the language, as proposed by the Miller-Chomsky requirement? The answer relies on analyzing the questions grammars have traditionally been constructed to answer. In fact, grammars are associated with a certain range of questions, and these are not readily associated with the different questions of performance theory, as I have taken them to be, above.

Indeed, a great many linguistic descriptions have the purpose of revealing the framework within which linguistic forms are related to each other. This tradition extends back many centuries. Transformations as conceived originally in Chomsky[4] and Harris[5] explicitly relate sentence structures of different types; for example, the structure of negative sentences to that of kernel sentences. The rules of transformation that accomplish these relationships are taken to reveal the structure of the language, i.e., the framework within which the types of sentences of the language are related. The modifications of transformational grammar that have occurred since 1957 have all remained inside this traditional domain. For example, Chomsky[6] defined transformations as the rules that relate internal (deep) structures to external (surface) structures, again a conception of linguistic structure that depends on the interrelation of forms. The further changes brought forth by the generative semanticists also stay within this framework (e.g., Lakoff[7]).

It is a simple matter to demonstrate the truth of this description of grammars by examining the form of linguistic argumentation. The process is devoted to revealing the relationships among structures. Rosenbaum,[8] for example, established that complements, italicized in (1), are a kind of Noun Phrase, since if they were not, the passive sentence (2) could not be derived by the passive transformation as usually stated, which operates only on Noun Phrases.

(1) Columbus demonstrated *that the world is not flat.*
(2) *That the world is not flat* was demonstrated by Columbus.

His argument, that is, hinges on the relationship between passive and nonpassive sentence types, and is directed toward segmenting complements so that this relationship between sentence structures can be stated. The argument, then, is directly adapted to the goal of revealing the framework in which sentence structures and other forms are related.

Notice, however, how far we have drifted from the goals given above for a theory of linguistic performance; that is, to describe and explain the mental operations that take place during actual occurrences of speech recognition and production. These goals have no obvious connection with the conception of grammatical structure just described. The structural descriptions of sentences that permit the rules of the grammar to relate sentence structures to other sentence structures within a systematic framework have no obvious bearing on the processes whereby the structures of single utterances are organized or interpreted. It may be shocking, incredible, or annoying to realize that there is no necessary or even plausible connection between two domains that feel as if they should be connected, but in fact there is no special reason to suppose that the interrelation of sentence structures and the mental processes involved in producing or recognizing utterances are connected, let alone connected in the precise way described by the Miller-Chomsky requirement. Not only is there no obvious way to connect grammar and performance, but if we force a connection the result is absurd. Should an explanation of how an utterance with a passive sentence structure is integrated during speech, for example, include an explanation of how the passive sentence is related to other sentences not uttered, in this case the active counterpart?

Nor is it particularly clear in what sense linguistic performance can be said to involve a grammatical parsing into such constituents as Sentence, Noun Phrase, Verb Phrase, etc. From a grammatical point of view, the meaning of these categories is clear. Part of the structural description of a passive sentence, according to Rosenbaum's treatment described above, for example, includes a NP that dominates an internal S. Clearly, one function of this bracketing is to permit one expression of the framework in which the active and passive sentence structures are related, i.e., the passive transformation in this case. Other functions similarly have to do with the interrelations of linguistic forms. For example, if *that the world is not flat* is a Noun Phrase, then it can be placed in other Noun Phrase contexts, as in *John remembered NP* (John remembered that the world is not flat), but this also is an interrelation of sentence structures. As far as I can tell, the parsing of sentences into grammatical constituents such as NP, VP, etc. always is done so as to make possible structural interrelations within a grammatical framework. Hence, there is no reason to assume, now applying the above conclusion, that a parsing into grammatical constituents plays any part in the psychological processes involved in the production or recognition of single utterances.

The elements in this process, in fact, seem to take a basically different form in which sound and meaning form a psychological unity. Kozhevnikov and Chistovich[9] referred to these units as "syntagmas," meanings that can be heard and meanings that can be spoken. Lashley[10] presented a similar idea in his seminal paper on the problem of serial order in behavior. If grammatical categories such as NP, VP, S, etc. play any part in the organization of syntagmas, this part would be basically different from the one played in a grammatical description and could not be considered as meeting the Miller-Chomsky requirement.

If grammatical terms are used in the descriptive vocabulary of an account of linguistic performance, this is a kind of pun. The terms S, NP, VP, etc. have a definite meaning in the framework that relates sentence structures to other sentence structures. These terms have a quite different meaning (and in fact a rather obscure one) in the context of the mental processes involved in recognizing or producing single utterances without regard to their relationships to other utterances. Indeed, the occurrence of the same terms in the vocabulary of both kinds of descriptions, gammatical and performance, would seem to be a fact of little or no significance unless one is willing to say that performance with single utterances actually includes a stage in which distinct sentence structures are interrelated. (Psycholinguists have not been beyond actually doing this, as described below.)

At this point one might reasonably suppose that, surely, any two things as generically similar as the framework in which sentence structures are related and the processes whereby sentences are recognized or produced must be somehow associated. Indeed, they are. The question is whether they are directly connected, or whether they are associated because each is connected to some third entity. It appears to me that the most plausible view is the latter one. I find it not plausible that the structure of anything as complex and ephemeral (considering actual speech) as language would ever be grasped as a whole within the limits of a single method, such as the interrelating of sentence structures. In fact, descriptions of the mental processes that take place during performance bring additional perspectives onto the true structure of language. It is useful to consider these further perspectives exactly because they are not directly connected to the grammatical perspective. There is no reason a priori to expect the grammatical framework of language and the mental processes of speakers or listeners to have any more in common than a generic resemblance due to each being a perspective view onto the same third thing, which is the true structure of language. And a generic resemblance seems to be the case.

The question of competence arises from a consideration of the epistemological foundations of a linguistic framework and of linguistic performance. It is not reasonable to dismiss grammar a a purely formal arrangement of linguistic objects. A grammatical description has validity as a partial characterization of linguistic competence, as is confirmed by many observations. Nonetheless, the grammatical framework in which sentence structures are interrelated is only a partial view of the underlying true structure of language. Surely, no one would disagree with this. My claim is that considerations of the actual operations of performance provide a different and also incomplete view of the true structure of language. Each view makes its contribution to the scientific understanding of language, but this addition of views is cancelled if, as has been the case, performance is required to converge on linguistic descriptions as in the Miller-Chomsky requirement.

Of course, one might question the terminological accuracy of referring to a grammar as a description of *competence*, if it is just one perspective view among others onto the true structure of language. If there is a true structure of language, different glimpses of which one obtains according to the method adopted, this true structure would be the individual's competence, this word being understood in its ordinary meaning. Competence, from this point of view, never comes fully into view, although we see more and more of it the larger the variety of perspectives we bring to bear.

Taking the Miller-Chomsky requirement to heart has led more than one psycholinguistic theory into the absurd position of trying to describe the mental operations that take place during the recognition of single sentence structures with a conceptualization of the problem that is fundamentally the comparison of two or more sentence structures. Illustrative examples are the kernelization hypothesis of Mehler,[11] the clausal hypothesis of Fodor et al.,[3] and the verification hypothesis of Clark and Chase.[12].

In each of these, it is necessary to posit a stage of processing, presumably reflecting the actual mental operations of the subject, that incorporates a sentence structure that is related to the sentence structure actually being processed. This hypothetical stage exists for no other reason than to meet the Miller-Chomsky requirement. For example, in Mehler's kernelization hypothesis, transformed sentences (passives, questions, negatives) are supposed to be understood by reducing them to the nontransformed sentences (kernels) to which they are related in the 1957 Chomsky theory Mehler used. In the clausal hypothesis of Fodor et al., all sentences are understood by relating them to one or more internal clauses (sentoids), the structure to which surface structures are related in the 1965 Chomsky theory that Fodor et al. use. In the Clark and Chase verification theory, negative sentences are understood by reducing them to propositions in which the affirmative version of the sentence appears as the argument and False appears as the predicate, this being the structure to which negative sentences are related in the semantic theory that Clark and Chase use.

These theories differ in the linguistic model to which they pledge allegiance, but they are as one in absurdly inserting a new structure that is related to the sentence structure actually being understood, just because it appears within the framework of a particular linguistic model.

Psycholinguistic processing needs to be described directly on its own terms. The connections to various grammatical descriptions will then come into view by themselves. Relative clauses, for example, can be described as utterances understood in a single pass without recovering internal sentences (Wanner and Maratsos[13]). Nevertheless, the semantic structures built up during this process contain the same internal relationships of meaning as an embedding of one sentence into another contains. The latter description is designed to show how sentences with relative clauses are related to other sentences not with relative clauses. In other words, there is a generic and somewhat impenetrable connection between grammar and performance descriptions as if they were related no more than that they are different views of the same third thing. Having these two perspectives onto relative clause structures is obviously more useful than having only one supplemented with a "performance device." For example, in the case of the Wanner-Maratsos theory, we can use aspects of the performance processing to explain aspects of the relative clause structure itself (such as why the relative pronoun is inflected to agree with the case assignment inside the relative clause). Our understanding of relative clauses is thereby deepened.

One might argue that the gap between performance and grammar is simply a temporary zone of obscurity due to our current limited understanding of language and language processing. Eventually, continuing this argument, a more general theory of cognition will be developed in which both linguistic performance and the interrelation of linguistic structures will find a place. This appears to be the position adopted by Pylyshyn.[14] Surely, no one would wish to object to such an attitude. However, it seems to be completely visionary. Either it reduces to a faith that, since everything is ultimately interconnected, why not grammar and performance too? or trying to be explicit, to the Miller-Chomsky requirement. The latter, in fact, is endorsed by Pylyshyn:

If the suggestion is that a model of the language user must, in describing a wider data base, also account for the type of structure captured by a generative grammar, then we are in agreement. [This is so because . . .] the development of a more general theory of cognition should proceed by attempting to account for the structure which is the output of a competence theory, together with other kinds of psychological evidence, rather than to incorporate the competence theory as formulated. (pp. 45–46)

Falling short of a universal theory of human intelligence in which grammar and the syntagmatic aspects of cognition are coherently integrated, Pylyshyn's view reduces to a reaffirmation of the principle that has already guided psycholinguistics for 15 long years, a principle, moreover, that leads to absurd results.

Nothing I have said should be construed as meaning that linguistic theory is irrelevant to the problem of explaining language performance. On the contrary, it follows from what I have said that in order to consider any question of performance, the relevant linguistic facts must be taken into account. It should not be construed as meaning, either, that linguistics as a science is concerned only with the interrelation of linguistic forms. In fact, much recent work by linguists is directed toward different goals, particularly the work on linguistic variation in social contexts. The interrelation of forms, nonetheless, is a traditional goal of linguistics and appears to be the goal most directly involved in the problems of competence and performance under discussion.

My concern in this paper has been with the difference in the level of analysis between grammar and linguistic performance and the correlated distinct goals of these two perspectives. Each is a special and partial view of linguistic competence. It seems unreal to assume, as has been done, that a particular method, that of relating linguistic structures to each other within a systematic framework, encompasses the entirety of the true structure of language. A multiplicity of approaches seems unavoidable. Following this line of thinking, we are led to reject the Miller-Chomsky requirement in which performance is viewed as a kind of aberration of grammar and to seek accounts of performance that stand on their own. In this way our depth of understanding of language and human cognition will be increased.

REFERENCES

1. MILLER, G. A. & N. CHOMSKY. 1963. Finitary models of language users. *In* Handbook of Mathematical Psychology. Vol. II. R. D. Luce, R. R. Bush & E. Galanter, Eds. John Wiley & Sons. New York, N.Y.
2. WATT W. C. 1970. On two hypotheses concerning psycholinguistics. *In* Cognition and the Development of Language. J. R. Hayes, Ed. John Wiley & Sons. New York, N.Y.
3. FODOR, J. A., T. G. BEVER & M. F. GARRETT. 1974. The Psychology of Language. McGraw-Hill Inc. New York, N.Y.
4. CHOMSKY, N. 1957. Syntactic Structures. Mouton. The Hague, The Netherlands.
5. HARRIS, Z. 1951. Methods in Structural Linguistics. Univ. Chicago Press. Chicago, Ill.
6. CHOMSKY, N. 1965. Aspects of the Theory of Syntax. MIT Press. Cambridge, Mass.
7. LAKOFF, G. 1970. Linguistics and Natural Logic. Studies in Generative Semantics No. 1, Department of Linguistics. Univ. Michigan. Ann Arbor, Mich.
8. ROSENBAUM, P. S. 1967. The Grammar of English Predicate Complement Constructions. MIT Press. Cambridge, Mass.
9. KOZHEVNIKOV, V. A. & L. A. CHISTOVICH. 1965. Speech, Articulation and Perception. Joint Publications Research Service, National Technical Information Service. Washington, D.C. (JPRS 30,543)
10. LASHLEY, K. S. 1951. The problem of serial order in behavior. *In* Cerebral Mechanisms in Behavior. L. A. Jeffress, Ed. New York: John Wiley & Sons. New York, N.Y.
11. MEHLER, J. 1963. Some effects of grammatical transformations on the recall of English sentences. J. Verb. Learning Verb. Behav. 2: 346–351.

12. CLARK, H. H. & W. G. CHASE. 1972. On the process of comparing sentences against pictures. Cognitive Psychol. 3: 472–517.
13. WANNER, E. & M. MARATSOS. An Augmented Transition Network Model of Relative Clause Comprehension. Dept. of Psychology. Harvard Univ. Cambridge, Mass. Unpublished.
14. PYLYSHYN, Z. W. 1973. The role of competence theories in cognitive psychology. J. Psycholinguistic Res. 2: 21–50.

ARE THEORIES OF COMPETENCE NECESSARY?

Kurt Salzinger

Biometrics Research Unit
New York State Psychiatric Institute
New York, New York 10032

Polytechnic Institute of New York
Brooklyn, New York 11201

Pick up almost any book on language and immediately you are confronted with the term "competence" followed by the injunction: You will make no progress in the study of language without taking competence into account. What is the meaning of this all-important term? According to Chomsky (Ref. 9, p. 4), competence refers to the "speaker-hearer's knowledge of his language," and performance (the other side of the coin) refers to "the actual use of language in concrete situations." Furthermore, he tells us: "Linguistic theory is concerned primarily with an ideal speaker-listener, in a completely homogeneous speech-community, who knows its language perfectly and is unaffected by such grammatically irrelevant conditions as memory limitations, distractions, shifts of attention and interest, and errors (random or characteristic) in applying his knowledge of the language in actual performance" (p. 3). While actual language use may provide some evidence regarding the mental reality underlying language behavior, he continues, it "surely cannot constitute the actual subject matter of linguistics, if this is to be a serious discipline" (p. 4).

A first reading of this enumeration of topics to be avoided, namely, memory, motivation, attention, and assorted social psychological, personality, and other psychological variables, suggests that this pronouncement is the preamble of some kind of nonaggression pact between the fields of linguistics and psychology: Linguistics promises not to infringe on the territory of psychology by studiously avoiding any attempt to explain anything that a psychologist might find of even remote interest, in exchange for which psychology promises to return the favor. However, as everybody knows, this is not true, for Chomsky (Ref. 9, p. 9) declares, "No doubt, a reasonable model of language use will incorporate, as a basic component, the generative grammar that expresses the speaker-hearer's knowledge of the language."

Then, having stated that he is interested in a mentalistic linguistics, Chomsky (p. 193) explains: "Mentalistic linguistics is simply theoretical linguistics that uses performance as data (along with other data, for example, the data provided by introspection) for the determination of competence, the latter being taken as the primary object of its investigation." In other words, although he is not interested in actual performance, with all its ugly obtrusive variables, he will use it to investigate competence. Elsewhere (Ref. 8, p. 36), we are warned that we must restrict our sense of performance data to those situations in which we may do so in "devious and clever ways." Although admitting behavioral data of some sort into his area of study, he nevertheless disposes of the behaviorists' opposition to mentalism by saying (Ref. 9, p. 193): "The behaviorist position is not an arguable matter. It is simply an expression of lack of interest in theory and explanation."

It might be well to make clear at the outset that behaviorists are indeed interested in theory—I shall assume nobody believes that behaviorists lack interest in explaining their data and will therefore not comment on that any further. Perhaps the

178

point can be made clearer by explaining that the behaviorist objection is only to theories that place the significant problems beyond the reach of empirical investigation. Skinner's[69] objection in his paper "Are theories of learning necessary?" (from which the title for my paper stems) was to the use of another dimensional system, such as psysiology or mental events, to explain something that was happening on a behavioral level. Whether a theory using physiological dimensions will become acceptable is a matter of obtaining the requisite data both in physiology and in behavior. A theory employing mental terms, however, gives rise to no data and therefore cannot become acceptable in the future, either.

But let us return to the problem of using some carefully selected segment of performance data to shed light on the competence of the speaker-hearer. Essentially such a procedure consists of the linguist deciding what part of the performance data to explain. It reminds me of Vonnegut's recent explanation of his published interview.[74] He describes it in the following way: "It is what I *should* have said, not what I *really* said . . . I went to work on the transcript with pen and pencil and scissors and paste, to make it appear that speaking my native tongue and thinking about important matters came very easily to me." (p. xxii)

I assume that in these introductory remarks I have made clear to those unacquainted with my views and work that my answer to the question posed in the title is a resounding "NO." I hope, in this paper, to catalogue the reasons for eliminating the concept of competence—at least for the psychologist, if not for the linguist. But even in linguistics, it is fair to say that the concept of competence is getting a bit frayed. Hymes, to take one outstanding linguist, has created the concept of communicative competence.[25] He rejects the idea that one first does an analysis of the structure of a language and then adds the knowledge of sociology to arrive at the area of sociolinguistics. Hymes (pp. 132–133) tells us: "There is no internal linguistic makeup that would lead one to group together 'See you later, alligator,' 'Ta Ta,' 'Au revoir,' 'Don't take any wooden nickels,' 'Glad you could come' . . . as leave-takings." He gives further reasons[25] for the necessity of broadening what he calls the restricted concept of grammatical competence, by including such social factors as would explain utterances by a secretary on the telephone, e.g. "May I say who's calling?" For here the appropriate answer as given by the generative grammar approach would be just "Yes" when the linguistic competence called for is the translation into the question "Who's calling?", with "May I say . . ." to be responded to as a polite form.

Hymes also comments on Chomsky's concept of creative language use. A sentence called novel solely by internal criteria may be inappropriate or bizarre when the context is taken into account, whereas a sentence not regarded as novel by internal criteria may indeed be so because it occurs in a novel context. Finally, in a demand for the "liberation" of the concept of competence from being simply a synonym of the word "grammar," Hymes (Ref. 25, p. 205) asks that the concept of competence refer to "abilities actually held by persons." Those abilities are not distributed equally among all people, nor are they so distributed among situations. Hymes wants to restore the old meaning to the word "competence," that is, a summary statement about the behavior that the individual is likely to emit at some future time. Other sociolinguists make the same point that Hymes makes; they maintain that there is no such thing as linguistics without the social part: There is only sociolinguistics.

Generative grammar has also been criticizd by those linguistics not yet convinced of the wisdom of sociolinguistics. Derwing[13] makes a detailed study of Chomsky's system. His book should be read by linguistics and psycholinguistics alike, for he has carefully analyzed Chomsky's writings and those of his students, pointing out both the contradictions in their work and the ultimate lack of testability of the theory.* Derwing's summary statement (p. 321) is worth quoting: "The chief argument of this book has been that contemporary linguistics has gone fundamentally astray, both conceptually and methodologically."[13]

For those who feel that linguistics must have something to contribute to the psychology of language, there is some solace to be had. One needs to look for those linguists who view the empirical examination of real language behavior as the cornerstone of their work. One such linguistic approach is called form-content analysis. Originated by William Diver at Columbia University, it has been applied to Spanish by Garcia[18] and to German by Zubin,[75] to mention but two examples. The approach is diametrically opposed to Chomsky's basic assumptions that one should exclude human factors from attempts to understand language. Garcia points out the difference between the two systems by showing that Chomsky postulates a nonrandomness of signals to be explained by a formal system of rules regarding the signals in terms of the criteria of simplicity of description; Diver speaks of nonrandomness of vocal movements in people who are trying to communicate with signals that have meaning. Thus for Diver and his students, the dichotomy of competence and performance is simply not possible. They use such human functions as memory, laziness (cf. Zipf's Law of Least Effort), and avoidance of complexity as factors to explain the use of certain words, in particular, grammatical classes.

Zubin[75] tested the hypothesis, in the German language, that the greater the causality of a noun, the greater the probability that it will be in the dative rather than in the accusative case after verbs of avoidance. He verified this hypothesis by constructing different situations for the native German speakers who were asked to construct sentences describing what happened. To give only one example, when Zubin described a person as avoiding a car because it stands in his way, the subjects summarized the situation using the dative 14% of the time, but when he described the same person as avoiding a car that is driving toward him, the subjects used the dative 100% of the time. Clearly the dative morphological signal connotes more activity in the noun it is applied to than does the accusative morphology. This is only an example, but it shows both the usefulness of including nonlinguistic factors in considering the reason for grammatical structure, and the empirical nature of the validation procedure that can be applied to grammatical problems.

Before presenting my catalogue of reasons for the elimination of the concept of competence, allow me to refer you to some papers in which I deal with the generative model as a whole[46,50,51] (see also Ref. 55, introduction), so that I will be able, here, to concentrate on the concept of competence.

Competence as a Long, Complicated Promissory Note

The time is long overdue for that performance model that Miller and Chomsky[37] promised us will contain the competence model as an essential part. There are a number of reasons for the nonfulfillment of the promise. To begin with, there is the abyss that exists between competence and performance. Repeatedly we are warned that competence merely contains the rules of the system that accounts for the sentences that English speaker-hearers *could* construct—if only they were perfect—and that what we need is a performance model that would account for the failings in the human being that prevent him or her from manifesting the perfection of the

---

*Many of the points that I will make in this paper are also made in Derwing's book. Even though I came across this book late in the writing of this paper, it was a delight to find it. I thank David Zubin for pointing it out to me.

competence model. The performance model is a device that shows how we forget and are distracted and thus are unable to embed forever, as the competence model tells us we must. The competence model is simply a logical system. As a consequence, it is very difficult indeed to know where to begin to connect it to something real, such as speech.

In addition to ruling out all those things that psychologists study in human behavior, the competence model begins with a unit that is quite arbitrary, namely, the sentence; there are, after all, a great many other possible units,[52] and there are a great many things that people actually say that are not sentences (cf. Hymes, above.[25]) Perhaps we would be better off having an *incompetence* model in addition to the competence model to take care of all the nonsentences and the nongrammatical utterances that serve to cause trouble, since the competence model is only about those grammatical sentences that a generative grammarian considers so. In a commentary on a paper by Chomsky,[10] Black[2] spoke of the sentence as a "grammarian's artifact," pointing out that speaking an indefinitely long sentence is about as far removed from actually talking as walking an indefinitely long distance is from actually walking. Black also objected to the procedure of verification of the grammaticality of the sentences. Comparing the verification of Chomsky's system with that of Kepler's Laws of the Planetary Motions, Black[2] says: "We cannot ask a planet how it thinks it ought to be behave in situations that don't arise: yet this seems to be what we are doing when we consult a native 'informant'." (p. 454) In response, Chomsky[11] maintains that in Kepler's case a telescope has the same role as an informant has in Chomsky's. He insists that there is no difference in principle between the two verification procedures.

However, when I criticized Chomsky for being unable to show that grammaticalness can be reliably judged by native speakers of English, as his system requires,[46] he responded (Ref. 12, p. 93): "Obviously, the failure [to find a reliable division between grammatical and nongrammatical strings] indicates nothing more than that the tests were ineffective. One can invent innumerable tests that would fail to provide some given classification. Surely the classification itself is not in question. Thus, Salzinger would agree, quite apart from any experimental test that might be devised, that the sentences of this footnote share an important property that does not hold of the set of strings of words formed by reading each of these sentences, word by word, from right to left." This statement makes clear that Chomsky does indeed wish to impose a principle for the verification of grammar different from that for the verification of the Laws of Planetary Motion, for it is hard to conceive of asking for the validation of Kepler's Laws by appealing to judgments of certain extreme values only. If we find it difficult to agree on some sentences but easy on others, then Chomsky wishes to appeal only to the simple ones to verify the theory. In sum, the promissory note has not been redeemed because the basic model does not lend itself to the explication of behavior which Chomsky calls by the derogatory term "performance."

Competence as an Idealization

One argument that Chomsky gives for the great discrepancy between the competence model and behavior is that the competence model is an idealization. But we must ask: An idealizaton of what? If it is an idealization of language behavior, why does it exclude from consideration so many sentences and so many nonsentences that we know to occur? On the other hand, if it is an idealizatoin of an underlying neurophysiological system to explain how language is produced and understood— something often implied by the generative grammarians—why are all the terms basically behavioral and the verification procedure one of intuition? The answer to both questions appears to be that the idealization is restricted to that of a generative grammarian as speaker-hearer when at work on the model.

The idealization of competence fails as an attempt at reductionism for the following reasons: For reductionism to succeed, it must formalize both the reducing and the reduced sciences. The competence model that we are presented seems, on the contrary, to do neither, for it deals with a level that is neither behavioral nor neurophysiological, although it is closer to the behavioral level, and the terms are of such a nature as to make translation into the neurophysiological science no easier. In addition, not only is it true, even by Chomsky's own admission, that we have not yet formalized language behavior (performance, if you must call it that) but we do not yet have the knowledge, never mind the formalization, in biology, the reducing science, for the reduction. Luria,[34] one of our foremost biologists, in an article eager to show how biology can help to explain language behavior, says, after stating that the justification for treating language as a biological phenomenon comes from Chomsky's "observation" that all human language is based on innate grammatical and syntactic structures (p. 28): "How to approach the biology of human language and thereby also the biology of the human mind is not yet easy to see." In other words, reductionism as an approach to the study of language is beset by only two problems: 1) We do not know enough to formalize language behavior, and 2) we do not have enough data in biology to begin the formalization there. Turner (Ref. 73, p. 334) says: ". . . reductionism as an article of faith in the absence of a well-structured secondary science (psychology) is a trivial thesis." The idealization cum reduction that Chomsky presents us then fails on the grounds that reductionism is not possible under the present circumstances.

In his book on Psychological Explanation, Fodor states (Ref. 15, p. 134): "A theory that predicts the observational data but fails to predict correctly the relevant counterfactuals is a false theory, whatever the area of science in which it may be entertained." The model or theory or idealization must predict not only behavior that is observed, but it must also *not predict* behavior that does *not* occur. The interesting fact about the competence model is that it predicts grammatical sentences unlimited in length (let us, for the sake of argument, agree that we know what they are) and it shows quite clearly that it cannot generate ungrammatical strings. The model then fails on both counts. First, it fails to generate the nongrammatical strings that we can observe to occur, and then it predicts the generation of infinitely long sentences with infinite embeddings that we know cannot occur.

It is interesting to quote Miller (Ref. 36, p. 88) in this context: "Chomsky's achievement was to prove rigorously that any language that does *not* restrict this kind of recursive embedding contains sentences that cannot be spoken or understood by devices, human or mechanical, with finite memories." Miller uses that as an argument for the distinction between competence and performance; that is, between the idealization and the real behavior. But should we not conclude that any model predicting behavior so obviously absurd both logically (as proved by Chomsky) and empirically (as shown by many experiments, if not by common sense) ought to be abandoned? I have not yet had the opportunity to study the recent book by Fodor et al.,[16] but in their discussion of sentence perception, I find that they are in agreement with my view. They say (p. 279): "Any model of the ideal speaker-hearer which is incompatible with whatever is known about the rest of human psychology is ipso facto disconfirmed."

Let us turn to another aspect of the competence model. It assumes that one model is sufficient for both the speaker and the hearer. The question that I would like to raise about this turns on both the logical and the empirical grounds for the assumption. Fraser et al.[17] performed an experiment in which they thought they had shown that children understand more than they can speak, and that therefore the acquisition of language could not take place through the reinforcement of speech. Of course, behavior theory does not assume that language is acquired through one mechanism only. Nevertheless, Fernald[14] showed that their experiment did not prove the precedence of comprehension to production, since the comprehension measure had had a contaminating statistical advantage not present in their production measure.

Shipley et al.,[67] also interested in language as stimulus, performed an experiment in which children were given certain verbal directions. The children did better in following directions presented in well-formed structures than in telegraphic form, even though they could not at that age produce such well-formed structures. Again it looked as if the children's comprehension, which is assumed in these studies to better reflect competence, exceeded their production. Brown,[4] however, interpreted the findings to mean that the children responded in a puzzled way to the telegraphic speech of their mothers because their mothers did not ordinarily speak that way. What looked like superior performance in response to the well-formed sentences was better explained by poorer performance in response to telegraphic speech.

Luckily, we have another study bearing directly on this question. Kramer[26] repeated the study with some improvements. She presented anomolous sentences to children, that is, sentences that asked them to do things which are peculiar, or at least unusual, such as "Sit on the telephone." The children responded to these kinds of structures by essentially correcting them semantically. They *spoke* on the telephone rather than sitting on it. Furthermore, when addressed in telegraphic speech—that is, with commands minus function words—they did as well in following the instructions as when they were given the same directions in well-formed sentences. Again we find that comprehension does not exceed performance. But perhaps more important, the study shows that the child, like the adult, makes use of whatever information he or she is given or has available in responding. The concept of response bias seems to explain a great deal here. Having learned earlier that one *speaks* on the telephone, the child on hearing the word "telephone," does what he or she has been reinforced to do in the past. Thus, while the child appears to follow some complicated, well-structured sentence-form requiring the knowledge of an arcane system of rules, the child is in fact merely following the surrounding stimuli in the only way he or she has learned. The issue then is not whether the child comprehends before speaking, or vice versa, or does both at the same time; the issue concerns what stimuli control the behavior of the child. The concept of the functional stimulus cannot be ignored in this area any more than in any other. What the speaker-hearer model gains in simplicity by proposing one system for both, it loses in real life where organisms respond in the most direct way possible. The normal redundancy of an utterance is usually strengthened by its redundancy with the environment, the past history of communication, the facial expression, other gestures, and so on. Thus, conversation always involves a multiplicity of stimuli, only some of which are verbal, and only a subset of those are grammatical.

Competence as a Flight from Simplicity

It sounds simpler to have one system for both comprehension and production, but the step left out is the required analysis-by-synthesis to achieve understanding. I have commented on such models in detail elsewhere.[51] The behavioral model, on the other hand, says that the organism responds to the stimulus that has the greatest evoking power at that time and place. It is for that reason that when we read or hear, we often make a mistake in interpretation, or we understand something correctly even though it is stated in a misleading way when analyzed carefully but in the absence of the environment in which it was emitted. The above studies with children simply show the same tendency in them, namely, to interpret puzzling utterances in a familiar way rather than to spend time worrying about the ambiguity of the utterance.

Although generative grammarians have always emphasized ambiguity, it has been a concept of importance only in their system and not in actual speech. Real people always take into account stimuli around them: stimuli that precede the utterance, the speaker, the hearers, etc. The compound stimulus then functions to evoke a response that allows the conversation to continue. Furthermore, unlike the generative grammarian who can only reread the same isolated puzzling sentence, the real speaker or hearer has the option of asking "What?" or "What do you mean?", or the like. The fact that ambiguity is not to be tolerated in actual social intercourse is at least partially demonstrated by some of our studies in which we have found that hospitalized schizophrenic patients speak in an ambiguous way and that the more ambiguous or the less understandable they are, the longer their stay in the hospital.[61-63]

Another case where we are faced with the choice of a simpler vs. a more complex model is with respect to the perception of clicks and language stimuli simultaneously presented. The idea was that the subject would be able to perceive clicks more readily between than within units of the sentence and would therefore report the occurrence of the click at the boundaries, thus supplying us with information concerning the existence of the units. Ingenious as this technique is, it fails to exclude those basic variables which enter all experiments in perception. There are what Reber[43] calls "response biases" and the subject's general attentional priorities that also control his "placement" of the click. To be sure, Bever[1] has responded to these criticisms, but it is not yet entirely clear what kind of variable of what particular level of unit[72] the phenomenon of click migration reflects. It is one thing to make experiments "clever and devious," as Chomsky suggests; it is another altogether to show exactly which variable controls the outcome. The fact that speech is not orinarily devoid of accompanying stimuli directing the hearer suggests that the study restricted to the utterances only may well be an impossible task.

The notion of responding to simpler rather than more complex stimuli is fortified by what we know about the behavior of animals. Such seemingly complex responses as movement toward an environment of high humidity, as in the woodlouse, can be explained by what ethologists call "kinesis," an undirected movement varying with the intensity of stimulation. Thus, although the end product of the movement in the woodlouse that moves more in dry than in wet environments is to bring it into wet environments, it is clear from empirical study that this is not movement toward or away from environments of particular humidity. The mechanisms organisms have that allow them to achieve certain ends are very often quite different from what a superficial inspection might suggest. The mechanism underlying a particular act need not contain within it the end which is in fact achieved. From what we know about the evolution of animals, the idea that human beings should have been given a particular device somewhere in the brain for recognizing sentences or for separating grammars from one another seems rather far-fetched when one considers the kinds of slow and small changes that take place over time and yet that have rather profound effects on the interaction of the organism with its environment.

Although it has been argued for some time, and most persuasively, by Lenneberg[30] that speech in human beings is unique among the animals now extant and that only a discontinuity theory of language evolution could explain human speech, recent research[19,20,41,42,44] has shown that the nonhuman primates are capable of learning language as long as we do not try to make them vocalize, a response that is difficult for them to execute for peripheral-musculature and vocal-cavity reasons, rather than because of some deficit in the brain, as Lenneberg would have us think.[30] And so while Chomsky and his students tell us that language is species-specific and everybody dutifully repeats it, some psychologists have proceeded to examine the question empirically despite its logical absurdity. At this point, those who were surprised that nonhuman primates could learn to communicate in ways quite similar to ours have retreated by quickly adjusting their definition of what constitutes language; the final point of retreat, I imagine, will have to be the ability to say what Noam Chomsky says about language. If one of the nonhuman pimates can be trained to say that, then perhaps we will have to accept the notion that the human being is not the one and only possessor of true language.

Competence as a Modifier in Noun's Clothing

It is my contention that when we make a noun of an adjective, we run the danger of reification. We all know what happened when the adjective "unconscious" was turned into a noun: People began to speak of *the* unconscious and to look for things inside it; they began to speak of taking things out and they even paid specialists to remove things. Now, with respect to competence, we seem to have the same problem. It is one thing to say that an individual is competent or even that his or her behavior appears to be competent, but when one begins to speak of a person's competence, one comes just a little closer to the notion of asking for its location and its content. After all, if you have a competence, you must have it somewhere, and if you have it somewhere, you must have something in it. It is for this reason that Chomsky did not content himself with the word "grammar" to describe what he means by competence. For grammar, in our experience, already has an external referent, as in grammar books, and so would not have done for Chomsky's model. The fact that this competence now lies inside the body also means that one need not examine real verbal interchange to study it, since all the necessary information is internalized. And finally, this change of part of speech allows one to hide in the competence attic all the problems that one would ordinarily have to examine downstairs in the living room where the performance takes place.

Competence as a Concept in Fact's Clothing

Once the competence was located inside the organism, it was not long before people started to speak about explaining the facts of competence. Even at this conference, the speakers of this session were assigned the task of examining *how*, not *if*, the notion of competence could be used to account for linguistic performance. Since when does the investigator holding to one theory have to account for the concepts which the holder of another theory uses to explain his or her data? But this is how far we have come. It is my hope that after you have read this paper, it will be quite clear that competence is a model, not a fact. For after all, the only thing which any investigator has to account for is data, not theory. We are virtually surrounded by logical and so-called "common-sense" arguments for the necessary existence of competence. The richness of language itself has been used to show that there must be some built-in device that makes it possible for us to acquire it "so quickly"; and yet we have very little measurement of the rapidity of language acquisition; on the other side, we have an increasingly greater accumulation of data showing that the acquisition of language behavior continues for a much longer period of time than was originally suggested.

We are regularly confronted with the "obvious impossibility" of having children learn language word by word without the rules that the competence model says we have built into our language-acquisition devices. But this is a straw child. For no behavior theorist maintains that any response, including the lowly bar press of the rat or even the more circumscribed pecking response of the pigeon, is acquired without the mechanism of response generalization hard at work, without, that is, the concept of response class.[46] In addition, and contrary to the assertions of generative grammarians, psychologists are not reduced to dealing with behavior sliced in arbitrary ways, with one atrophied unit size. On the contrary, because of their use of functional definitions of responses, they are not in any way tied down to any preordained unit size. Behavior theory is quite comfortable with the idea that in the presence of one set of stimuli, one unit size may be the crucial one, while in the presence of another, another unit size may be appropriate. Furthermore, the idea of different-size units at the same time is also acceptable. A great deal of rather interesting research has been in progress for some time concerning concurrent responses in behavior theory,[6] and a full discussion of the problem of unit size in verbal behavior appears elsewhere.[52]

It is clear that under some circumstances unit size may be very small, such as the phoneme, whereas under others it may be the word, phrase, clause, sentence, paragraph, story, essay, argument, or description. The importance of the flexibility of such unit-size definitions is that they reflect the actual functional relationship of the stimuli surrounding the responses in question.

To review, language behavior is considered by behavior theorists to consist of varying unit sizes. The responses are also always considered as members of various response classes. Thus, to give an example, members of the same response class may differ in length but may be evoked by the same stimulus, e.g., a fire. That kind of event may evoke the responses, "Oh!" "Help!" "There's a fire here!," and the making of a telephone call, running away, an increase in heart rate, etc. The problems involved in the definition of response classes are discussed in detail in Reference 46.

Competence as a Roadblock to Language Modification

This brings us to the problem of whether language behavior is assumed to have been acquired by a process of learning or whether it is viewed primarily as the result of an unfolding process. If it is primarily the latter, then we must face every deficit in language behavior as something built in by competence; on the other hand, if we assume that language behavior is learned and maintained through the variables of behavior theory, then we are at least in a position to try to improve the behavior. I am not trying to say that the basic assumption that language behavior is learned makes it true—although I shall contend that we have much data to defend such a view. I am saying that by making the opposite assumption, that language is almost completely a matter of maturation, we forestall investigation into the possibility of modification.

The facts of history are that operant conditioners simply ignored Chomsky's so-called devastating review[7] of Skinner's *Verbal Behavior*. [70] Beginning with Greenspoon's experiment in 1955[21] based on previous work by Skinner, on the conditioning of plural nouns, an onslaught of verbal conditioning studies was unleashed [45,48,27,23] which showed the possibilities of this paradigm in many fields of psychology, including social, developmental, and especially abnormal psychology. Response classes of various kinds, and units of different lengths, were used in the experiments. Some of these studies were diverted by an uninformed determination to be precise, with the unfortunate result of reducing the operant conditioning of verbal behavior to a rote memory experiment consisting of the pairing of one of three pronouns with a single past-tense verb, all printed on little 3 X 5 index cards. Such experiments, set up essentially as problem-solving tasks for sophomore students, deteriorated into controversy over whether or not there can be any conditioning without awareness. Much of this material is well summarized by Krasner,[28] so I shall comment only that there are indeed situations in which verbal conditioning is possible without the subjects being aware of it.

In our experiments on self-referred affect statements in normal and schizophrenic patients,[58-61] we conditioned subjects while they were even unaware that an experiment was going on, never mind that they were being conditioned. In another experiment we demonstrated response generalization from positive to negative affect and vice versa.[40] We[64] found that the conditioning of plural nouns was possible in the context of continuous speech, with plural nouns ending in the /z/ sound being more conditionable than those ending in the /s/ sound. The subjects' reinforcement history clearly interacted with their current conditioning. While response class membership is thus a matter for empirical investigation, conditioning does take place. These basic experiments made clear that operant conditioning can be applied to verbal behavior.

In an experiment in which a papier maché clown served as the source of reinforcement by turning on his light-bulb nose and delivering candy, S. Salzinger and others in our laboratory[65] conditioned young children to speak at various rates by using different schedules of reinforcement. Of interest with respect to the concept of response class was the fact that children reinforced for the emission of general self-references showed an increase, not only in the self-references, but also in their total amount of speech, because most of their speech dealt with themselves. Again we find an interaction between the reinforcement procedure and reinforcement history.

The application of reinforcement procedures to children with little or no speech was attempted in our laboratory in 1965[47,56] as well as in others about the same time (e.g. as summarized by Lovaas in 1973[31]). Many children without speech can, by means of well-planned schedules of reinforcement and by programming various situations appropriate to the emission of verbal responses desired at each stage of learning, be trained to speak. This kind of conditioning situation provides not only the possibility of helping children to acquire language who more often than not are left unhelped because of the implication that they are suffering from brain damage the effect of which cannot be altered, but also provides the observer with the opportunity to watch the acquisition of language in slow motion, so to speak. In our observations of one four-year-old boy, whom we conditioned, we noticed, after he had learned to name objects in his environment, that the introduction, by imitation training, of an utterance of more than one word gave him a very useful tool for the further utilization of language. In one session he was reinforced for saying "Give me candy" instead of, as before, for simply saying "candy." Having learned that the emission of the full utterance "Gimme (we accepted this approximation to "give me") candy" resulted in his getting candy, he generalized the use of the frame "Gimme_____".to anything else that he wanted. This use resembled the pivot-open construction that is now in some disrepute, but obviously it was a construction strengthened by its specific reinforcing property, the kind of verbal response that Skinner[70] called a mand. Here, the critical variable was the reinforcing consequence.

In contrast to the competence model, the behavior-theory model would also try to improve the language behavior of those children who do not get the appropriate kind of training to use their language in such a way as to be reinforced by the establishment in society. Staats treats this problem particularly with respect to reading,[71] but many additional studies have been done and are to be found in the *Journal of Applied Behavior Analysis*. Studies of this kind are also reviewed in Salzinger.[78]

The general point to be made with respect to competence is that by assuming that it is innate without specific evidence for it, except in terms of such generalities as the common time of language acquisition—which could, after all, be explained by common types of environments, especially early in life when all human infants depend to a large extent on an adult—an obstacle is set up in the path of helping people. The history of operant conditioning is replete with instances in which we were told that a particular behavioral deficit is psychologically determined and therefore cannot be modified, when a judicious application of behavior modification found this to be untrue. It is important that we not blame the faults in our environment on the children through the making of unwarranted assumptions.

Competence as a Roadblock to a General Theory of Behavior

Just how special is the human being? The evolution of science is punctuated by periods of controversy about the centrality of *homo sapiens*. First we had to give up the centrality of our world, then we were forced to admit our relationship to other primates, at least with respect to our anatomy and physiology, then we ungraciously admitted that at least some of our responses resembled those of the animals, then we granted that we did not always know what we were doing, and finally, we allowed that at least some, if not all, of our behavior was determined by the environment. We are still trying to sequester unto ourselves the notion that only human beings think, and we are fighting at our last bastion to claim that only human beings have language. The data are nevertheless assailing us here also. I have already alluded to them. The fact is that chimpanzees have already constructed utterances with plastic forms, by means of sign language, or by pressing buttons on a computer. Furthermore, these responses have the productive or creative aspect that linguists have for so long attributed solely to human beings. At least Washoe, the signing chimpanzee of the Gardners, was found signing to herself while "reading" a picture book, although, to be sure, she was doing it while up in a tree.

What are the advantages in considering a human being as an animal? There are many. We have much data about animals under a variety of circumstances, with and without invasion of their neurophysiological and biochemical systems. We find a great deal of order in these data. In the course of our research we have found that it is fruitful to extrapolate to human beings, in terms of both the data and the generalizations drawn from them. The experiments applying behavior theory to human beings have also been successful (see Ref. 49). Thus when we speak of stimulus control, we have a concept that has proved itself useful not only in describing the behavior of animals but also the behavior of people in a variety of situations. Behavior theory has been successfully utilized in education whether through programmed instruction or more effective teaching techniques, in abnormal psychology in the more humane control of psychotic behavior and in the more effective treatment of neurotic behavior, in social psychology in the more precise description of social interaction, in psychophysics in the elucidation of the concept of threshold, with signal-detection theory to give it a mathematical foundation, in psychopharmacology in the precise and effective pretesting of drugs and their effects on behavior, in developmental psychology in the better handling of children and the gaining of a surer understanding of their behavior, in physiological psychology by providing the precision of behavior control against which physiological theories can be effectively tested, and in the better understanding of the interaction of the behavior within the skin and that without.

Given a theory of behavior as powerful as that, it seems foolish to avoid using it to shed light on the language behavior of human beings. To insist that human beings must be different and that they cannot be traced through the history of evolution seems like a willful attempt to leave unused the most powerful tool we have in psychology for uncovering the sources of our language behavior. Embracing a competence model based on the premise of exclusivity seems foregone to be a failure on that count alone.

The caricatures that pass for descriptions of behavior theory in the area of psycholinguistics accuse behavior theorists of failing to believe in the organism. This is not justified. Behavior theorists view psychology as a biological science, and therefore view the neurophysiology and the biochemistry determined by the genes and the somatoplasm of the organism as variables. The competence model, on the other hand, views the organism as a constant. Current findings suggest that both the inside and the outside of organisms are conditionable by the same general paradigms.

In contrast to the competence model, behavior theory looks for those properties in the organism that make it sufficiently flexible to acquire language. A few years ago I made up a list of five such properties for language as stimulus and language as response.[53] If we need a concept like competence, then those are the properties we should examine.

The first property is *language-learning potential*. Essentially, this property suggests the investigation of the various response systems of an organism to determine if any of these systems could be efficiently accommodated to serving the function of language. Assuming that something needs to be learned in order to have a language such as human beings have, we would turn our attention to the modifiability of the response systems—whether they can be modified by imprinting, by respondent conditioning, or by operant conditioning.

The second property is *general learning capacity*. Any animal that can, in general, be only minimally influenced by its environment would not be expected to develop a language dependent on the kinds of modification which must be mediated by the environment. We have a large literature on the learning ability of various animals.

The third critical property for language development is *verbal response availability*. Recent investigators of language in chimpanzees made a breakthrough because they looked for a response system that had a high-enough rate. Essentially, we are saying that the response allowing the organism to communicate must have an operant level high enough for the process of reinforcement to act on it. An individual incapable of producing sounds cannot be expected to develop language by vocalizing, but may acquire it through signs.

The fourth property necessary for language is the *relative verbal response conditionability*. In human beings, verbal behavior is eminently conditionable. In selecting an animal's response for language, one must select a system that has already been shown to respond to conditioning procedures.

The fifth property is the *regulating function*. Generative grammarians and modern psycholinguists have shown a singular lack of interest in this very important function. An outstanding theoretical treatment has come from Luria.[32,33] He was able to show a regular progression over age of verbal control over nonverbal responses. It seems to me that no matter how convoluted your grammatical system, if it does not reveal how language guides nonverbal and verbal behavior, the model is incomplete.

Before leaving the issue of the blocking effect of the competence model on a general theory, I would like to describe the inadequacies of the attempts by psycholinguists to discredit the behavior theory model in the area of language behavior. In 1966, McNeil[35] presented the following anecdote to demonstrate the futility of employing behavior theory to explain the acquisition of language: The mother is trying to get the child to stop using the double negative in "Nobody don't like me." Despite the mother saying "No" and repeating to the child "Nobody likes me" some ten times, the child finally says, "Oh, Nobody don't likes me." (p. 69) It is peculiar that the mother should have chosen to correct the *grammar* of this very self-abnegating statement. One possibility is that in this interchange the mother's repetitive statements are positive reinforcers that keep the child going. Mother and child may be playing a game.

If the mother was being serious, however, it mght be well to point out that a change in this behavior could be brought about by other methods. One would use shaping procedures along with repetitions of parts of the desired phrase or sentence. In addition to the use of an inefficient modification procedure, the mother was also hampered by a lack of supporting environmental stimuli. There is no obvious discriminative stimulus for the statement involved, and the constant repetition, in the absence of an appropriate stimulus, appears to be an insufficient condition for learning even when language learning is viewed as a learning of rules. Moeser and Bregman[38,39] showed that the rules for a miniature language system were not learned in the absence of pictures corresponding to each of the sentences, even when 3,200 trials were presented, although class membership of new words could be learned through verbal context alone, once the rules based on the sentences with pictures had been acquired. Thus the fact that the child seemed unable to dispense with the double negative did not provide evidence for a "stage" in language maturation. Rather, it reflected inadequate learning conditions.

In another attempt to show that behavior theory does not explain the acquisition of language, Brown and Hanlon[5] investigated what they call "communication pressure" at a time when the children are supposedly acquiring new grammatical structures. They classified the child's questions into well-formed ones and into non-well-formed ones, and the interlocutors' responses into "sequiturs" and "nonsequiturs." By their definition, the answer "We ate them all" to the question"Where Christmas cookies?" was a sequitur (an answer that showed that the question was understood) to a question not well formed; the answer "Your spoon?" to the question "Where my spoon?", on the other hand, was considered to be a nonsequitur, since it consisted of a question, not an answer. They found no significant differences in the number of sequiturs or nonsequiturs to the child's well-formed or non-well-formed questions, and concluded that there was no selective communication pressure.

This study fails to show a lack of communication pressure in children, not because there is none, but because of a number of methodological errors. The sampling of the consequences evoked by the questions is unduly restricted. Presumably, a sequitur ought to have some positively reinforcing properties—but how can it, when, while showing comprehension of the question, it informs the child that he may not have the cookies? Furthermore, it is not at all clear that the partial repetition of the child's statement (the nonsequitur in the analysis) might not be functioning as a positive reinforcer even though it does *not* show full comprehension of the question. At times, merely giving the child attention by making a verbal response may suffice as a reinforcer. At other times, presenting a discriminative stimulus—

that is, a stimulus in the presence of which a response is positively reinforced—may evoke another utterance of the same kind. At some times, the critical reinforcer may be nonverbal—a smile, a look, a cookie, a toy; at others, it may be verbal—repetition of what the child said, agreement, praise, or the telling of a story. Only observation of a good deal of behavior and its consequences can make clear what responses are being reinforced and what the reinforcers are in each case. The classification system that Brown and Hanlon used to decide that no communication pressure toward more grammatical speech existed, partially confounded their classification system with the classification system of positive reinforcer, negative reinforcer, and punisher.

Brown and Hanlon tested the relevance of behavior theory in another way as well. They related syntactically correct and incorrect speech to contingent approval and disapproval. Within the former category, they included statements such as "That's right," "Correct," "Very good," and "Yes"; in the latter category, they included statements such as "That is wrong," "That's not right," and "No." They found relatively few occurrences of these kinds of approval and disapproval. Among those few occurrences that they did find, the parents did not approve more often of the syntactically correct structures than of the others. Here are some examples of the data they found (p. 49): "Child: 'Draw a boot paper.' Mother: 'That's right. Draw a boot on paper.' Child: 'Mama isn't boy, he a girl.' Mother: 'That's right.'"[5] What can we make of this?

First, we must remember that these conversations by no means include all the reinforcers or even the significant ones in these situations. Food, cookies, attention, hugging, smiling, opportunity to draw are all positive reinforcers of which we have no record from the tapes that were studied by Brown and Hanlon. Second, it is quite true that parents mostly reinforce the content, not the form of verbal behavior, and that is because language is communication, not a protracted lesson in grammar or syntax. Third, the mother was very likely reinforcing the child for drawing, not for speaking, at the time of the child's remark, "Draw a boot paper." In addition, however, the mother was clearly correcting the child's grammar as well by the repetition in altered form. All in all, Brown and Hanlon do not present impressive data to test the relevance of behavior theory in the acquisition of language.

Typically, generative grammarians accuse behavior theorists of oversimplifying. In this case, it is the grammarians and grammarophiles who are doing the oversimplifying. To find out whether an acquired response is reinforced, you must observe its occurrence and its consequences, not by preselecting some series of events *thought* to act as positive or negative reinforcers, but by observing all the consequences—verbal and nonverbal, conditioned and primary. The Brown and Hanlon study simply does not test the hypothesis it sets out to test. For an example of a much better effort at observing the contingent relationship between events in the environment and the child's speech, we recommend Horner and Gussow,[24] who analyzed the complete tape recording of two full days' worth of verbal behavior. The contingencies in that case were quite clear.

We come to the conclusion that it is better to make use of a general theory of behavior than one specially constructed for human beings and that on that count alone we should eliminate the concept of competence.

Competence in the Guise of a Theory of Language

It is clear that what Chomsky talks about is grammar, but what he wishes to generalize about is *language*. I think the time has come to say that the emperor has no clothes. We have already talked about the social variables that Chomsky is determined to exclude, and we have already shown how misguided that approach is.

Now, I would like to point out that an increasing number of investigators have rightfully become discontented with a theory of language that is restricted to grammar. There are theoretical questions, such as what the deep structure is filled with, being raised by linguists who want to fill it with semantics, and there are the more psychological questions being raised by such investigators as Schlesinger,[66] who tries to derive a structure of meaning. He puts into the deep structure the intentions of the speaker: what he or she wishes to say. While this is still putting inside the organism what resides outside, it does show a progression from grammar to meaning.

Also of interest in recent years is the greater appeal that the external environment has had for developmental psychologists. This is what Brown has called "rich interpretation"[4] and has been used by Bloom[76,77] and Bowerman.[3] Bowerman (p. 11) argues: ". . . many additional clues to competence can be found in the nonlinguistic contexts of speech events, the linguistic interaction between parent and child, the relationship between successive utterances of the child, and the comparison of the child's speech to that of his parents." She states that Chomsky's model of transformational grammar is not equipped to provide "an explicit account of the semantic functions of sentence elements" and therefore "may be basically unable to reflect children's linguistic knowledge adequately." (Ref. 3, pp. 14–15.)

We were able to show in our laboratory that the extent to which an individual understands another depends on psychopathological and social variables. We have already mentioned that schizophrenic patients are more difficult to understand than are normal individuals. We have also investigated how social contact patterns affect the extent to which people understand one another.[22,57] The degree to which one person knows another and the centrality of the individual in the group are very important indeed in explaining how well people understand each other.

Krauss and Glucksberg[29] tested a number of children for communicative competence. Children were required to name unique graphic figures so that adults could correctly apply the names to those same figures. The results showed that even at age 14, children still had not yet acquired the same competence that adults had in communicating in this way. The authors argued that one should make a distinction between Chomsky's grammatical competence and the communicative competence that interests psychologists.

Finally, it might be worth while to mention one more study done in our laboratory. Taking Chomsky at his word that one can have grammar without meaning, we[54] constructed two types of sentences out of function words and nonsense syllables. One type was the simple declarative sentence in the active mood; the other, the complex sentence, which, according to Chomsky, ought to require transformations for proper processing, was the passive negative question. We also presented the elements of every sentence in random order. We had a number of interesting findings, but most germane to this discussion is the fact that it was no more difficult to memorize the more complicated structure than the simpler one. In a clear test of material devoid of meaning, the grammatical structure of sentences has no effect at all. The role of grammar, it seems, is not to be independent, but rather to be the overly dependent appendage our common sense has always told us it must be.

I wish to end my paper with a puzzle. The puzzle is this: When is behavior not performance? The answer that Chomsky and his colleagues give us is, "When it is competence." I believe that behavior theory can more meaningfully deal with the problem that underlies the distinction between competence and performance. The distinction came about because people behave differently on different occasions;

they speak differently and they respond to speech differently. My suggestion is that we study the conditions that provide us with differences in behavior, without worrying about which one reveals the real underlying ability of the individual. This means that we must define in precise ways the reinforcement contingencies that apply to language as behavior and to language as stimulus. It simply does not follow that a child who "knows" something in one situation will know it in another.[68] This is a familiar problem in all psychological tests where one must generalize from the test situation to school or job conditions. If we can solve the problem with respect to language, we might be making a contribution to testing as well. Only after studying language in relation to conditions of emission will we be on the way to gaining an understanding of the psychology of language.

It is my belief that we are ready for this approach, for we have come a long way from the *Sturm und Drang* of competence to the *Ach und Weh* of its nontestability.

Acknowledgment

The author is grateful to R. S. Feldman for his assistance with the manuscript.

References

1. BEVER, T. 1973. Serial position and response biases do not account for the effect of syntactic structure on the location of brief noises during sentences. J. Psycholinguistic Res. **2**: 287–288.
2. BLACK, M. 1970. Comment. *In* Explanation in the Behavioural Sciences. R. Borger & F. Cioffi, Eds. Univ. Press. New York, N.Y.
3. BOWERMAN, M. 1973. Early Syntactic Development. Cambridge Univ. Press. London, England.
4. BROWN, R. 1973. A First Language: The Early Stages. Harvard Univ. Press. Cambridge, Mass.
5. BROWN, R. & C. HANLON. 1970. Derivational complexity and order of acquisition in child speech. *In* Cognition and the Development of Language. J. R. Hayes, Ed.: 11–53. John Wiley. New York, N.Y.
6. CATANIA, A. C. 1966. Concurrent operants. *In* Operant Behavior. W. K. Honig, Ed.: 213–270. Appleton-Century-Crofts. New York, N.Y.
7. CHOMSKY, N. 1959. Review of Skinner's *Verbal Behavior*. Language **35**: 26–58.
8. CHOMSKY, N. 1964. Formal discussion. *In* Monographs of the Society for Research in Child Development. U. Bellugi & R. Brown, Eds. Vol. **29**: 35–39. Antioch Press. Yellow Springs, Ohio.
9. CHOMSKY, N. 1965. Aspects of the Theory of Syntax. M.I.T. Press. Cambridge, Mass.
10. CHOMSKY, N. 1970. Problems of explanation in linguistics. *In* Explanation in the Behavioural Sciences. R. Borger & F. Cioffi, Eds. Univ. Press. New York, N.Y.
11. CHOMSKY, N. 1970. Reply. *In* Explanation in the Behavioural Sciences. R. Borger & F. Cioffi, Eds. Univ. Press. New York, N.Y.
12. CHOMSKY, N. 1972. Language and Mind. Enlarged edit. Harcourt Brace Jovanovich. New York, N.Y.
13. DERWING, B. L. 1973. Transformational Grammar as a Theory of Language Acquisition. Cambridge Univ. Press. Cambridge, England.
14. FERNALD, C. D. 1972. Control of grammar in imitation, comprehension, and production: Problems of replication. J. Verbal Learning Verbal Behav. **11**: 606–613.
15. FODOR, J. A. 1968. Psychological Explanation. Random House. New York, N.Y.
16. FODOR, J. A., T. G. BEVER & M. F. GARRETT. 1974. The Psychology of Language. McGraw-Hill. New York, N.Y.
17. FRASER, C., U. BELLUGI & R. BROWN. 1963. Control of grammer in imitation, comprehension and production. J. Verbal Learning Verbal Behav. **2**: 121–135.

18. GARCIA, E. C. The Spanish Pronoun System. North Holland Press. Amsterdam, The Netherlands. In Press.
19. GARDNER, B. T. & R. A. GARDNER. 1971. Two-way communication with an infant chimpanzee. In Behavior of Nonhuman Primates. A. M. Schrier & F. Stollnitz, Eds. Vol. 4: 117–184. Academic Press. New York, N.Y.
20. GARDNER, R. A. & B. T. GARDNER. 1969. Teaching sign language to a chimpanzee. Science 165: 664–672.
21. GREENSPOON, J. 1955. The reinforcing effect of two spoken sounds on the frequency of two responses. Amer. J. Psychol. 68: 409–416.
22. HAMMER, M., S. POLGAR & K. SALZINGER. 1969. Speech predictability and social contact patterns in an informal group. Human Organization 28: 235–242.
23. HOLZ, W. C. & N. H. AZRIN. 1966. Conditioning human verbal behavior. In Operant Behavior: Areas of Research and Application. W. K. Honig, Ed.: 790–826. Appleton-Century-Crofts. New York, N.Y.
24. HORNER, V. M. & J. D. GUSSOW. 1972. John and Mary: A pilot study in linguistic ecology. In Functions of Language in the Classroom. C. B. Cazden, V. P. John & D. Hymes, Eds.: 155–194. Teachers College Press. New York, N.Y.
25. HYMES, D. 1974. Foundations in Sociolinguistics. Univ. Pennsylvania Press. Philadelphia, Pa.
26. KRAMER, P. E. 1973. Young children's responses to commands differing in length, structure, and meaning. Ph.D. Dissertation. Yeshiva Univ. New York, N.Y.
27. KRASNER, L. 1958. Studies of the conditioning of verbal behavior. Psychological Bulletin 55: 148–170.
28. KRASNER, L. 1967. Verbal operant conditioning and awareness. In Research in Verbal Behavior and Some Neurophysiological Implications. K. Salzinger & S. Salzinger, Eds.: 57–76. Academic Press. New York, N.Y.
29. KRAUSS, R & S. GLUCKSBERG. 1969. The development of communication: Competence as a function of age. Child Devel. 40: 255–266.
30. LENNEBERG, E. 1967. Biological Foundations of Language. John Wiley & Sons. New York, N.Y.
31. LOVAAS, O. I. 1973. Behavioral Treatment of Autistic Children. General Learning Press. Morristown, N.J.
32. LURIA, A. R. 1967. The regulative function of speech in its development and dissolution. In Research in Verbal Behavior and Some Neurophysiological Implications. K. Salzinger & S. Salzinger, Eds.: 405–427. Academic Press. New York, N.Y.
33. LURIA, A. R. 1969. Speech development and the formation of mental processes. In A Handbook of Contemporary Soviet Psychology. M. Cole & I. Maltzman, Eds. Basic Books, New York, N.Y.
34. LURIA, S. E. 1974. What can biologists solve? The New York Review of Books. 21(1): 27–28.
34. McNEILL, D. 1966. Developmental psycholinguistics. In The Genesis of Language. F. Smith & G. A. Miller, Eds.: 15–84. M.I.T. Press. Cambridge, Mass.
36. MILLER, G. A. 1967. The Psychology of Communication. Penguin Books. Baltimore, Md.
37. MILLER, G. A. & N. CHOMSKY. 1963. Finitary models of language users. In Handbook of Mathematical Psychology. R. D. Luce, R. R. Bush & E. Galanter, Eds. Vol. 2: 419–491. John Wiley & Sons. New York, N.Y.
38. MOESER, S. D. & A. S. BREGMAN. 1972. The role of reference in the acquisition of a miniature artificial language. J. Verbal Learning Verbal Behav. 11: 759–769.
39. MOESER, S. D. & A. S. BREGMAN. 1973. Imagery and language acquisition. J. Verbal Learning Verbal Behav. 12: 91–98.
40. PORTNOY, S. & K. SALZINGER. 1964. The conditionability of different verbal response classes: Positive, negative and nonaffect statements. J. Gen. Psychol. 70: 311–323.
41. PREMACK, D. 1970. A functional analysis of language. J. Exp. Anal. Behav. 14: 107–125.
42. PREMACK, D. 1971. On the assessment of language competence in the chimpanzee. In Behavior of Nonhuman Primates. A. M. Schrier & F. Stollnitz, Eds. Vol. 4: 185–228. Academic Press. New York, N.Y.
43. REBER, A. S. 1973. What clicks may tell us about speech perception. J. Psycholinguistic Res. 2: 286–287.
44. RUMBAUGH, D. M., T. V. GILL & E. C. VON GLASERSFELD. 1973. Reading and sentence completion by a chimpanzee (Pan). Science 182: 731–733.

45. SALZINGER, K. 1959. Experimental manipulation of verbal behavior: A review. J. Gen. Psychol. **61:** 65-94.
46. SALZINGER, K. 1967. The problem of response class in verbal behavior. *In* Research in Verbal Behavior and Some Neurophysiological Implications. K. Salzinger & S. Salzinger, Eds.: 35-54. Academic Press. New York, N.Y.
47. SALZINGER, K. 1968. On the operant conditioning of complex behavior. *In* Research in Psychotherapy. J. M. Shlien & H. Hunt, Eds. Vol. **3:** 122-129. American Psychol. Assoc. Washington, D.C.
48. SALZINGER, K. 1969. The place of operant conditioning of verbal behavior in psychotherapy. *In* Behavior Therapy: Appraisal and Status. C. Franks, Ed.: 375-395. McGraw-Hill. New York, N.Y.
49. SALZINGER, K. 1969. Psychology: The Science of Behavior. Springer. New York, N.Y.
50. SALZINGER, K. 1970. Pleasing linguistics: A parable. J. Verbal Learning Verbal Behav. **9:** 725-727.
51. SALZINGER, K. 1973. Inside the black box, with apologies to Pandora. A review of Ulric Neisser's Cognitive Psychology. J. Exp. Anal. Behav. **19:** 369-378.
52. SALZINGER, K. 1973. Some problems of response measurement in verbal behavior: The response unit and intraresponse relations. *In* Studies in Verbal Behavior: An Empirical Approach. K. Salzinger & R. S. Feldman, Eds.: 5-15. Pergamon Press. New York, N.Y.
53. SALZINGER, K. 1973. Animal communication. *In* Comparative Psychology. D. A. Dewsbury & D. A. Rethlingshafer, Eds.: 161-193. McGraw-Hill. New York, N.Y.
54. SALZINGER, K. & C. ECKERMAN. 1967. Grammar and the recall of chains of verbal responses. J. Verbal Learning Verbal Behav. **6:** 232-239.
55. SALZINGER, K. & R. S. FELDMAN. 1973. Studies in Verbal Behavior: An Empirical Approach. Pergamon Press. New York, N.Y.
56. SALZINGER, K., R. S. FELDMAN, J. E. COWAN & S. SALZINGER. 1965. Operant conditioning of verbal behavior of two young speech-deficient boys. *In* Research in Behavior Modification. L. Krasner & L. P. Ullmann, Eds.: 82-105. Holt, Rinehart & Winston. New York, N.Y.
57. SALZINGER, K., M. HAMMER, S. PORTNOY & S. K. POLGAR. 1970. Verbal behaviour and social distance. Lang. Speech **13:** 25-37.
58. SALZINGER, K. & S. PISONI. 1958. Reinforcement of affect responses of schizophrenics during the clinical interview. J. Abnormal Soc. Psychol. **57:** 84-90.
59. SALZINGER, K. & S. PISONI. 1960. Reinforcement of verbal affect responses of normal subjects during the interview. J. Abnormal Soc. Psychol. **60:** 127-130.
60. SALZINGER, K. & S. PISONI. 1961. Some parameters of the conditioning of verbal affect responses in schizophrenic subjects. J. Abnormal Soc. Psychol. **63:** 511-516.
61. SALZINGER, K. S. PORTNOY & R. S. FELDMAN. 1964. Verbal behavior of schizophrenic and normal subjects. Ann. N.Y. Acad. Sci. **105:** 845-860.
62. SALZINGER, K., S. PORTNOY & R. S. FELDMAN. 1966. Verbal behavior in schizophrenics and some comments toward a theory of schizophrenia. *In* Psychopathology of Schizophrenia. P. Hoch & J. Zubin, Eds.: 98-128. Grune & Stratton, New York, N.Y.
63. SALZINGER, K., S. PORTNOY, D. B. PISONI & R. S. FELDMAN. 1970. The immediacy hypothesis and response-produced stimuli in schizophrenic speech. J. Abnorm. Psychol. **76:** 258-264.
64. SALZINGER, K., S. PORTNOY, P. ZLOTOGURA & R. KEISNER. 1963. The effect of reinforcement on continuous speech and on plural nouns in grammatical content. J. Verbal Learning Verbal Behav. **1:** 477-485.
65. SALZINGER, S., K. SALZINGER, S. PORTNOY, J. ECKMAN, P. M. BACON, M. DEUTSCH & J. ZUBIN. 1962. Operant conditioning of continuous speech in young children. Child Devel. **33:** 683-695.
66. SCHLESINGER, I. M. 1971. Learning grammar: From pivot to realization rule. *In* Language Acquisition: Models and Methods. R. Huxley & E. Ingram, Eds.: 79-89. Academic Press. New York, N.Y.
67. SHIPLEY, E. F., C. S. SMITH & L. R. GLEITMAN. 1969. A study in the acquisition of language: Free responses to commands. Language **45:** 322-342.
68. SIGEL, I. E. 1974. When do we know what a child knows? Human Devel. **17:** 201-217.
69. SKINNER, B. F. 1960. Are theories of learning necessary? Psychol. Rev. **57:** 193-216.
70. SKINNER, B. F. 1957. Verbal Behavior. Appleton-Century-Crofts. New York, N.Y.

71. STAATS, A. W. 1968. Learning, Language, and Cognition. Holt, Rinehart & Winston. New York, N.Y.
72. TOPPINO, T. C. 1974. The underlying structures of sentences are not the primary units of speech processing: A reinterpretation of Bever, Lackner, and Kirk's findings. Percep. Psychophysics 15: 517–518.
73. TURNER, M. B. 1967. Philosophy and the Science of Behavior. Appleton-Century-Crofts. New York, N.Y.
74. VONNEGUT, K., Jr. 1974. Wampeters, Foma, and Granfalloons. Delacorte Press. New York, N.Y.
75. ZUBIN, D. A. 1974. Experimental validation of a linguistic analysis. Paper presented at the Linguistic Society of America. Amherst, Mass.
76. BLOOM, L. 1970. Language Development: Form and Function in Emerging Grammars. The M.I.T. Press. Cambridge, Mass.
77. BLOOM, L. 1973. One Word at a Time. Mouton & Co. The Hague, The Netherlands.
78. SALZINGER, K. Language behavior. In Analysis of Behavior: Social and Educational Processes. A. C. Catania & T. A. Brigham, Eds. In press. Irvington/Naiburg. New York, N.Y.

THE RELATION OF COMPETENCE TO PERFORMANCE

D. Terence Langendoen

Brooklyn College, Brooklyn, New York 11210
Graduate Center of the City University of New York
New York, New York 10036

This paper is concerned with the relation of linguistic competence to linguistic performance, and with the epistemological status of what the systems of competence and performance represent. I hold that what both competence and performance represent is knowledge; competence represents knowledge of the structure of language and performance represents knowledge of the conditions of use of tokens of linguistic structures. This view of competence is standard;[1,2] this view of performance, perhaps, is not. The utility, and hence desirability, of this view of performance, however, will become apparent below.

I take the relation of competence to performance to be that competence is a component of idealized performance. Certainly, this view has much to recommend it. Consider such behaviors (aspects of performance in operation) as conscious punning and paraphrasing one's remarks. There is no way to describe punning behavior without assuming that the punner has available the literal meaning of what he says, which is one aspect of his knowledge of linguistic structure, and similarly for the behavior of paraphrasing. If we examine even the most fundamental aspects of linguistic performance—speech perception and speech production—we find, again, that the most plausible descriptions of the systems involved require the availability of purely linguistic knowledge. The problems to which a theory of speech comprehension must address itself are the speed and accuracy with which listeners determine the meaning of what is said in their presence, and whatever divergence there is between this utterance meaning and the literal meaning that the utterance type has by virtue of its linguistic structure. We will discuss the first problem later; let us now look more closely at the second of these two problems. First of all, the divergence in question is not simply an artifact of the claim that utterances are tokens of utterance types that have literal meanings as a consequence of their linguistic structures. Everyone who understands a language is aware of this divergence, and is in fact capable of exploiting it for various communicative purposes. Let me now introduce a couple of technical terms that will help to clarify the nature of the problem, and its theoretical solution. A semantically well-formed linguistic construction is said to be *meaningful*, whereas a semantically appropriate token of a linguistic construction in a particular situational context is said to be *significant*. Thus, an example like "Energy is equal to the product of mass times the square of the speed of light" is meaningful, but a token of it used by a teacher to nursery-school children would not be significant. On the other hand, an example like "Golf plays John" is not meaningful, but a token of this semantically ill-formed sentence used by John's golfing partners to describe his poor performance might be fully significant.

We can now address ourselves directly to the problem of accounting for the divergence of significance from meaningfulness, as it is systematically related to the contexts in which utterance tokens of sentence types are used. Consider an example such as "We certainly have a genius in the White House now." The literal meaning of this expression is that the inhabitant of the White House at this time is endowed with extraordinary intellectual ability, but we can easily imagine contexts in which the significance of this expression would be exactly the opposite. Our ability to compute

197

the relation of meaningfulness to significance as a function to context can be expressed informally as $F (S, C) = S'$, where S is a structural description of utterance type as provided by the theory of competence, C is a full specification of the relevant contextural information about the utterance token, and S' is a representation of the significance of this token in the specified context.[3] Note that we can now take S', the representation of the significance of the utterance token, to be the structural description of some expression different from the type represented by this token. Thus, in the contexts in which the expression "We certainly have a genius in the White House now" has a significance opposite to its literal meaning, we can take the significance to be represented by the literal meaning of the sentence-type "We certainly have a moron in the White House now." In other words, we can consider the theory of the internalized system that determines the significance of utterance tokens, like a grammar, to be a system of establishing sound-meaning correlations, only not ones for the language, but ones for particular utterance-context pairs. This very plausible model of one aspect of speech comprehension thus takes the availability of knowledge of linguistic structure as one of its crucial inputs.

The view that performance represents a system of knowledge, like competence, was first proposed to provide the basis for the claim that the systems of competence and performance interact: that properties of the system of knowledge of linguistic structures constrain the properties of the system of knowledge of the use of structures and vice versa.[4,5] Together with the view that performance theory incorporates competence, this view puts us in a position to give a more precise account of how it is that there are sentences in each natural language that no human being that knows that language can possibly use.

It is well known that grammars that have been written to describe the competence of native speakers of particular languages overgenerate in the sense that they characterize as part of these languages structures that none of those native speakers recognize as structures of those languages. For example, the regular grammatical processes in English that enable us to form relative-clause modifiers of nouns generate structures such as that found in the sentence "The man that the woman that the child that the dog that the cat that the mouse feared chased bit hugged saw screamed," which no speaker of English recognizes as such. This has sometimes led to skepticism regarding the adequacy of such grammars, and of the theories that permit them;[6] but if the inability of language users to deal with such sentences can be accounted for within the theory of performance, there is no reason to reject the theory of competence solely on the basis that it provides for the possibility of grammars that generate sentences that no native speaker recognizes.[7]

As we have already argued, a generalized theory of performance, one that is neutral with respect to acts of speaking, listening, or introspection, may be thought of as a function $F(S, C) = S'$, where S and S' are linguistic structures, and C is a representation of the relevant context in which a token of S is used, and F determines what a token of a given linguistic structure may be used to signify in a given context. If the external context is null, and if the structure S has no special significance to the individual who uses it, we represent the context as C_o; C_o consists of just those performance principles that are systematically used in the direct comprehension of linguistic structures. If S is structured in such a way that the performance principles in C_o permit it to be understood, it follows that $F(S, C_o) = S$, and we may say that the individual who has internalized the grammar that generates S, and the performance principles of C_o, knows that he knows that S is a structure of his language that relates a particular meaning to a particular sound sequence. This is so because that individual knows that S may be used to express a particular meaning solely by virtue of the fact that he knows that S has that meaning by the rules of his internalized grammar.

Now consider the case of a structure generated by the grammar that cannot be understood under any circumstances (excluding those involving direct instruction in the application of the rules of grammar to obtain that structure). Such a case may be represented by $F(S, C_o) = \emptyset$. This means that the sound-meaning correlation that the individual knows by virtue of his internalized competence to be associated with S is not available to that individual, even when he is introspecting about S. We conclude that while he knows that S is a structure of the language by virtue of his competence, he does not know that he knows it, by virtue of his performance.

The converse case, in which the performance system assigns an interpretation to a structure not generated by the grammar in the context C_o, is apparently much rarer, but does arise.[8] In such a case, we would say that the individual who uses that structure knows that it is not part of his language (again by virtue of his internalized grammar), but that he does not know that it is not.

As Miller and Chomsky have argued,[7] there is no reason to believe that the devices for constructing sentences that exceed the performance capacities of individuals who have internalized those devices, should disappear as languages evolve. There is reason to expect, however, that grammars should contain or develop devices for paraphrasing unintelligible structures in intelligible form. In many cases, syntactic transformations are such devices, as has been repeatedly noted.[1,7,9] In particular, transformations such as extraposition in English[10] have the effect of converting center-embedded structures (which tend to be unacceptable) into right-branching ones (which tend to be acceptable). However, even left- and right-branching structures ultimately cannot be comprehended,[11] and interestingly enough, grammars also provide devices for eliminating left- and right-branching structures in favor of coordinate-like structures, which turn out to be the most easily comprehended. [1,11] That grammars are organized in part to facilitate the operation of performance devices argues strongly for the view that competence and performance are describable as systems of knowledge that interact in the minds of individual speakers.

In conclusion, I should like to address myself directly to the major arguments that have been raised against the view that one's knowledge of a language is represented in the mind in the form of a generative, i.e. formal, grammar, and that this grammar is a component in the mental representation of performance (the mental structures that underlie performance). In the oral presentation of this paper at the conference on which this annal is based, I myself raised the objection that since formal grammars of natural languages contain infinitely many rules, they cannot directly be represented in the mind. But, being formal objects, grammars containing infinitely many rules can be finitely represented by a system of meta-rules, or *rule schemata*, as they are customarily called.[1] We may assume that what is mentally represented are meta-grammars, containing rule schemata, effective procedures for enumerating the infinitely many rules that these schemata abbreviate, and also effective procedures for computing the derivations of the sentences of the language given the rules of grammar.[12] Thus, the fact the grammars of natural languages are infinite objects does not provide the basis for objecting that competence cannot be mentally represented, and still be a formal representation of knowledge of language.

Second, it has been argued that if derivations of sentences are actually computed in the course of speaking and listening to speech, there should be some measurable consequence of that mental activity. It has been claimed that no such consequences have been found, and hence that the activity is not engaged in. The fallacy in this line of reasoning should be immediately apparent, but let me spell it out, just in case it isn't. Suppose we have two distinct grammatical sentences of a language, S_1 and S_2, whose derivations are identical, except that S_2 has undergone an optional syntactic transformation that S_1 has not. Suppose we find that under any behavioral measure of complexity we can think of, S_2 is never more complex than S_1 (t may even be the case that on some of these measures, S_1 is more complex than S_2). It does not follow that therefore users of S_1 and S_2 do not compute the derivations of those sentences on the occasions of their use, since the computations may be performed so quickly that we have no measurement device subtle enough to record the difference between them, or that even if we do, the effects of computation are swamped by other factors, such as that the surface structures may differ in perceptual salience (recall that one of the effects of transformations is to simplify surface-structure representations).

Third, it has been argued that if our knowledge of linguistic structure is represented in the form of a generative grammar, it should take longer than it does for people to produce and to recognize sentences of their language. In fact, such arguments are directed only against the specific claim that we produce and recognize sentences using a grammar by the technique of "analysis-by-synthesis."[13] But this is not the only technique for performing speech production and recognition using a grammar. Suppose, instead, we view the speech production and recognition devices in the head as general-purpose finite-state devices. The states and instructions of those devices can be directly constructed from the rules (or meta-rules) of grammar; in fact, algorithms for such constructions (assuming the theory of context-free phrase-structure grammar, which is known to be inadequate, but which can be taken as a first approximation to a true theory of grammar), have been developed.[11,14] Hence the observation that we speak and comprehend sentences with great speed and accuracy in itself does not rule out the possibility that we use our internalized grammars in the course of speaking and listening to speech.

References

1. CHOMSKY, N. 1965. Aspects of the Theory of Syntax. MIT Press. Cambridge, Mass.
2. PYLYSHYN, Z. 1973. The role of competence theories in cognitive psychology. J. Psycholing. Res. 2: 21–50.
3. KATZ, J. J. & D. T. LANGENDOEN. Pragmatics and presupposition. To be published.
4. BEVER, T. G. & D. T. LANGENDOEN. 1971. A dynamic model of the evolution of language. Linguistic Inquiry 2: 433–463.
5. BEVER, T. G., J. J. KATZ & D. T. LANGENDOEN, Eds. An Integrated Theory of Linguistic Ability. T. Y. Crowell. New York, N.Y. In press.
6. REICH, P. 1969. The finiteness of natural language. Language 45: 831–843.
7. MILLER, G. A. & N. CHOMSKY. 1963. Finitary models of language users. In Handbook of Mathematical Psychology. II. R. D. Luce, R. R. Bush & E. Galanter, Eds.: 419–491. John Wiley & Sons. New York, N.Y.
8. LANGENDOEN, D. T. & T. G. BEVER. 1973. Can a not unhappy person be called a not sad one? In A Festschrift for Morris Halle. S. Anderson & P. Kiparsky, Eds.: 392–409. Holt, Rinehart & Winston. New York, N.Y.
9. LANGENDOEN, D. T. 1970. The accessibility of deep structures. In Readings in English Transformational Grammar. R. A. Jacobs & P. S. Rosenbaum, Eds.: 99–104. Ginn-Blaisdell. Waltham, Mass.
10. ROSENBAUM, P. S. 1967. The Grammar of English Predicate Complement Constructions. MIT Press. Cambridge, Mass.
11. LANGENDOEN, D. T. Finite-state parsing of phrase-structure languages and the status of readjustment rules in grammar. To be published.
12. LANGENDOEN, D. T. The performance of competence. To be published.
13. HALLE, M. & K. N. STEVENS. 1964. Speech recognition: A model and a program for research. In The Structure of Language: Readings in the Philosophy of Language. J. A. Fodor & J. J. Katz, Eds. 604–612. Prentice-Hall. Englewood Cliffs, N.J.
14. CHOMSKY, N. 1959. On certain formal properties of grammars. Information and Control 2: 137–167.

SOME COMMENTS ON COMPETENCE AND PERFORMANCE

George A. Miller

*Department of Psychology
The Rockefeller University
New York, New York 10021*

If you are ever asked to be a discussant, I'll tell you how you do it. You go off and gather your own thoughts; then you hope that somebody says something that will make one of those thoughts relevant to the occasion. It will turn out that some of the things I'll have to say now will be relevant to what you've already heard, but that's just my good luck.

How can we best understand the notion of linguistic competence in order to account for linguistic performance? In collecting my thoughts about competence and performance, I began with a strong suspicion that these words mean different things to different people, and that much of the disagreement that this distinction has inspired in recent years could be understood if we thought in terms of people who believed they were talking about the same thing but really weren't. So, as a first step, I began listing alternative uses of the terms "competence" and "performance." Without even trying very hard, I got up to eight different versions of the distinction. I will review them for you briefly.

Two of them, I believe, are historically established. At the time Chomsky formulated his version, and cast it in terms of competence and performance, these were precedents that he could (and in fact did) cite. The principle precedent was a *linguistic* one. Sometime before 1910 de Saussure had distinguished between *langue* and *parole*, i.e., language and acts of speaking, in terms of a distinction between a social norm and individual manifestations of that norm. His purpose was to give primacy to the study of language as a way to unify a diverse range of physical, social, and psychological facts. I've always wondered to what extent de Saussure was influenced by the sociological distinction, current in Paris in those days, between collective representation and individual representation. But I don't know any historian of science who has dug into that.

Another precedent that existed was what I would call a *cognitive* version. Lashley, as early as 1929, and Tolman many times through the 1930s, distinguished knowledge and performance in terms of what an organism had learned versus what he might be motivated to do with his knowledge on any particular occasion. That is, a rat could have learned where the food bin was and, in some sense of the word "know," could know where the food bin was, but not go there if he wasn't hungry. I think their purpose was to deepen some rather superficial behavioristic theories that were popular in their day by introducing theoretical variables that could not be directly observed in the behavior but, perhaps, could be abstracted or inferred from it.

Chomsky's inspiration was largely from Saussure, but he was aware of the cognitive distinction as well, and I think he tried to subsume them both in his own view of the matter. I would call Chomsky's view a *rationalistic* view of the distinction.

This distinction was initially developed in our chapters in the *Handbook of Mathematical Psychology* (1963). In those chapters Chomsky distinguished between competence and performance, between the language that a person knows and the speech acts that a language user performs. This was done in terms roughly analogous to the distinction between, say, an axiom system and various realizations of such a system.

201

This made the problem of providing grammars of a particular language comparable to the problem of providing an axiom system. Consequently, this led to a peculiar relation between what you can observe and the theory you're talking about. You can't test a grammar in terms of errors committed by any particular language user on any particular occasion, just as you can't test an axiom system in terms of the errors someone makes in applying it. The point is that Chomsky's rationalistic formulation, I think, captured both the linguistic and the cognitive distinctions, and at the time it seemed to be a significant advance in theorizing.

Since then there has been, as we're all well aware here, a great deal of discussion of this distinction and attempts to invoke it in one way or another in other areas. There is a version that I think of as *developmental*, because it's frequently observed that children can understand linguistic constructions that they don't use spontaneously. Among students of child language it's become fashionable to phrase this observation in terms of the children's competence exceeding their performance. I don't like this usage. The source of this disparity is probably the fact that the listener's task is easier than the speaker's; so this developmental view seems to make competence equal to listening and performance equal to speaking, which certainly was not my understanding of what was involved.

This view is related to a view that I would call a *situational* version of competence. It is frequently observed that performance varies according to the situational context. A child may, in a school situation, seem to be totally incompetent and then, put into a certain play situation, may demonstrate that he really did have all the relevant knowledge, after all. Consequently, this has led some psychologists to distinguish two kinds of competence; that which is the basic knowledge of the language itself and some other kind of competence that has to do with the competence of using this basic knowledge in particular situations.

On the other hand, there are the views of those who are critical, not just of the competence-performance distinction but of the whole way in which Chomsky tried to formulate a theory of competence. Let me call this the *critical* version. These people, the critics, tend, I think correctly, to see this distinction as a defense of mentalism. Now, if you reject the implication that the competence-performance distinction is mentalistic, then it just seems to boil down to the traditional, and rather uninteresting distinction, between a theory and the data. Viewed in this way, if that's your view of it, what Chomsky seems to be saying is that his axiomatic kind of grammatical theory is impervious to any kind of disproof by empirical observation, since the language users' deviations from the theory can be dismissed as computational errors, or perhaps the experiment can be dismissed as being irrelevant to the theoretical question. Since a theory that can't be tested is worthless, many critics rejected the distinction and, along with it, the theory that inspired it.

Another view of the distinction is one I would call *methodological*. The fact is that transformational and generative linguistic theories are *not* immune to test. Their frequent revisions are evidence that they can be tested and revised. The problem was that the tests relied on linguistic intuition as data. So some workers (I think it's fair to say that T. G. Bever takes a line at least parallel to this) defended a reformulated version of the competence-performance distinction: Theories of competence were distinguished from theories of performance in terms of a reliance on linguistic intuitions versus a reliance on empirical and experimental observations. Intuitive judgments are certainly mentalistic, so that aspect of the original distinction is preserved. Nevertheless, the methodological version shifts the battleground to what I consider an even less interesting piece of real estate. Since linguists use intuitive judgments as data and psycholinguists use experiments as data, this seems to suggest that the competence-performance distinction is identical to the distinction between linguists and psycholinguists, a view that Dr. McNeill disavowed, I believe.

My eighth and last version is the notion that competence and performance are *autonomous*. It seems that the next step would be to abandon any effort to characterize the relation between competence and performance. Linguistics has its goals and its methods; psychology has its goals and methods. They are just two different ways of looking at the same thing, much as a logician and a psychologist might both have useful but unrelated things to say about reasoning. Since they are autonomous sciences, we shouldn't expect either to verify the theories of the other. I think this view preserves, in a rather unattractive form, the observation that misuse cannot invalidate an axiom system.

There are probably many other versions of the competence-performance distinction. But since any number larger than seven is effectively infinite to me, I gave up that approach and tried to think instead about my own ideas of what the distinction *should* be. Fortunately, Zenon Pylyshyn has written an article called "The Role of Competence Theories in Cognitive Psychology" that was published in the *Journal of Psycholinguistic Research*, Vol. 2, no. 1, in 1973, that expresses my opinion better than I could. It's a rather long article, so I can't read it to you. But I can recommend that if you have a serious interest in my views of the competence-performance distinction, you should read Pylyshyn's article.

There is a part of his article that seems to me to give the correct answer to the question that this morning's speakers were asked to answer, so I'm going to take the liberty of summarizing that part of it for you.

Pylyshyn points out that a competence theory, in Chomsky's sense, can be thought of as a machine that computes a certain recursive function. If there is one machine that can compute this function, there must be an infinite variety of machines that could compute it. So one problem the theorist faces is to characterize the simplest machine that can do it.

The criteria that a theorist will use in selecting what he considers to be the simplest, most parsimonious, best-integrated, and esthetically most pleasing machine, are not easy to capture. But the point he makes, and that I would like to endorse, is that "what this means is that one must not make too much of the exact form of the competence theory in the related task of building a broader psychological theory."

This is really rather obvious, but the failure to recognize this point has led to confusion among psychologists about the role of competence theory in the construction of a broader theory of cognition. Indeed, the linguists have caused some of this confusion by the way they have talked about the relation. For example, Saussure, in his famous distinction between language and acts of speaking writes as follows: "But what is language? It is not to be confused with human speech, of which it is only a definite part, though certainly an essential one." If the phrase "a definite part" is not misleading, it is at least ambiguous. Chomsky often speaks in a similar way. In 1965, in *Aspects*—I think this has already been quoted by Dr. Salzinger—he wrote that, "No doubt, a reasonable model of language use will incorporate, as a basic component, the generative grammar that expresses the speaker-hearer's knowledge of the language."

Here the phrase is "incorporate the generative grammar as a basic component." Dr. Langendoen, our one certified linguist in the group this morning, again reaffirmed this position that a theory of competence is a component of an idealized theory of linguistic performance.

It is at this point that Pylyshyn says, "If the suggestion is that a model of the language user must, in describing a wider data base, also account for the type of structure captured by the generative grammar, then we are in agreement. If, on the other hand, it is meant to suggest that a model of the language user must in some corner of the model contain a context-free rewriting system generating a base component in a given sequence (from S to a terminal string) followed temporally by the application of cyclically ordered transformation, then we must disagree." I think even Dr. Langendoen disagrees.

The point is that the form of the grammar is settled on for very good reasons, but for reasons that do not attempt to take account of any data other than primary linguistic intuitions. If the grammar had been developed to account for these data plus other evidence, it would probably have taken a very different form. A theory that is most parsimonious in describing data X can take a very different form from a theory that is most parsimonious in describing data X *and* data Y.

So, Pylyshyn concludes, "This argument suggests that the development of a more general theory of cognition should proceed by attempting to account for the structure which is the output of a competence theory, together with the other kinds of psychological evidence, rather than to incorporate the competence theory as formulated."

As someone who spent several years trying to incorporate Chomsky's theory of competence, as formulated at that time, into a theory of performance, I must say in my own defense that it was an approach we had to try. The fact that you can't simply tack a psychological tail onto a syntactic kite was not initially obvious—it was something we had to learn by trying to do it.

My own version of this insight was that a linguistic theory of competence is not a component of, but an *abstraction from* the cognitive theory that I wanted to construct. But the sense I give to this phrase, "an abstraction from," is very similar to that expressed by Pylyshyn, since I want a theory that will account both for the linguistic intuitions and for many other psychological facts.

So, the answer to the question "How can we best understand the notion of linguistic competence in order to account for linguistic performance?" is very simple. The exact form of the competence theory should not concern us too much. It may change next month. But the data it accounts for must also be accounted for in our broader psychological theories. In that sense we should understand it as setting some of the central problems that a broader theory must account for.

To those who complain that Chomsky's theory of competence has not solved all our problems, I would certainly give strong support. But then I would add that we wouldn't even have known what our problems were without Chomsky's theory to guide us.

It should be obvious that the more data a theory must account for, the more complicated the theory is going to be. I believe that our optimal strategy, however, is the same as the strategy pursued so successfully in theoretical linguistics: to formulate a *competence* theory that accounts for more data, particularly for data relating to the temporal aspects of speech production and perception. This broader competence theory should also be formulated as a machine that can compute a certain recursive function, but one that comes close to representing actual cognitive processes while still accounting for the data that the transformational generative grammars account for. This will clearly be a much more difficult theoretical task. It may take a long time to discover how to do it.

If we are so lucky as to succeed, however, and if I should live long enough to see it—I will be personally very interested to see whether or not linguists will also adopt the broader model. That should be the real test of whether theoretical linguistics is a branch of cognitive psychology.

DISCUSSION

Doris Aaronson, *Chairperson*

Department of Psychology
New York University
New York, New York 10003

DR. WALBURGA VON RAFFLER ENGEL (*Vanderbilt University, Nashville, Tenn.*): I have a question for Dr. McNeill, or any of the previous speakers. Why do they make an equivalence of linguistics with transformational linguistics? Many criticisms of linguistics have been of linguistics as if it were transformational linguistics. These criticisms have been raised by our group, which has never been transformational even from the start of transformational linguistics. It was hard for us to get this publicized, because papers were turned down by the linguistic societies. We had to publish largely in Europe. We have now a little group that is called "The Linguistic Association of Canada" in the United States, where we gather together all those people who have never accepted transformational grammar. All I would ask is not to say "linguistics equals transformational grammar," because then what are we—chemists? So please, when you speak about people who make this very awkard association between competence and performance—we did make a distinction, we clarified it as long as five or six years ago. It took me two trials to get the paper on competence and performance that was critical of Chomsky's approach to the Linguistic Society of America. It had to be published in Belgium. But all I ask is that you please state what type of linguistics you criticize.

DR. AARONSON: Dr. McNeill, would you like to comment on that?

DR. MCNEILL: No, I don't especially want to comment on it. The only claim I made for linguistics in general, which I think is correct, is that it's the science of comparing structures. And that's been true since the Greeks. I hope that it was clear that I was mentioning the particular case of transformational grammar because it is in that context that the competence-performance distinction has been most discussed. But I have to slight practically every other school of thought. I mean that there are too many to mention.

DR. ENGEL: Yes, but then say "transformational grammar." I'm not speaking as much to you as to yesterday's speakers. It's just going too far, because there are some linguists who have never accepted this approach.

DR. RACHAEL FALMAGNE (*Clark Univ., Worcester, Mass.*): Dr. McNeill, if I didn't misunderstand you, one of your last points was to identify the difference between linguistics and psycholinguistics with the study of competence versus performance.

DR. MCNEILL: No, I just want to distinguish competence and performance, not psycholinguistics and linguistics. I see why I might have misled you when I said that you can't specify the relationship between linguistics and psycholinguistics any more precisely than you can the relationship between competence and performance. So the focus here is competence and performance, not the two fields. They might go in any direction, unpredictable by us all.

DR. R. FALMAGNE: Yes, I was going to question that. I'd like to mention a distinction that seemed important to me, simply, that there are two ways to conceive of competence. You can have a competence model, which seems basically a description of the language as an external object, where you forget the speaker as much as you can. That's the domain of linguistics.

On the other hand, in psycholinguistics you may have another type of competence notion, where you put competence in the speaker's mind. Therefore, it's a hypothetical construct, as in any other psychological theory. There the relation between competence and performance is tighter than otherwise because competence is part of the speaker's knowledge, and performance specifies how it is retrieved, and so forth.

DR. McNEILL: I had trouble finding someone to attribute the second view, which is that competence is a purely formal description devoid of any psychological interpretation. Now I can attribute it to you. You apparently hold that view. But I believe you maybe unique. Clearly my description of the theory of competence is very different from that. I'm claiming it has psychological validity. There are really relationships among sentences which you can see when they are presented to you, and you can describe them in some kind of grammatical framework. There really are processes of producing sentences. These two processes are intimately related; but they're not related in a way that appears to be particularly interesting to describe. Because it's changeable, it's general, vague or—they're quite different perspectives. That's the point I'm making.

DR. JACK BLOOM: I'm the Head of the Speech and Hearing Department at the Rockland Children's Psychiatric Hospital in New York State. Some of our staff have been using behavior modification, and we get the child to talk. Now, the only thing is that when he talks he doesn't sound like you and me when we speak. In other words, what happens is that although he says the word or phrase, he doesn't say it with an appropriate intonation, with appropriate volume, or with appropriate pitch. Now, my question to you, Dr. Salzinger, is: Is he talking when he says it in a bizarre way? Or is talking simply the utterance of the word?

DR. KURT SALZINGER: The virtue of taking a child who has no speech and providing that child with the possibility of speaking seems to me to be unassailable. I have worked with such children. I think that anybody who has done it will realize that this is a profound change you have produced, because these children now have a way of responding to other people that they didn't have before, and that makes those other people respond to them in ways that did not occur before. As to the possibility of inappropriate intonation or peculiar volume control in originally speech-deficient children who have acquired speech through operant conditioning, I know of no evidence stating that this inappropriateness is a product peculiar to systematic operant conditioning. Were I confronted with such children as you describe, then I would try to condition appropriate intonation patterns by making reinforcement contingent on them.

However, I'm not trying to sell any miracle drug here. Behavior modification does not instate speech in all people. It does so in some. I think in those that it helps, it does a job, and it is preferable to sitting on one's hands and saying "I can't help this child."

DR. HOWARD FISHER (*City University of New York, New York, N. Y.*): This is a comment for Dr. Kurt Salzinger. His talk seems to have, for me, the title "The final solution to the competence question," and in that regard, if it weren't so sad it would be humorous to try to point out the number of absurdities in the presentation.

First, however, I find that there is a great deal of absurdity in the ethics of his comparative ethology, in which Washoe the chimpanzee is given the privilege of the power to create language or to generate it and the human being is denied the same privilege. The second absurdity is the general nature of reductionism itself, which I won't comment on. The third is the substitution of one reductionism for a presumed other. I'll make that my last comment. Dr. Salzinger found it easy to refer to the evoking power of stimuli, which I would regard as an absurd situation, of one mysticism for a presumed other: namely, the description of generative structures.

DR. AARONSON: We have some negative reinforcement here for Dr. Salzinger. Will that increase or decrease his vocal utterance responses?

DR. K. SALZINGER: Considered to be a punisher, it might have a temporary suppressing effect, but as a negative reinforcer, it makes a number of escape responses possible, and I shall attempt some of these.

Language is not a privilege. Furthermore, I'm not denying the existence of language. What I am suggesting is that we look at language as a biological function. This makes a good deal of sense to me, because we have evidence along the phylogenetic scale for language being a biological function. I have not given a paper here on the behavior-theory model for language (for that see my Reference 78). I have suggested that we should look at a behavior theory as a first step. We may want to modify it as we learn more, but as a first step we wish to use a theory that explains the largest number of facts about the largest variety of organisms. I think we should push that as far as we possibly can, and not invoke new concepts until they are absolutely necessary. I believe that there is a continuity between Washoe and human beings. I also believe there are differences. I had thought this so obvious that I should not have to say it.

In contrasting Chomsky's notions of competence with the concepts of behavior theory, I tried to make the point that the latter's power stems from its many applications to animal behavior in general, not just to the study of language. Because of the general power of behavior theory, I am saying that one should apply it to language behavior. Now, if you want to use a different model, that's all right. But I object to the imperialism of the generative grammarians who claim that they have logical proof that behavior theory doesn't work. The logical proof maintains that behavior theory cannot be applied to language, but the empirical proof—that is, experiments—show that both human and at least some nonhuman primates can be conditioned to communicate. As for the power of discriminative stimuli, it must be pointed out that it is far from mysticism. The concept of discriminative stimuli is an entirely empirically verifiable concept. In that sense it is the exact antithesis to the generative grammarian's concept of competence.

DR. ROGER SHY (*Georgetown University, Washington, D.C.*): I'm from the Center of Applied Linguistics. I have a clarification, rather than a question. As a sociolinguist, I thought I would come here and observe, and not have anything to say. But since sociolinguistics was brought in, I do feel obliged to clarify a matter regarding the use of sociolinguistics, and Hymes in particular, to support—whether implied or stated, I'm not clear which—your feeling that no theory of competence is necessary, along with the more or less implied support of empirical rather than intuitive data in such matters as that.

Because Hymes and some others feel that a competence defined by abstract grammar is not as adequate as we'd like to have it, one should not conclude that this means that we feel that no theory of competence is necessary. I don't think, really, that you can use that as support for the conclusion that no theory of competence is necessary and that sociolinguists support this. I think that sociolinguists are looking at a much broader concept of competence than we used in the past, and that's not really saying the same thing.

DR. K. SALZINGER: I agree. What I tried to say about Hymes was that he believes that one cannot simply accept the competence model of generative grammar and then graft onto it the social variables. He has said very clearly that he rejects competence in that sense.

He wants what he calls "communicative competence," which takes the other variables into account from the very beginning. That's a very important point. Last night Tom Bever was doing some grafting when he suggested that we ought to take the social variables, and put them all together by some process of simple addition. I don't think that it can be done in that piece-meal manner. I think this is where Hymes and I are very much in agreement.

DR. HANS FURTH (*Catholic University, Washington, D. C., and Sussex University, London, England*): I thought Dr.Salzinger's point, the positive points, were very well taken; however, I think it is time to be limited in one's claim. I mean, you are just as imperialistic in your claim as you claim other people are being. You say, "Look how powerful the behavioral method is; we have been able to condition a few children." But what is this, compared to the millions of children who are readers and to the millions of deaf children whom you can't condition to learn language? You have said you have had it as your goal for the past 20 years, and the success is so small that it is pitiful that you bring up these few children whom you conditioned to make a few grunts or speak a few sentences. So don't make exaggerated claims that you can condition speech when you can't do it.

Now, Chomsky's model of language performance has also helped children. I can quote your reports of children whose language performance has been improved because the generative model of language was used by having a language curriculum that was more realistic, based on linguistic competence.

I know you are smiling at this, but this is nothing compared to these little conditioned responses. I mean that the deaf children have been around for the last 15 years, and if your model is so powerful, by all means go ahead. I know many schools that would be only too happy to use your model. So let's be a little realistic.

Let me say just one more thing. I agree with you that Chomsky's model has been very inadequate. I think it has been inadequate not because he has used the model of competence, because I think competence is a psychological reality that we have. We have a linguistic competence, just as we have competence to know the world. I think Chomsky has neglected the competence of knowledge in general. He has tried to build a psychology of the child based only on linguistic competence. And, of course, this is a vacuum. If one would try to see linguistic competence within the framework of the general competence of a human being, then we could make some progress. I certainly have no objection at all to using behavioral methods, but let's be a little modest about it.

DR. K. SALZINGER: The power of behavior theory does not stem from the conditioning of speech alone. On the other hand, I think we agree that a number of children, and adults for that matter, have been conditioned with respect to speech. Those people learned to speak, not to grunt. When a child's speech manifests peculiar intonation patterns, then we must use an appropriate reinforcement contingency to modify that.

As far as the deaf are concerned, just about five years ago (SALZINGER, K., 1970. Behavior theory and problems of the deaf. A. A. D. **115**: 459-468), I was invited to a conference to give a talk on behavior theory and problems of the deaf. There were three other behavior theory-oriented psychologists there. The impression I got at that time was that they were just beginning to apply behavior theory to deaf children. Therefore, if there are only a few deaf children conditioned to speak, we must attribute that to the small number of such attempts.

But my point on behavior theory is that it has worked in many studies, that it has been applied to animals up and down phylogenetically, that it has been used successfully in psychopharmacology, that it has been used fruitfully in abnormal psychology, and so on. I don't think we can quarrel about that. And I believe that the vacuum produced by the failure of generative grammar theory can be elucidated by the studious application of behavior theory. At the very least, we ought to entertain the possibility of using such a powerful model to elucidate the language function of human beings.

DR. BEVER: Terry, [D. Terence Langendoen] as I understand it, what you're saying is that competence is something that individual human minds converge toward in their representation of linguistic knowledge, but since the grammars that are the embodiment of competence are, according to you, infinite, no individual mind actually contains competence.

You also made the point that the reason one studies linguistics in the face of that is that one wants to know what the true structure of language is. Now, the question is: on that view, where do linguistic universals come from? If competence is some kind of spiritual grail toward which the child's mind grasps and reaches but never quite attains, how did it acquire the linguistic structure that it has in the first place?

DR. LANGENDOEN: You are exactly right in observing that it is the existence of linguistic universals that most strongly supports the view that grammars are internalized by the human mind. My objection that generative grammars *per se* cannot be internalized is a purely technical one: one cannot internalize infinite objects. I assume, therefore, that one internalizes a finite meta-grammar of the language one knows, along with the principles that enable one to compute the rules of the grammar, given the schemata of the meta-grammar. Note that these principles are themselves presumably universal. I hope to have something substantive to say about them before long.

DR. RIEBER: What, specifically is a mental structure?

DR. LANGENDOEN: I can answer this question only with respect to language. I currently take the mental structures that represent the schemata of meta-grammars of languages to be the states and instructions of the enriched finite-state devices that are used in speech production and perception (i. e., performance). Technically, this is only a model or theory of mental structures, not a substantive claim about how they are realized chemically or neurologically.

DR. JACK CATLIN (*Cornell Univ., Ithaca, N. Y.*): It's sort of a friendly comment to Professor Langendoen. It has two parts. First of all, it seems to me that perhaps the whole competence-performance bugaboo is historically a conceptual confusion about certain facts that we know to exist about the language. This includes facts about relations between sentences, like active and passive, versus the particular descriptive systems that linguists have used to represent those facts. A lot of heat is raised because we worry about whether the particular linguistic system that transformational grammarians use to represent certain structural regularities has anything to do with psychology. Instead, what's needed, and I think this is really where Professor Langendoen may be going also, is an exploration of the variety of descriptive systems that not only will account for the structural regularities of language, but in addition can be integrated into a language-processing system.

The second aspect of the comment is that in fact one likely possibility may be "augmented transition networks," because they really are clever enough, for example, to express relations between active and passive. You can do things that look transformation-like with them, and formally they have the same power as the transformational grammar. This also means they are too powerful, just as a transformational grammar is, and we have to worry about getting constraints on both of them.

DR. LANGENDOEN: As Jack said, that was a friendly comment, and I appreciate it.

DR. RIEBER: I would like to take a stab at Dr. Miller's question regarding the source of Saussure's influence. Many authorities indicate Durkheim's influence upon Saussure in his distinction between individual and collective representations. I believe the influence can be traced back to the work of Auguste Comte. The Positive Philosophy and Psychology of this period was passed on to anthropologists who were interested in psychic unity and then was picked up by men like Durkheim, Saussure, and Chomsky.

One of the interesting things about this chain of influences is that when you take a look at the life-style performance of these men, they have some very important things in common. They were interested in social and intellectual reforms and revolutions of one type or another, and they were also interested in universals. I do believe that it would be a fruitful area to dig into, in terms of historical research.

THE CRITICAL PERIOD FOR LANGUAGE ACQUISITION AND ITS POSSIBLE BASES

Stephen D. Krashen*

English Language Institute
Queens College, College of the City of New York
Flushing, New York 11367

THE CRITICAL PERIOD HYPOTHESIS FOR HUMAN LANGUAGE

The idea of a critical period for learning derives from studies by Hess[1] and by Lorenz,[2] who observed that greylag goslings "imprinted" on certain moving objects only during a certain limited developmental stage (a few hours after hatching). Lenneberg[3] (see also Ref. 4) has hypothesized that a critical period may exist for human language as well, and suggests that first language may be completely and naturally acquired only between the ages of about two and puberty. Two important arguments implicate puberty as the time of the close of the critical period. The first of these (pp. 142–150) is based on an analysis of recovery from aphasia in children: Lenneberg notes that "the chances for recovery from acquired aphasia are very different for children than for adult patients" (p. 142). In the adult, according to Lenneberg, recovery may occur fairly rapidly (within three to five months). However, "symptoms that have not cleared up by this time are, as a rule, irreversible" (p. 143). Yet, "if language had developed before the onset of [this] disease and if the lesion is confined to a single hemisphere, language will invariably return to a child if he is less than nine years old at the time of the catastrophe" (p. 146). Aphasias that develop around puberty or after will "commonly leave some trace behind which the patient cannot overcome" (p. 150). To the extent that recovery from aphasia involves actual relearning of the first language, to that extent does this data directly support the notion of a critical period.

The observations of Lenneberg et al.[4] of language learning in Down syndrome children also provide direct evidence of a reduced first-language learning capacity after puberty. For these mentally retarded children, their slow progress in language acquisition continues only until puberty, an observation that indicates that "even in the absence of gross structural brain lesions, progress in language learning comes to a standstill after maturity" (p. 155).

THE CRITICAL PERIOD HYPOTHESIS AND SECOND LANGUAGES

Although the critical period hypothesis is directly concerned with first language, it makes certain predictions about second language learning in both children and adults. These predictions will be considered in this section, and research testing these predictions summarized.

It is not unreasonable to expect that if a critical period exists, second-language learning before the close of the critical period would proceed in the same manner as first; such learning would also be "acquisition." A strong version of the critical period

*Present address: Department of Linguistics, University of Southern California, Los Angeles, Calif. 90007

TABLE 1

PREDICTIONS MADE ABOUT SECOND LANGUAGE LEARNING BY A STRONG CRITICAL
PERIOD HYPOTHESIS

	Second Language Acquisition	
	Before Puberty	After Puberty ("learning")
Similar to first language acquisition	yes	no
May be learned without instruction	yes	no
Presence of foreign accent	no	yes
Native competence in syntax, semantics	yes	no

hypothesis predicts that language learning should proceed quite differently and involve different mechanisms after puberty. In addition, second language learning before puberty, one would expect, could proceed "naturally," without formal instruction, while after puberty, as Lenneberg notes, "automatic acquisition from mere exposure seems to disappear...and foreign languages have to be taught and learned through a conscious and labored effort" (p. 176).

Another prediction is that "...foreign accents cannot be overcome after puberty" (p. 176). In fact, a strong critical-period hypothesis predicts that language learning after puberty will never reach native speaker level competence, while that which occurs earlier may. TABLE 1 summarizes these predictions.

Since the publication of *Biological Foundations of Language*,[3] evidence has been gathered that addresses many of these points. In some cases, this new evidence is consistent with the predictions in TABLE 1. In others, the predictions are not fully supported, and these cases force some reevaluation of the nature of child-adult differences presumed by the strong version of the critical period hypothesis. Each prediction will be discussed separately.

(1) (a) Second-language acquisition that takes place before puberty will be similar in process to first-language acquisition, but (b) second-language learning occurring after puberty will not.

There seems to be little doubt thus far that second-language acquisition in children is similar in important ways to first-language acquisition. Similarities in the acquisition of wh-questions,[5] and negation,[6] and in the evolution of perceptual strategies[7] have already been noted. Also, Dulay and Burt[8,9] have reported that children learning English as a second language have an invariant difficulty ordering for English function words, suggesting a common order of acquisition and the use of similar acquisition strategies to first-language learners. The actual difficulty order found by Dulay and Burt was not the same as the invariant order found in first-language acquisition studies;[10,11] to explain this difference, Dulay and Burt note that the order of acquisition posited for older learners is not influenced by the cognitive deelopment that the first-language learner undergoes while acquiring his first language.

The first half of prediction 1, then, is thus far confirmed. What of adults? Much of language-teaching methodology assumes that the process of learning a language during adulthood is very different than it is during childhood. Systems that emphasize repetition and rote learning, and attempt to control learners' utterances in the target language to prevent errors ("bad habits") assume that second-language learning during adulthood is not a "creative process"; that is, it does not involve the constant formulating and altering of hypotheses about the target language. Although reseach on children learning both first and second languages indicates that such a process is involved for them, and that child language acquisition proceeds in many respects in stages that are invariant across all children, it has recently been assumed that adults learn by forming correct "habits" (all the while resisting the habit strength of their first language) and that the order of acquisition of rules and lexical items is determined by the particular syllabus employed.

Richards[12] has summarized recent studies in error analysis and concludes, however, that errors made by adults are to a large extent "intralinguistic"; their origins are "found within the structure of English itself" (p. 98). Such overgeneralizations and overextensions of rules to wrong environments cannot be interpreted as due to interference from the first language, because they are common to learners of different linguistic backgrounds. Such errors may also be termed "developmental," according to Richards, since they reveal the presence of interim grammars, just as children's errors reveal their progress in ariving at the adult set of rules for first-language acquisition.

Moreover, an analysis of adult learning of English function words has revealed a striking similarity between pre- and postpuberty second-language learning. Bailey et al.[13] analyzed utterances produced by adult learners of English as a second language (ESL) in a test of oral production[14] for the appropriate use of eight function words in obligatory contexts[11] (-ing, third person singular -s, contractable copula, plural -s, articles, irregular past, possessive -s). They found that despite differing levels of English competence among the subjects, different amounts of exposure to English, and different native languages, there was a very consistent order of relative difficulty for all subjects (TABLE 2 presents correlations between classrooms of ESL students in the two programs tested). This result confirms, along with the work in error analysis cited above, that adults make many syntactic errors that are not simply the result of interference from the first language.

In addition, Bailey et al.[13] found that the relative difficulty order shown by the adults was not significantly different from that found by Dulay and Burt[8, 9] for five-to-eight-year-old children learning English as a second language. The adult order did not correlate significantly with relative accuracies for function words reported in children learning first language;[15] interestingly, de Villiers' cross-sectional data for adult nonfluent aphasics reveal a difficulty order nearly identical to that found in Bailey et al. for those items covered in both studies.[16]

Moreover, the differences between the groups investigated in various studies becomes even smaller if one considers NP- and VP-related function words separately. Such an analysis (suggested by Eileen Nam) shows complete agreement for NP-related function words, and reveals that first-language learners differ from the others mainly

TABLE 2

CORRELATIONS BETWEEN GROUPS OF ESL STUDENTS FOR FUNCTION WORD ACCURACY*

	ELI 1	ELI 2	ELI 3	ELI 4	CON ED 1	CON ED 2A	CON ED 2B
ELI 2	.85[b]						
ELI 3	.53	.79[b]					
ELI 4	.93[b]	.82[b]	.51				
CON ED 1	.78[a]	.83[b]	.43	.69[a]			
CON ED 2A	.93[b]	.86[b]	.49	.88[b]	.90[b]		
CON ED 2B	.84[b]	.68[a]	.16	.78[a]	.84[b]	.93[b]	
CON ED 3	.71[a]	.80[b]	.52	.69[a]	.84[b]	.63[a]	.94[b]

*ELI = English Language Institute (intensive); CON ED = Continuing Education program; a = p < .05 (one-tailed); b = p < .01 (one-tailed). From Ref. 13.

in that the contractable copula and contractable auxiliary are acquired later. Whatever principles are able to predict the child's order with therefore probably go a long way toward predicting a second language and aphasic order as well. TABLE 3 lists difficulty orders found in the studies discussed here.*

Although this data clearly forces some alteration in the critical-period hypothesis (strong version), the following pieces of counter-evidence must be considered:

(1) The order of difficulty found for adult learners of English was not matched in Hakuta's longitudinal study of a single Japanese girl learning English.[17] While the order he found for the VP-related function words agrees with the second-language order found in Bailey et al., his subject's overall order does not.

(2) In a recent study by Bever, Nam & Scholes using Spanish-speaking adults learning English, the stage in which the NP that was first in the sentence was considered the actor was present from the beginning, the tendency gradually getting weaker as proficiency increased. For first-language learners and for children learning English as a second language, such a stage was found at the intermediate stage of language acquisition.[18]

(2) (a) Second languages acquired before puberty may be learned without formal instruction, but (b) second languages learned after puberty will require formal instruction.

There is some evidence supporting part (a). Hale and Budar[23] compared junior high school students learning English as a second language who (1) had extra ESL classes and extensive contact with speakers of their first language, and (2) learners who had no extra ESL classes but who were relatively isolated from speakers of their own language. Greater English proficiency was found for the second group. Also, Fathman[20] found no difference in English proficiency among young (age 6–15) learners who did and did not have formal ESL training. She did, however, find that those who had lived in the U.S. longer were more proficient.

If (b) is interpreted to mean that formal instruction is, in general, of more benefit to the adult language learner than is exposure, it is most likely true. Even if some adults are able to "pick up" languages by use and exposure, it has been shown that the classroom has, in general, a consistent and positive effect on adult language learning, but exposure does not. A series of studies performed at Queens College in New York has confirmed that when the effects of practice (defined as a function of years of exposure and language use) and years of formal instruction are compared, it is reliably the case that more instruction means more language learning, whereas more practice may or may not mean more proficiency in the target language. Moreover, this effect was found to be consistently present for fairly large numbers of different groups of students, using a variety of measures of proficiency.

---

*It should be pointed out that Bailey et al. and Dulay and Burt used a "partial credit" scoring system, with some credit given for misformed function words. Brown and the de Villiers tallied only presence and absence of function words. De Villiers[16] notes, however, that errors of commission were rare for her subjects. There is always the possibility that the adult learner gets his order because of the syllabus. Bailey et al.[13] attempted to handle this possibility by testing students from different classes and programs and comparing their results, assuming that teachers and texts would differ with respect to the sequence of instruction used. A forthcoming study, however, by Byrd and Dumicich, in which professional ESL teachers were asked to rank order structures according to their intuitions about difficulty, revealed an order not significantly different from the one found in Bailey et al. It is thus possible that many teachers do indeed teach the order found in the study. It would be interesting to test function word acquisition in adults who have learned or are learning English informally.

TABLE 3

DIFFICULTY ORDER OF FUNCTION WORDS: COMPARISON OF CROSS-SECTIONAL STUDIES*

Adults (ESL)[13]	Adults (aphasic)[16]	Children (ESL)[8]	Children (ESL)[9]	Children (L1)[10]	Children (ESL)[20]
ing	ing	plural	articles	plural	ing
con cop	plural	ing	ing	ing	
plural	con cop	con cop	(con) cop	part irreg	articles
articles	articles	con aux	con aux	articles	
con aux		articles		con cop	
past irreg	past irreg	past irreg	past irreg	poss	poss
third per s	third per s	third per s	poss	third per s	third per
poss		poss	third per s	con aux	
NP: pl	NP: pl	NP: pl	NP:	NP: pl	NP:
art	art	art	art	art	art
poss		poss	poss	poss	poss
VP: ing	VP: ing	VP: ing	VP: ing	VP: ing	VP: ing
con cop	con cop	con cop	con cop	past irreg	
con aux		con aux	con aux	con cop	
past irreg	past irreg	past irreg	past irreg	third per	third per
third per s	third per s	third per s	third per	con aux	

*Rank order correlations with adult ESL: adult aphasic = .90 (p < .05); child ESL[8] = .90 (p < .01); child ESL[9] = 89 (p < .01); child L1 = .57 (ns).

TABLE 4

FORMAL INSTRUCTION VERSUS EXPOSURE

Does "practice" have an effect?

	A	B
practice =	15	10
yrs study =	5	5

Prediction: A more proficient than B
Results: ELI—true of 6/14 pairs (ns)
Con Ed—true of 10/21 pairs (ns)

Does formal instruction have an effect?

	A	B
practice =	10	10
yrs study =	6	2

Prediction: A more proficient than B
Results: ELI—true of 7/9 pairs (T = 5.5, p < .025, one-tail)
Con Ed—true of 8/11 pairs (T = 7.5, p < .025, one-tail)

test	corr. with years in English-speaking country		corr. with reported years of study	
	r	p (one-tail)	r	p (one-tail)
Michigan	.18	.05	.50	.001
Comp.	−.22	.025	−.34	.005
Cloze (E)	.24	.01	.47	.001
Cloze (A)	.25	.01	.45	.001

The first two studies (Krashen & Seliger,[21] Krashen et al.[22]) compared instruction and practice by matching pairs of foreign students on one of these variables and seeing whether the student who excelled on the other was more proficient in English (TABLE 4).† For both studies combined, 16 out of 35 pairs matched for instruction were consistent with the hypothesis that more practice means more proficiency; that is, in about half the cases did the student with more practice outperform his partner with less. When students were matched for practice, however, it did prove to the the case that more instruction meant more proficiency. This was so for seven of nine cases in one study and for eight of eleven cases in the other, a result that in each study was statistically significant.

In the most recent study of this series, Krashen et al.[23] correlated placement examination scores for 116 students of ESL enrolled in the Queens College Continuing Education Program with students' reports of years of English study and years spent in

†In these studies, formal instruction was operationally defined as the students' report of the number of years of English study in school. No attention was given to matters such as methodology used, hours per week the class met, or whether the student had seriously pursued his studies. The only exception made was that one semester in the Queens College English Language Institute (300 contact hours) was counted as one year. In the first study[21] practice was defined as the product of years spent in the U.S. and how much English the student reported that he spoke each day (on a scale of one to ten). In the second study[22] students were asked to indicate years spent in U.S. and also to indicate how much English they spoke each day on a scale of one to four; subjects with the same number of years in the U.S. and the same report of speaking were matched. The measure of English proficiency in Ref. 21 was teacher ranking, and in Ref. 22 it was the Michigan "Examination in Structure."

English-speaking countries. The results (TABLE 4) confirm the earlier studies in that formal instruction was shown to be a better predictor of English proficiency and extended this result to a wider variety of testing devices. In this study, exposure, as measured by years in an English-speaking country, was shown to have a significant effect, but accounted for relatively little of the variation in test scores.

Prediction 2 is supported, then, to the extent that in general, instruction is useful for adult second-language learning in that it has a more consistent effect on proficiency than does exposure.

What does formal instruction do for the adult? It has been argued elsewhere[24] that the essential features of formal language instruction are the isolation of rules and lexical items and the presence of feedback (error detection and/or correction). These two features seem to be common to all language-teaching methods and seem not to be necessary for language acquisition before puberty. If this analysis is correct, these features may be just those that are needed by the adult learner and fill in "areas" where the Language Acquisition Device (LAD) is "weakened" at puberty.

Such features of formal instruction are, of course, available to the adult outside of the classroom through dictionaries, grammars, and helpful native speakers. In fact, recourse to rules and feedback may *always* characterize the successful "informal" learner and may explain how highly motivated individuals are able to improve in second-language mearning outside the classroom, even, in some cases, outperforming less-motivated students attending classes. Such cases are reported in Upshur[25] and in Mason.[26]

(3) Foreign accents cannot be overcome easily after puberty.

Since the publication of *Biological Foundations of Language*,[3] three studies have been done that confirm that prediction 3 is basically correct. Asher and Garcia[27] and Oyama[28] studied groups of Spanish- and Italian-speaking immigrants, respectively. In both studies, speech samples were tape-recorded and played for native speakers of English who rated the samples with respect to degree of foreign accent. Both Asher and Gracia and Oyama conclude that those who arrived in the United States earlier have more convincing American accents in English.

Our study[29] was a pedagogical exercise: Linguistics students at UCLA, Queens College, and Bar Ilan University were asked to interview immigrants to the United States or Israel as a class assignment. Subjects were asked whether they felt most ordinary speakers of their target language could tell they were not native speakers of English or Hebrew. The results were consistent with those of Asher and Garcia and Oyama and are given in TABLE 5.

As in Oyama's study, there was no significant effect of years in the United States (Asher and Garcia found time in the U.S. to be significant only in the case of those who arrived before puberty.)[30]

American subjects were also asked two questions related to type of motivation. To avoid a possible confound with age of arrival, answers were analyzed only for the group who arrived between ten and fifteen. It was found that those who reported a convincing accent said that significantly fewer of their friends spoke their native language; also, they tended to consider themselves "more American." Seliger et al.[29] interpret these results as consistent with the hypothesis that an "integrative" motivation[31] assists in successful language learning. Consistent with Oyama's finding that initial motivation did not relate to accent learning, Seliger et al. also found that those in the 10–15 year old group who reported a "conscious effort" to lose their foreign accent were not significantly more successful than those who made no such effort.

Labov[32] has suggested that similar constraints exist with respect to the acquisition of a second dialect: New York speech, he claims, is acquired by non-New Yorkers if they move to the New York area before puberty. Such a phenomenon, if true, extends and confirms prediction 3 as well as drawing an interesting parallel between dialect and language learning. In a design similar to that used by Seliger et al., Krashen and Seliger[30] asked linguistics students to interview people living in the New York City area who were not born in New York. Subjects were asked whether they recognized "New York Speech" (all did, confirming Labov's claim that there is a well-agreed-upon dialect spoken in New York), and whether, when they traveled outside New York, non-New Yorkers took them for New Yorkers from their speech. The results of this survey are given in TABLE 5, which shows trends similar to those in the foreign-accent survey, but with less sharp "breaks" between the groups. Again, there was no effect of years lived in New York. The data thus confirm Labov's suggestion and further implicate puberty as an important turning point in language learning.

(4) Full native-like competence in syntax and semantics may be achieved in second languages acquired before puberty, but not in second languages acquired after puberty.

TABLE 5

INTERVIEWS WITH IMMIGRANTS

Responses to the question: Do you think most ordinary Americans (or Israelis) think you are a native speaker of English (Hebrew)?*

Target Language	Age of Arrival	No	Don't Know	Yes
English	9 and under	4	3	26
Hebrew		2	3	30
English	10–15	17	4	21
Hebrew		9	1	20
English	16 and older	72	4	6
Hebrew		50	1	5

Responses to the question: When you travel outside the New York City area, do non-New Yorkers take you for a New Yorker by your speech?†

Age Moved to New York	Yes	No
3–9	40	27
10–15	27	40
16 and older	15	65

*From Ref. 29.
†From Ref. 21.

A small amount of data bearing on this prediction has been gathered since 1967, the most ambitious being included in Oyama's dissertation.[28] In addition to the accent test described above, Oyama's subjects, Italian-born immigrants to the United States, also took several tests involving the syntactic and semantic components of the grammar. In two of these (a "sentences through noise" task and a test in which subjects were asked to make grammatical acceptability judgments), a clear effect for age of arrival was observed; those who arrived in the United States at younger ages did best, and there was no effect for years spent in the U.S. Oyama's data thus confirm that age of arrival, as in the case of accent, is related to ultimate success in syntactic and semantic areas of linguistic competence, and prediction (4) is supported for her subjects taken as a group.

POSSIBLE BASES OF THE CRITICAL PERIOD

Evidence cited here on second-language acquisition in general supports the existence of the critical period: adults profit more from formal language instruction than they do from exposure to a second language, and probably do not attain native-like levels of proficiency in the target language. The effects of puberty on language learning, however, may not be entirely devastating. The adult LAD still functions in some ways similar to those of the prepuberty learner, as evidenced by the occurrence of overgeneralization errors and the Bailey et al.[13] result of invariant difficulty ordering of function words in learners of English as a second language. When certain crucial elements of formal instruction are made available to the adult, his LAD is apparently able to function, at least to some extent, in ways not totally dissimilar to the child's.

What happens at puberty to cause a change in language learning? In *Biological Foundations of Language*, Lenneberg[3] claims that there is a neurological basis for the difference in language learning capacity seen between children and adults. According to Lenneberg, underlying the child's ability to learn language naturally and completely is the fact that the development of cerebral dominance is not yet complete: The infant brain is "equipotential" for language; that is, either hemisphere can assume the language function successfully in the case of injury to the other side, and "dominance" is first detectable at around two, becoming fully established at puberty. Related to this picture of the development of lateralization is Lenneberg's claim that "transfer" of the language function, that is, the right hemisphere's "taking over" language in the case of injury to the left hemisphere, is completely successful only before puberty. This "interhemispheric plasticity" has been associated with the plasticity necessary to learn a second language.[33]

Since 1967, work in the area of cerebral dominance has shown that the picture of development of lateralization is somewhat different from that given by Lenneberg. Although no evidence has been presented to disconfirm the hypothesis that the infant brain is equipotential, cerebral dominance has nevertheless been detected in the neonate[34-36] (see also Ref. 37 and Kinsbourne, this annal).

Another change in the theory of the development of cerebral dominance, and one with more relevance to the critical period hypothesis, is the finding that the development of lateralization is complete much earlier than at puberty and thus may have nothing to do with the critical period.

Krashen[38] reexamined clinical data used by Lenneberg to support his claim that lateralization was established by puberty (cases of unilateral brain damage resulting in language disturbance) and concluded that the same data was consistent with the stronger hypothesis that lateralization is completely developed by five. Additional cases of unilateral damage in older children were examined and were found to be consistent only with the lateralization-by-five hypothesis: the percentage of cases of aphasia due to left-hemisphere lesions is about the same in children over five as it is in adults. In addition, no clear evidence was found to support the hypothesis that the minor hemisphere can completely take over the language function ("transfer") after five.

Data from dichotic listening also supports the lateralization-by-five hypothesis. Krashen and Harshman[39] reanalyzed previously preformed dichotic listening studies that used children as subjects and concluded that no significant change in degree of lateralization took place after five. Also, studies by Berlin et al.,[40] Goodglass,[41] and Dorman and Geffner[42] concur that the right-ear advantage in dichotic listening is fixed by five. Krashen and Harshman conclude that the completion of the development of lateralization may, in fact, have more to do with the acquisition of first language, a process that is also complete at around five (for detailed discussion, see Krashen[43]). Thus, the completion of the development of lateralization may represent the acquisition of language, rather than the establishment of a "biological barrier" to further natural language learning.‡

What, then, might be the basis for the close of the critical period? A possibility Rosansky and I are considering at present is that the close of the critical period is related to Inhelder and Piaget's stage of formal operations, which begins around puberty. It is at this time that the child begins to formulate abstract hypotheses to explain phenomena and becomes interested in general, rather than *ad hoc*, solutions to problems. This "general tendency of adolescents to construct theories" (Inhelder and Piaget,[44] p. 336) may inhibit "natural" language acquisition: the person who has reached the stage of formal operations may have not only the ability but also the need to construct a conscious theory (a grammar) of the language he is learning. This may make him unwilling to approach language more than one rule at a time, hence the presence of rule isolation in language teaching systems. Feedback may become necessary for the adult to be able to confirm his own conceptions of the rule he is learning.[45]

Children learning first language do not have the capacity or need for these general hypotheses and thus are not able to have and are not concerned with having a conscious knowledge of individual linguistic rules. The first-language acquisition literature also indicates that immediate feedback is less important for children than for adults.[46] It would be interesting to see whether error correction has any positive effect of prepuberty second-language acquisition; this hypothesis predicts it would not.

The adult's desire to have a conscious understanding of language may be just what prevents him from attaining full competence; it is quite difficult to express all of a natural language in terms of isolated rules. Thus, the adult may be limited by his ability to describe language to himself. The formal operations hypothesis thus predicts both the "incompleteness" and "unnaturalness" of adult second-language learning. A possible problem, however, is that this hypothesis also predicts that mentally retarded Down syndrome children also enter the stage of formal operations at the same time that their linguistic development "freezes."

Several scholars have linked the close of the critical period to so-called "affective variables."[47, 48] It may be the case, however, that certain of these personality changes occurring at puberty may themselves be a consequence of formal operations; their effects on language learning could then be considered indirect effects of formal operations, the direct effects being those described above. According to Elkind,[49] the ability to think abstractly, a characteristic of formal operation, leads the adolescent to "conceptualize his own thought...[and] to take his mental constructions as objects and reason about them" (p. 66). Above, I have suggested that this new ability leads to the capacity and perhaps the requirement to create an abstract grammar of a second

---

‡If the development of lateralization is complete by about age five, and if Lenneberg's observation that complete recovery from aphasia is possible before nine is correct, then one must conclude that the mechanisms for complete recovery after five do not include "transfer" of the language function to the minor hemisphere (unless the right hemisphere can retrain itself for language despite specialization for other functions). Cases of "ipsilateral" recovery in adults, that is, cases in which undamaged language dominant tissue is thought to take on language functions, are described in Roberts (1958). The capacity for complete ipsilateral recovery may be a function of age, children tending to be more able to utilize what are normally non-language areas of the dominant hemishere than are adults.

language. Another consequence, according to Elkind, is that the adolescent can now also "conceptualize the thought of other people."

> ...this capacity, however, is the crux of adolescent egocentrism. This egocentrism emerges because, while the adolescent can now cognize the thoughts of others, he fails to differentiate between the objects toward which the thoughts of others are directed and those which are to focus of his own concern. The young adolescent, because of the physiological metamorphosis he is undergoing, is primarily concerned with himself. Accordingly, since he fails to differentiate between what others are thinking about and his own mental pre-occupations, he assumes that other people are obsessed with his behavior and appearance as he is himself. *This belief that others are preoccupied with his appearance and behavior constitutes the egocentrism of the adolescent.* (p. 67)

The adolescent's resulting self-consciousness, his reluctance to reveal himself, his feeling of vulnerability, may have a great effect on second-language learning. As in other forms of behavior involving other people, he may become very unwilling to make what *he* perceives to be an "error." He may thus be unwilling to trust his own hypothesis-generating and -testing abilities, and may instead prefer to rely more on rules that feel to him to be "correct," namely the rules of his first language. Even when second-language rules are made available to him on a conscious level (thanks to his new ability to think in terms of an abstract grammar), he may be unwilling to utilize them. In the domain of phonology, this gives rise to the foreign accent. In syntax, it results in "interference" errors, which make up a substantial proportion of adult errors (but not all; see discussion of Richards above), and which are largely absent in younger learners.[50]

What I have said here implies that the ability to "acquire" a language disappears completely with the onset of formal operations for everyone. Certainly the presence of rule isolation and feedback in all teaching systems presumes this is the case. (There is one exception: Newmark's[51] "Minimal Language Teaching System." Krashen and Seliger,[24] however, argue that students learning foreign languages with this system have some means of obtaining isolated rules and feedback.) Braine,[52] however, has obtained some evidence that some adults may still be able to engage in language acquisition. In his study, subjects listened to and were asked to repeat sentences in an artificial, meaningless language. On posttests, it was found that many subjects were able to distinguish "grammatical" from anomalous sentences with a high degree of accuracy. The experiment was actually designed to test the hypothesis that a small percentage of anomalous sentences in the primary data would not cause a serious learning deficit. Although this hypothesis was supported, what is of interest to us is Braine's comment that some of the subjects who did well on the posttest could not state the grammatical principles they used in deciding on well-formedness; rather, they relied on whether a given sentence "sounded right." It is possible that in these cases, some degree of language acquisition, rather than learning, took place, stimulated, perhaps, by the fact that the linguistic environment was basically that of exposure to primary linguistic data.

Reanalysis of studies that found that formal instruction was in general more beneficial for adults than exposure [21, 23] might reveal other indications of language acquisition in adults. Language testers distinguish two sorts of second language tests: discrete-point tests, which test knowledge of isolated rules and lexical items ("structure" and "vocabulary" tests), and integrative tests, which test functional abilities (e.g. composition).[53] If some adults are able to engage in language acquisition to some extent, and if rules acquired via acquisition are not consciously isolated in the mind of the acquirer, one would expect that the more integrative a test is, the lower the correlation with instruction and the higher with exposure. The data in TABLE 3 is suggestive in that direction; also, Eileen Nam has found some evidence for a higher than expected correlation with exposure for an oral test of English as a second language.

REFERENCES

1. HESS, E. 1959. Imprinting. Science **130:** 133–141.
2. LORENZ, K. 1970. Studies in Animal and Human Behavior. Harvard University Press. Cambridge, Mass.
3. LENNEBERG, E. 1967. Biological Foundations of Language. John Wiley & Sons, New York, N.Y.
4. LENNEBERG, E., I. NICHOLS & E. ROSENBERGER. 1964. Primitive stages of language development in mongolism. *In* Disorders of Communication. Vol. XLII: Research Publications, A.R.N.M.D. Williams and Wilkins. Baltimore, Md.
5. RAVEM, R. 1968. Language acquisition in a second language environment. Intern. Rev. Appl. Linguistics. **6:** 175–185.
6. MILON, J. 1974. The development of negation in English by a second language learner. TESOL Quart. **8:** 137–143.
7. BEVER, T. & N. DENTON. The perceptual system of speech may be learned separately for each language in young bilinguals. Unpublished paper.
8. DULAY, H. & M. BURT. 1973. Should we teach children syntax? Language Learning **23:** 235–252.
9. DULAY, H. & M. BURT. 1974. Natural sequences in child second language acquisition. Language Learning **24:** 37–53.
10. DE VILLIERS, J. & P. DE VILLIERS. 1973. A cross-sectional study of the acquisition of grammatical morphemes in child speech. J. Psycholinguistic Res. **2:** 267–278.
11. BROWN, R. 1973. A First Language. Harvard University Press. Cambridge, Mass.
12. RICHARDS, J. 1971. A non-contrastive approach to error analysis. English Language Teaching **25:** 204–219; also *in* Focus on the Learner: Pragmatic Perspectives for the Language Teacher. J. Oller and J. Richards, Eds. Newbury House. Rowley, Mass.
13. BAILEY, N., C. MADDEN & S. KRASHEN. 1974. Is there a "natural sequence" in adult second language learning? Language Learning **24:** 235–243.
14. BURT, M., H. DULAY & C. HERNANDEZ. 1973. The Bilingual Syntax Measure. Harcourt, Brace, Jovanovich. New York, N.Y.
15. DE VILLIERS, J. & P. DE VILLERS. 1973. A cross-sectional study of the acquisition of grammatical morphemes in child speech. J. Psycholinguistic Rec. **2:** 267–278.
16. DE VILLIERS, J. 1974. Quantitative aspects of agrammatism in aphasia. Cortex **10:** 36–54.
17. HAKUTA, K. 1974. A preliminary report on the development of grammatical morphemes in a Japanese girl learning English as a second language. Working Papers in Bilingualism **3:** 18–38.
18. BEVER, T. 1970. The cognitive basis for linguistic structures. *In* Cognition and the Development of Language. J. Hayes, Ed. John Wiley & Sons. New York, N.Y.
19. HALE, T. & E. BUDAR. 1970. Are TESOL classes the only answer? Modern Lang. J. **54:** 487–62; also *in* Focus on the Learner: Pragmatic Perspectives for the Language Teacher. J. Oller and J. Richards, Eds. Newbury House. Rowley, Mass.
20. FATHMAN, A. 1974. The relationship between age and second language productive ability. Paper presented at the winter meeting of the Linguistic Society of America. Dec. 1974. New York, N.Y.
21. KRASHEN, S. & H. SELIGER. The role of formal and informal environments in second language learning: a pilot study. Intern. J. Psycholinguistics. In press.
22. KRASHEN, S., H. SELIGER & D. HARTNETT. 1974. Two studies in adult second language learning. Kritikon Litterarum. 2/3: 220–228.
23. KRASHEN S., C. JONES, S. ZELINSKI & C. USPRICH. How important is instruction? English Language Teaching J. In press.

24. KRASHEN, S. & H. SELIGER. 1975. The essential characteristics of formal instruction. TESOL Quarterly **9:** 173–183.
25. UPSHUR, J. 1968. Four experiments on the relation between foreign language teaching and learning. Lang. Learning **18:** 111–124.
26. MASON, C. 1971. The relevance of intensive training in English as a foreign language for university students. Lang. Learning **21:** 197–204.
27. ASHER, J. & R. GARCIA. 1969. The optimal age to learn a foreign language. Modern Lang. J. **53:** 334–41.
28. OYAMA, S. 1973. A sensitive period for the acquisition of a second language. Ph.D. dissertation. Harvard Univ. Cambridge, Mass.
29. SELIGER, H., S. KRASHEN & P. LADEFOGED. 1975. Maturational constraints in the acquisition of a native-like accent in second language learning. Lang. Sciences **36:** 20–22.
30. KRASHEN, S. & H. SELIGER. Maturational Constraints in the acquisition of a second language and a second dialect. Lang. Sciences. In press.
31. GARDNER, R. & W. LAMBERT. 1972. Attitudes and Motivation in Second Language Learning. Newbury House. Rowley, Mass.
32. LABOV, W. 1970. The Study of Nonstandard English. Nat. Council Teachers Eng. Urbana, Ill.
33. SCOVEL, T. 1969. Foreign accents, language acquisition, and cerebral dominance. Lang. Learning **19:** 245–254.
34. WITELSON, S. & W. PALLIE. 1973. Left hemisphere specialization for language in the newborn. Brain **96:** 641–646.
35. MOLFESE, D. 1972. Cerebral asymmetry in infants, children, and adults: auditory evoked responses to speech and music stimuli. Ph.D. dissertation. Pennsylvania State University. University Park, Pa.
36. GARDINER, M., C. SCHULMAN & D. WALTER. 1973. Facultative EEG asymmetries in babies and adults. Brain Information Service Conference Report no. 34. Unversity of California at Los Angeles. Los Angeles, Calif.
37. HARSHMAN, R. & S. KRASHEN. 1973. On the development of lateralization. Brain Information Service Conference Report no. 34. University of California at Los Angeles, Los Angeles, Calif.
38. KRASHEN, S. 1973. Lateralization, language learning, and the critical period: some new evidence. Lang. Learning **23:** 63–74.
39. KRASHEN, S. & R. HARSHMAN. 1972. Lateralization and the critical period. Working Papers in Phonetics (UCLA) **23:** 13–21.
40. BERLIN, C., L. HUGHES, S. LOWE-BELL & H. BERLIN. 1973. Dichotic right ear advantage in children 5 to 13. Cortex **9:** 393–402.
41. GOODGLASS, H. 1973. Developmental comparison of vowels and consonants in dichotic listening. J. Speech Hearing Res. **16:** 744–752.
42. DORMAN, M. & D. GEFFNER. 1974. Hemispheric specialization for speech perception in six year old black and white children from low and middle socioeconomic classes. Cortex **10:** 171–176.
43. KRASHEN, S. 1973. Mental abilities underlying linguistic and non-linguistic functions. Linguistics **115:** 39–55.
44. INHELDER, B. & J. PIAGET. 1958. The Growth of Logical Thinking from Childhood to Adolescence. Basic Books. New York, N.Y.
45. CORDER, S. 1967. The significance of learner's errors. Intern. Rev. Appl. Linguistics **4:** 161–169.
46. CAZDEN, C. 1965. Environmental assistance to the child's acquisition of grammar. Ph.D. dissertation. Harvard University. Cambridge, Mass.
47. TAYLOR, B. 1974. Toward a theory of language acquisition. Lang. Learning. 23–35.
48. STEVICK, E. 1974. Why is a foreign accent? Linguistics and Psychoanalysis: Some Interfaces **1:** 1–2.
49. ELKIND, D. 1970. Children and Adolescents: Interpretive Essays on Jean Piaget. Oxford University Press. New York, N.Y.
50. DULAY, H. & M. BURT. 1974. Errors and strategies in child second language acquisition. TESOL Quart. **8:** 129–136.

51. NEWMARK, L. 1971. A minimal language-teaching program. *In* the Psychology of Second Language Learning. P. Pimsleur amd T. Quinn, Eds. Cambridge Univ. Press. Cambridge, England.

52. BRAINE, M. 1971. On two types of models of the internalization of grammars. *In* The Ontogenesis of Grammar. D. Slobin, Ed. Academic Press. New York, N.Y.

53. CARROLL, J. 1972. Some fundamental considerations in testing for English language proficiency of foreign students. *In* Teaching English as a Second Language. H. Allen and R. Campbell, Eds. McGraw-Hill. New York, N.Y.

PERCEPTION AND PRODUCTION IN A VISUALLY
BASED LANGUAGE*

Edward S. Klima

University of California at San Diego
San Diego, California 92115

Ursula Bellugi

The Salk Institute for Biological Studies
San Diego, California 92112

Whether or not speech is special (as some would argue), it seems to us that there remain questions of great theoretical import concerning the relationship between speech and language; namely, What would language be like without speech? What properties of the complex phenomenon we call language—including its production and perception—are due to the mode of expression, i.e., due to the channel in which the more abstract entities are realized as physical, perceptible stuff, and what properties are due to some broader lingusitic faculty or to cognition in general? What sort of stamp does sound itself put on language? What would be the effect of other possible modes?

Our small research group consisting of personnel at The Salk Institute and at the University of California at San Diego is approaching these questions by using an experimental situation provided by nature, that in which human beings are born deaf or become deaf during the prelingual period. We have purposely restricted our study to deaf people who are offspring of deaf parents and who learned as their first primary language the visual-gestural language called American Sign Language (ASL). By analyzing a language that utilizes a visual rather than an auditory mode of perception, and a gestural rather than a vocal mode of production, we can begin to address the problem of the relationship between language and its physical realization.

In this presentation we shall report on some of the findings of our studies including: 1) The status of sign language in terms of general visual symbolism and, in particular, the relationship between sign language and pantomime; 2) the way signs seem to be encoded and stored, according to results of experiments in the short-term memory paradigm and evidence from slips of the hand; 3) historical change in signs of ASL; and 4) the structure of sign language with special focus on the differences between sign language (ASL in particular) and spoken language (English in particular). Our emphasis will be on the interaction between the mode (in this case, the visual-gestural) and the more abstract linguistic and cognitive aspects of language.

To begin with, however, it is best to dispel some misconceptions that commonly arise concerning the sign languages of the deaf. First, there is no single universal sign language. Rather, there are many different sign languages, just as there are many different spoken languages. These differ from one another most obviously in the form of the signs which they use, but also in the kinds of grammatical devices employed. Thus, despite the common written language in America and Great Britain, the sign

*This research was supported in part by National Institutes of Health grant no. NS-09811, and by National Science Foundation grant no. GSOC-741780 to the Salk Institute for Biological Studies.

language used in America (ASL) is quite unrelated to the one used in Great Britain. The two sign languages are mutually incomprehensible. ASL is no more a universal gestural language than is any other individual sign language; nor is ASL either a derivative or a degenerate form of written or spoken English, although it has certainly been affected by its contact with English. ASL developed "naturally" in whatever way languages arise, change, and evolve.

Let us turn now to what might be expected of sign language in light of properties thought to be associated with visual symbols in general. In a provocative article, Roman Jakobson,[1] writing primarily about painting and film, differentiates the structural characteristics of the visual versus the auditory symbol. According to Jakobson, while a complex *auditory* symbol consists generally of successive serial constituents, a complex *visual* symbol involves a series of simultaneous constituents. (In later sections of this paper, we shall see that *simultaneity* is an important characteristic of sign language.) Another essential difference between visual and auditory symbols, according to Jakobson, is that with visual symbols there is a definite tendency to "reify"—to connect the symbols with objects, to ascribe mimesis to them, to view them as elements of an imitative art. On the other hand, Jakobson asserts, verbal and musical (i.e., auditory) symbols are characteristically resolvable into discrete, highly patterned components that do not exist as such in nature but are instead constructed ad hoc.

In his discussion, Jakobson happens to treat that part of visual semiotics which is nonlinguistic. But what is the situation when the sole *language* learned by an individual in a natural way is indeed *visual*, as is the case with sign languages learned by the congenitally deaf?

THE PANTOMIMIC ORIGIN OF SOME SIGNS

As de Saussure and many of his predecessors pointed out, the lexical items of spoken language are *essentially* arbitrary. The form of the English word "cat" has no direct relation to the form of a cat; the form of the word "bird" has no relation to any aspect of the representation of a bird; the form of the word "tree" has no relation to the actual appearance of a tree. In American Sign Language, we find, at first glance, that there is a considerable lack of arbitrariness in the form of many signs. Consider the following mimetic relations:

1) The sign CAT† representing the whiskers of a cat;
2) The sign BIRD representing the opening and closing of the beak of a bird; and
3) The sign TREE, using the arm and hand to represent the trunk and branches of a tree.

We must immediately add that few signs are so clearly transparent in their iconicity that a nonsigner can guess their meaning without some additional cues. Usually it is not possible for a nonsigner to guess even the topic of conversation in deaf communication, though, of course, this should be possible in pantomime. Nevertheless, many of the signs in a visual language like ASL appear to be far less arbitrary than the words of a spoken language.

It appears to us that (certainly from the point of view of their history) such signs are indeed motivated in the sense we have been describing: that is, they may well have begun from some sort of representation of objects, some sort of at-

---

†In this paper, we use an English translation-equivalent gloss to represent a sign. If more than one word is required to translate a single sign, the words are connected with hyphens. The form of the gloss has, of course, nothing to do with the form of the sign.

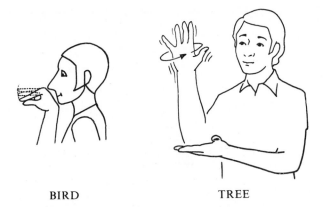

BIRD   TREE

tempt to act out, mime, imitate an object or action. We find that when new signs are invented on the spur of the moment, particularly new signs for concrete objects with distinctive shapes or typical movements, the iconic associations are often quite pronounced. This suggests that one possible way of analyzing the formational principles of ASL would be to consider the individual sign as an unanalyzable whole, a kind of *gestalt-like* unit. The obvious and very critical question, however, is *not:* How do a few novel signs appear to a naive hearing nonsigner? Rather, it is: How do *deaf* people whose primary native language is ASL process signs?

How Are Signs Coded? Evidence from Memory Experiments

As one means of approaching this question in an experimental context, we designed a series of short-term memory studies (reported in References 2, 3, and other forthcoming papers). On videotape we presented sequences of commonly known signs to deaf college students whose native language is ASL, and we required immediate, ordered recall. We then analyzed the many errors‡ our subjects made for clues to the way in which they had coded and processed the signs. We found that intrusion errors did not reflect, as they do for hearing subjects, the sound structure of the English words equivalent to the ASL signs (e.g., "cat" was never misremembered as "cot"). The errors also did not reflect the visual form of the equivalent English words in terms of the letters used to spell them, or their general shape (e.g., "cat" was never misremembered as "oat"). Nor did the errors reflect an essentially semantic organization in the processing and remembering of signs in this experiment (e.g., "cat" was not misremembered as "animal" or "dog").

Finally, the errors did not reflect, as might reasonably have been expected, the somewhat more iconic or representational character of the basic meaningful units of sign language. Rather, what we found was that a significant number of multiply occurring intrusion errors made by deaf subjects to signs were based on purely formational properties of the signs themselves. Let us consider the errors for the signs cited earlier:

1) The errors for the sign CAT, which seemed to represent the whiskers of a cat,

---

‡An "intrusion error" in our short-term memory experiments is a response that is not an item on the list presented nor on the immediately prior list. Intrusion errors in short-term memory are traditionally used to investigate the nature of the encoding processes. Conrad,[4] Sperling,[5] and others have shown that for hearing subjects verbal items (words or letters) are encoded in phonological form.

did not include "whiskers," "purr," "paws," "meow," "claws," "fur," or any other attributes that might be included iconically in the delineation of a cat along with its whiskers. But more than one deaf person misremembered the sign as INDIAN. The two signs—CAT and INDIAN—are each made with one hand only, each made on the cheek, and each made with the same handshape; in fact, they differ only in the particular movement involved, a brushing movement for CAT and two contact points for INDIAN.

2) The errors for the sign BIRD did not include "beak," "wing," "soar," "chirp," "feeder," or some other representational aspect of the referent. But more than one deaf person misremembered the sign BIRD as NEWSPAPER. The sign for BIRD and the sign for NEWSPAPER are each made with the same handshape and each involves the same movement; they differ only in the place of articulation—BIRD is made on the mouth and NEWSPAPER is made on the palm of the hand.

3) The errors for TREE did not include "trunk," "branch," or "leaf," but NOON was given by several subjects. The signs are similar in all respects except movement.

Sign   Error

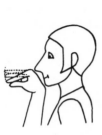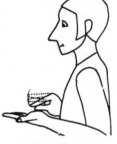

BIRD   NEWSPAPER

Sign   Error

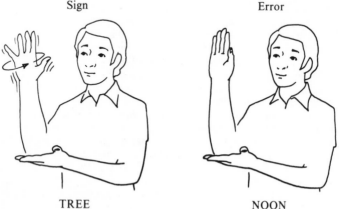

TREE   NOON

Indeed, most of the multiply occurring intrusion errors made by deaf subjects were visually similar to the original sign presented on the test, and visually similar in specific and predictable ways. The errors tended to preserve the relationship of the hands of the original sign presented; i.e., if the sign was a one-handed sign, the error was a one-handed sign, etc. But more significant than that, the majority of multiple errors differed from the sign presented in one aspect only. Our results were thus consistent with a theory that the signs of ASL are actually *coded* by the deaf in terms of a limited set of formational parameters, such as Hand Configuration, Place of Articulation, Orientation, and Movement§—parameters that in this context, are essentially *arbitrary* in terms of meaning.

How Are Signs Organized? Evidence from Production

There are also certain phenomena of everyday signing behavior (e.g., from production of signs in discourse) that support the results of these experiments, suggesting the functional independence of the parameters of ASL. Especially revealing is one class of spontaneous errors that occur in sign production, the "slips of the hand" that appear when some aspects of an intended message are transposed. (A similar phenomenon in spoken language, slips of the tongue, is discussed by Fromkin.[8])

If signs were stored as wholistic gestures, one might expect that the *only* errors would be transpositions of whole signs. Occasionally it does happen that entire signs in an intended message are interchanged. For example, one signer intended to sign TASTE-IT, MAYBE LIKE-IT, meaning "Taste it and maybe you'll like it," but she actually produced, LIKE-IT, MAYBE TASTE-IT. However, such global transpositions are very rare.

In most of the signing errors we have collected, it is not whole signs, but rather individual formational parameters of signs that are interchanged. The resulting gestures produced are often not actual signs of ASL at all. For example, one deaf person intended to sign SICK and TIRED. She transposed the Hand Configurations of the two signs, producing the first gesture with the Movement, Orientation, and Location of SICK, but with the Hand Configuration of TIRED; and the second gesture

Intended

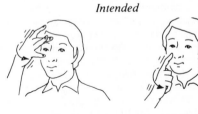

SICK   TIRED

Produced

"tick"   "sired"

§We use the term "formational parameters" to refer to those aspects described first by Stokoe[6,7] which make up the individual sign. He described three aspects of a sign: 1) the place where it is made, 2) the distinctive configuration of the hand or hands in making it, and 3) the action of the hand or hands. Later descriptions have added other parameters, such as orientation of the hands.

with the Movement, Orientation, and Location of TIRED, but the Hand Configuration of SICK. This is more or less analogous to "tick and sired" in English, but in the signed slip of the hand, the errors are not actual signs of ASL.

Although the most frequently interchanged aspects of signs are in Hand Configuration, slips of the hand involving Movement, Orientation, and Place of Articulation have also occurred in our data. This evidence further supports the hypothesis that the linguistic parameters posited for ASL are psychologically real for fluent deaf signers.

Let us consider again the more general question: Do signs of ASL have an iconic aspect? Undoubtedly many do, and this may be just what one should expect from primary visual symbols and our tendency to "reify" them. But at the same time, our memory studies and our observations of everyday behavior involving slips of the hand reveal that there is another, perhaps parallel, level of organization. At this other level, even those signs which retain some representational aspects appear to be processed by native signers as being constituted of a limited set of recurring elements that are themselves arbitrary in terms of meaning. The coexistence of the iconic and the arbitrary aspects may seem paradoxical. However, a study of recent historical change in signs may provide some clues to help resolve this paradox.

HISTORICAL CHANGE IN SIGNS: FROM ICONICITY TO ARBITRARINESS

In order to investigate historical change in signs, we have studied films of some elderly deaf signers made in the early part of this century, as well as certain sign language manuals published just after the turn of the century (cf. Long.[9]). In addition, we have interviewed (on videotape) elderly deaf signers, asking them for their recollections of signs that have changed during the past fifty years or so.

ASL has, in its contemporary form, lost a great deal of its transparency. Over time, signs have become less pantomimic or imitative and have assumed arbitrary shapes. The change is in the direction of more systematic aspects of the language. For example, in a 1913 film, the sign for BODY was made by moving both hands downward in parallel from the shoulders to the hips, outlining the contours of the body, as it were. The sign used today for BODY is made with the two hands in the same Orientation as before, but with two touches: one at the chest, and another above the waist. We note that there are many ASL signs made with two touches in one area, such as HOME, YESTERDAY, WE, QUEEN, BACHELOR. It is our assumption that the older ASL sign for BODY has become modified in a way that makes it like other contemporary ASL signs in terms of Movement.

Another example is the sign for SWEETHEART. According to elderly informants, this sign used to be made over the region of the heart with the two hands coming together at the edge of the little fingers in the shape of a valentine heart. No other ASL sign has this point of contact. The sign for SWEETHEART is now made on the center line of the body with the hands in contact at the knuckles. This is a type of contact occurring in a number of other current ASL signs (GAME, ACCIDENT, etc.)

Frishberg[10] notes an historical trend that limits the expression of lexical content to the hands. She has found many examples of signs that used to require a certain facial expression or body movement simultaneous with articulation by the hand. Over the years, the required body movement or facial expression dropped out or transferred to the hands. As a result, these signs are now made with the hands alone. For example, the old sign for PATIENT was made with the thumb at the lips as the head bowed downward. The bowing movement of the head is now performed by a movement of the hand—the thumb moves downward across the lips while the head

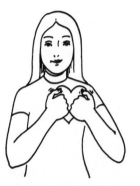 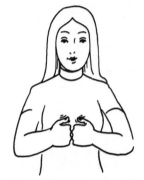

SWEETHEART—Old sign   SWEETHEART—Current sign

remains stationary. Similarly, the sign THINK originally involved resting an index finger on the forehead and moving the head in a circular motion. The present sign for THINK now involves a circular motion of the index finger near the forehead as the head itself remains still.

We see that historical change in signs gives some clues to what appear to be systematic pressures in ASL. The direction of change is often toward some recurring element or prime that is found in already existing signs of the language. Even those new signs coined on the spur of the moment which have marked iconic associations tend to constrain their iconicity to fit the system, by utilizing a limited set of recurring formational elements.

SIMULTANEITY IN SIGN LANGUAGE

What, then, is the nature of this set of recurring elements which figure in the internal organization of the individual sign, and how does the sign compare with the word of spoken language? In spoken language, even at the level of the word, the sequential arrangements of elements is paramount, both phonologicaly and morphologically. For example, "cats," the plural of "cat," consists of four phonological segments in sequence; /k/, /æ/, /t/, and /s/. At another level of analysis there are two morphological units in sequence, "cat" and the plural morpheme, which in this case has the shape "-s." (In some of their possible orderings, these phonological segments also render the English words "stack," "tax," "scat," "cast," "task," "acts," "axed," "sacked," and "asked.") Although simultaneity is also represented in the word—for example, tone and intonation occur at the same time as articulation—it is generally secondary.

But if the organization of the word in spoken language is primarily sequential, the organizational principle of the individual sign in sign language is primarily *simultaneous*. A sign is characterized by the simultaneous occurrence of: 1) one of a limited set of Hand Configurations, which have 2) a restricted set of Orientations and relations to other parts of the body, involved in 3) specific Movements, made in 4) specific Manners of Articulation, at 5) a restricted set of Places of Articulation.

Even the sorts of modulation of meaning that are often realized within the word of spoken language by affixation—i.e., sequential modification—are characteristically represented within the sign of sign language by some *simultaneous* change in Movement or in some other parameter. Take the following as an example of the difference between the modulation of meaning in English and in ASL. For instance, the modulation of the lexical item "blue" to achieve the meaning of "somewhat blue in color" consists, in spoken English, of the sequential addition of the morpheme "-ish" to the item "blue." In American Sign Language the parallel modulation to change BLUE to BLUISH is accomplished by the simultaneous superimposition of a lax-ness of Hand Configuration and a "suspendedness" in the quality of Movement on the citation form of the sign: BLUE.

But does the simultaneity that characterizes the structure of the individual sign and its regular morphological modifications also permeate higher levels of structure, such as syntax? Since two hands are available for signing, an extreme form of simultaneity is logically possible at the syntactic level; for example, one could sign GIRL with the right hand and, at the same time, EAT with the left hand for "the girl is eating." But in ordinary conversational signing, this type of simultaneity does not usually occur; i.e., the lexically specified subject or object of a predicate is not regularly expressed simul-taneously with the sign for the predicate itself. We do find use of a deictic sign like THERE (index finger pointing to a locus in sign space) occurring simultaneously with a lexical sign (e.g., GIRL), but two lexical signs do not ordinarily occur at the same time.

In other words, at the syntactic level sign language has a decidedly segmental aspect: one distinct sign follows another sequentially. But even here, other aspects of sign language syntax, such as those used to specify grammatical relations and pronominal reference, often rely not on the sequential order in which the signs oc-cur in the sentence, but rather on the articulated use of space. The ASL analogue of pronominal reference is accomplished by associating a specific locus in signing space with a noun in the utterance, which will subsequently be referred to by "point-ing" to that locus (as, for example, in the deictic sign THERE just mentioned). Sim-ilarly, verbs in ASL may actually incorporate these spatial loci in their form to in-dicate grammatical relations like subject and object.[11]

RESTRICTIONS ON THE FORM OF SIGNS: THE USE OF TWO ARTICULATORS

The fact that ASL has at its disposal the two hands but that in everyday signing the two hands are rarely, if ever, used to make two distinct lexical signs simultaneously raises a more general question. What are the effects of having, in the two hands, two distinct and independent articulators, and what are the restrictions on these pos-sibilities? The characteristics of ASL that follow seem to us to be reasonable candi-dates for exemplifying restrictions on the form or use of a language, restrictions that are directly related to production and perception.

Even in single signs that make use of the two hands, there are restrictions on the independence of the hands. By way of introduction, we note that there are three classes of signs in ASL, characterized by different arrangements of the hands. We have calculated the proportion of each of these classes in a corpus of more than 2,000 signs from the Dictionary of American Sign Language (Stokoe et al.[7]). About 40% of the signs are made with one hand only. The rest of the signs are made with two hands, but in two different kinds of arrangements. About 35% of ASL signs are made with both hands active, and sharing the same Movement. The other 25% are made with an active hand acting on the other hand, which is used as a base for the sign. It is in the signs made with two hands that restrictions on the independent use of the hands arise.

Consider first, the type of sign which is made with both hands active.¶ There are

¶ We note in passing that there are some minimal pairs of signs which differ only in that, say, sign A is made with one hand and sign B is made with both hands; in all other respects, the signs A and B are identical. Such pairs of signs include YELLOW and PLAY; PURPLE and PARTY.

significant restrictions on the form of individual signs of this class: the two hands must have the same Movement. Not only is there required symmetry of Movement, there is also in general a symmetry of Handshape as well. (The two hands may, however, be in different Places of Articulation, as in the signs NOTHING, SICK, or AWFUL.) The restrictions resulting in symmetry of Movement and Handshape in such signs are powerful ones, as is evidenced by certain historical facts. Frishberg[10] notes that when formerly one-handed signs become two-handed signs, both hands assume the same Movement and Hand Configuration as in the original sign. This is seen in the historical change which ANGRY, HURRY, and DIE have undergone in the past fifty years.

The second type of sign using the two hands involves an active hand operating on a base hand. In this class of signs, the Handshape of the two articulators may be (but need not be) symmetrical. But again we note an historical tendency toward such symmetry. Some signs of this class in which the hands originally had different shapes are now symmetrical in Hand Configuration (e.g., DEPEND, LAST, SHORT, WORLD). Facilitation of articulation certainly suggests itself in such cases.

There are no special restrictions on the Handshape of the active hand in signs involving an active and a base hand. The base hand, however, if not symmetrical in shape to the active hand, is restricted to a small set of six frequently occurring Handshapes, which account for 69% of all the entries in the Dictionary of ASL. In an experimental study of perceptual confusions of Handshapes under varying levels of visual "noise," these base Handshapes were found to be, on the average, more resistant to distortion by visual noise than were the other Handshapes of ASL.[12]

Thus we see that there are definite restrictions on the form of ASL signs with respect to the independence of the two hands. Whereas there are minimal pairs of ASL signs that differ only in the use of one hand as contrasted with two hands, in no case are there minimal pairs in which the two signs are distinguished only by the *particular* hand—right versus left—that is active in making the sign.

We can relate this to some informal observations we have made of deaf people in our research group. One young woman is distinctly left-hand dominant (Harris test); she invariably makes signs in citation form using her left hand as dominant or active. She also consistently uses her left hand as dominant in everyday signing. Her performance is in distinct contrast to the other deaf researchers in our group, who are right-hand dominant and use their right hand consistently as the active hand in signing. None of these signers show any tendency to alternate in the use of the hands in nonpoetic, nonnarrative signing. In other words, it makes no difference which hand is used as active in signing; the choice depends on the hand dominance of the individual signer. Of course, there remains the interesting question of whether this observed characteristic of the form of ASL signs represents a universal of sign languages.

CREATIVITY IN A TWO-HANDED LANGUAGE

We have now pointed out some physical possibilities in the production of signs that are *not* realized in everyday communication, including: 1) making two lexical signs simultaneously; and 2) alternating left and right hands in consecutive signs. Both of these possibilities depend on the existence of two independent articulators— the two hands—in producing sign language. Such possibilities, of course, do not arise in spoken language. In sign language they are allowed by the mode, and yet seem to be restricted in ordinary usage. However, we have found that these very possibilities are, in fact, realized in special self-conscious, preplanned, or rehearsed linguistic activities such as *plays on signs* and *sign-poetry*.[13]

We have made a collection of plays-on-signs by searching through our videotapes of deaf people signing and by noting instances as they occurred in everyday deaf communication among the members of our research group. Several processes of sign-play have come to light which are special to sign language itself, i.e., special to a visual-gestural language. Among these are the overlapping of two signs by making two signs at the same time or by holding a sign (or part of one) with one hand and making a second distinct sign with the other. As an example, one deaf person wanted to indicate an ambivalence of feeling about leaving for a new situation. He signed EXCITED and DEPRESSED at the same time, making "half" of each sign with either hand. Thus he compressed into one unit the expression of two contradictory—but simultaneously held—emotions.

Signs Made Simultaneously

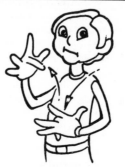

EXCITED/DEPRESSED

Through studies of poetic sign, or "art sign," created by members of the National Theater of the Deaf, we have been investigating a poetic tradition in sign language that is evolving in our own time. We have discovered several processes characteristic of poetic signing; among them are the overlapping of two signs (just as in sign-plays), and alternation in the use of right and left hands. The latter process results in a balance between the two hands and a more symmetrical use of the space in which the poem is produced.

SUMMARY

We have discussed aspects of production and perception in a visually based language, focusing on those properties of language that are due to the mode in which the language arose and on those which seem to be due instead to more general linguistic faculties. We asked specifically: What is the special effect of the visual-gestural mode on the form of sign language?

We described first the roots of sign language in pantomime and showed that signs are clearly less arbitrary than words of spoken language, as might well be expected with visual symbols. We gave evidence, however, that despite their iconic origin, signs are processed, coded, and organized by the deaf in terms of *recurring formational parameters*, essentially *arbitrary* with respect to meaning. Furthermore, we showed by studies of historical change in signs how the linguistic system affects the iconic gestures of the language, molding them into an organized, more arbitrary, system. Throughout this discussion, we emphasized the essentially different nature of the organization of a visual language, basically *simultaneous* rather than sequential. This difference in organization extends even to the modulation of meaning in signs.

Finally, we discussed some physical possibilities in the production of signs that are not realized in everyday communication. We pointed out that in self-conscious preplanned linguistic activities, such as plays on signs and art-sign, these possibilities—special to a language in a visual-gestural mode—are utilized. Our studies support what insightful observers have already noticed about the general differences between the visual and the auditory, and show that these general differences are strikingly evident in the special case of a language that has evolved for the eye instead of for the ear.

ACKNOWLEDGMENTS

The present members of our research group include: Dr. Carole Offir, Birgitte Bendixen, Bonnie Gough, Scott Liddell, Don Newkirk, Carlene Canady Pedersen, and Ted Supalla. Frank A. Paul made the illustrations for this paper. The films used in our investigation of historical changes in signs were lent to us by the Library Archives at Gallaudet College for the Deaf, Washington, D.C.

REFERENCES

1. JAKOBSON, R. 1967. On the relations between visual and auditory signs. *In* Selected Writings II. 338–344. Mouton. The Hague, The Netherlands.
2. BELLUGI U. & P. SIPLE. 1974. Remembering with and without words. *In* Current Problems in Psycholinguistics. F. Bresson, Ed.: 215–236. Centre Nationale de la Recherche Scientifique. Paris, France.
3. BELLUGI, U., E. KLIMA & P. SIPLE. Remembering in signs. Cognition: Intern. J. Cognitive Psychol. In press.
4. CONRAD, R. 1962. An association between memory errors and errors due to acoustic masking of speech. Nature **193**: 1314–1315.
5. SPERLING, G. 1963. A model for visual memory tasks. Human Factors **5**: 19–31.
6. STOKOE, W. 1960. Sign language structure. Studies in Linguistics. (Reissued Washington, D.C., Gallaudet College Press)
7. STOKOE, W., D. CASTERLINE & C. CRONEBERG. 1965. A Dictionary of American Sign Language. Gallaudet College Press. Washington, D.C.
8. FROMKIN, V. A. 1973. Slips of the tongue. Scientific American **229** (6): 110–117.
9. LONG, J. 1918. The Sign Language: A Manual of Signs. Athens Press. Iowa City, Iowa.
10. FRISHBERG, N. Arbitrariness and iconicity: Historical change in American sign language. *In* The Signs of Language. E. S. Klima and U. Bellugi, Eds. Harvard Univ. Cambridge, Mass. To be published.
11. FISCHER, S. & B. GOUGH. Verbs in American Sign Language. *In* The Signs of Language. U. Bellugi & E. Klima, Eds. Harvard Univ. Press. Cambridge, Mass. To be published.
12. LANE, H., P. BOYES-BRAEM & U. BELLUGI. 1975. Preliminaries to a distinctive feature analysis of American Sign Language. Salk Inst. Biological Studies. Unpublished.
13. KLIMA E. S. & U. BELLUGI. 1974. Wit and poetry in American Sign Language. Paper presented at Amer. Anthropological Assoc. Meetings. Mexico City, Mexico.

BALLISTIC CONTROL OF RHYTHMIC ARTICULATORY MOVEMENTS IN NATURAL SPEECH*

Samuel W. Anderson

Department of Communication Sciences
New York State Psychiatric Institute
New York, New York 10032

Before words come to me I get a sense of rhythm, something like a time schema. Before the words, I've had a sense of form, something into which the words as they appear can fit.[1]

Anyone capable of enjoying poetry will almost surely agree to the proposition that speech is rhythmic. But experimental questions concerning the nature of this rhythm have only recently been asked, and answers are slow in coming. Are rhythms physically measurable in natural speech? If so, how? In what units? What is the importance of speech rhythms in normal human communication? How is rhythm acquired?

Even clear formulations of the rhythm hypothesis are still quite tentative. Most advanced is the recent mathematical theory of dyadic conversion, presented by Jaffe and Feldstein,[2] but there is as yet no known link between models for human dialog and the data from early experiments dealing with the rhythmic cadences out of which individual utterances are ostensibly made. This paper is a first attempt at filling the gap.

Let us begin with a review of theories of speech rhythm based upon experimental results from phonetics and upon data collected and analyzed in our laboratory from samples of spontaneous talk. A preliminary ballistic control model that can account for the data will then be proposed and shown to be compatible with known control properties of the nervous system, both in the normal adult and developing child.

As many of us who are steeped in the faith all know, it was Lashley who prophesied that Chomsky was going to be right later on, even with respect to the action of the nervous system in controlling speech. Actually, it is Martin[3] who traces the origin of the speech rhythm hypothesis to Lashley,[4] and mounts a valiant programmatic attempt to reconcile two generative rules for stress assignment[5]† with a set of abstract "rhythmic trees." Martin's trees, constructed freely by the application of his rules and the use of null branches, supply a temporal structure for any accent pattern whatever, certainly guaranteeing effectiveness for whatever linguistic cadences may exist. He warns against the common "misconception. . that rhythm implies only periodic, repetitive behavior, like walking or breathing, and hence is too simple a concept to be of interest for speech behavior." (Ref. 3, p. 487). The difference is, of course, that those who propose a periodicity for speech do not claim that speech sounds, like footsteps or inhalations, occur repetitively. Rather, it is claimed that only a particular linguistic *feature*, the accent or stress, recurs more or less regularly.

Lehiste[6] sees Classe[7] and Abercrombie[8] as the original theorists of speech rhythm; Classe considers regular recurrence, or *isochrony*, of rhythmic units to be primarily a perceptual phenomenon, supported only by a *tendency* for regular pacing in speech production (Ref. 6, p. 1228). For Abercrombie, on the other hand, isochrony is a

---

*Supported by The Department of Mental Hygiene of New York State and a General Research Support Grant to the Research Foundation for Mental Hygiene, Inc.
†These are the nuclear stress rule and the compound rule.

property of the signal. He proposes as the periodic unit a "metric foot" made up of a group containing one, two or several syllables extending from one "stress pulse" to the next (Ref. 8, p. 217). We shall refer to the interpulse interval as the *stress period*.

In an experiment designed to test Abercrombie's hypothesis, Lehiste had two speakers recite each of seventeen sentences ten times each. She found that "the same foot types have remarkably similar durations . . ." (Ref. 6, p. 1230) in the intermediate sentence positions, but that each of the three disyllabic foot types analyzed had a different period. Because these differences were not perceived very accurately, Lehiste decided in favor of Classe. Unfortunately, Lehiste did not measure stress periods in the manner proposed by Abercrombie, but took measurements in terms of word boundaries instead. This criterion necessarily identifies a new word with each new stress (although not the converse). Its validity can be questioned with respect to polysyllabic words (e.g., "parenthetically," which receives at least two and perhaps three stresses). In any case, her result does not constitute a direct test of Abercrombie's notion of stress-period isochrony.

The perceived time of occurrence of stress beats has been examined by Allen.[9] He had his subjects synchronize their speech with finger tapping and with a series of equally spaced clicks, finding that the onsets of stressed syllables coincided closely with the beats. Except for syllables initiated by long consonantals, it was stressed vowel onsets that fell close to the beats. In the case of clicks, of course, stress period isochrony was *imposed*, but Allen shows that periodic stress timing is not impossible to achieve with considerable accuracy. Rapp[10] has obtained similar results, finding the period standard deviation to range between 20 and 45 milliseconds (p. 17).

It should be noted that Rapp found in this study that longer syllable-initial consonant clusters were followed by shorter stressed vowels and vice versa. Such a negative correlation between lengths of adjacent segments, i.e., *temporal compensation*, is often found, as will presently be seen. But Rapp's result is unusual, since it involves a CV interaction rather than a VC relationship, which is more common. It is perhaps an artifact of the need to adjust the tempo to an imposed pacing in this kind of experiment.

There is now emerging from the descriptive study of speech timing in various languages a set of coarticulatory relationships of sufficient generality that they may in fact indicate the basic timing characteristics of the human articulatory control process itself. This is not the place for a detailed review of universals in articulatory phonetics, and, indeed, it may be partly due to the fortuitous geography of phonology laboratories that most speech timing experiments are based on speakers of Russian, English, and Swedish. Hence generalizations to follow are of necessity abstractly interpreted and are to be regarded only to be presumptive universals at this time. Except where otherwise noted, experiments reported are based on the usual phonetician's method of having subjects recite specified utterances for subsequent analysis of either spectrogram or oscillogram.

Coarticulatory timing adjustment of consonants is usually small, being measured in tens of msec, rather than in hundreds as in the adjustment of vowels.[11,12] There are two principal consonantal effects: 1) shortening of a consonant when combined with other consonants in clusters;[11,13,14] 2) a positively correlated lengthening of consonants along with vowels in stressed syllables.[15]

In the case of vowels, coarticulatory timing effects are greater and more complex. Excluding those due to particular articulatory features, there are three types: 1) vowel-consonant (VC) interactions, 2) lengthening with stress, and 3) reduction with increasing speech rate. They will be taken up in turn.

1. A regularly reported VC interaction is the lengthening of vowels before voiced consonants and shortening before unvoiced ones.[13,14,16] It was proposed long ago by

Trubetskoy for many languages that VC articulations are of two types, "close contact" and "loose contact." (Ref. 16, p. 49). According to Lehiste, Fliflet demonstrated, by cutting time from tape-recorded V or C durations, that for German listeners, at least, *close* contact was signalled by a short vowel followed by a long consonant and *loose* contact by the opposite. Since Fliflet could obtain either effect by *cutting* time either from the beginning of the vowel or the end of the consonant, he was able to show that the contrast was based on the relative durations of vowel and consonant rather than on their absolute values. The voicing and contact phenomena are apparently independent, but both exhibit VC compensation.

2. It is claimed to be "established" that English stressed vowels are about 50% longer than their unstressed counterparts (Ref. 16, p. 36), and a similar degree of difference is reported for Swedish (Ref. 13, p. 11). In natural speech the proportional relation is not a constant, however, since it depends upon rate. As Lehiste puts it, "For certain languages, an increase in speech tempo is largely achieved by shortening unstressed syllables" (Ref. 16, p. 38).

3. By the spectral analysis of vowel reduction in Swedish, Lindblom[17] showed that the first two formants in a vowel begin normally and undergo transition (in directions appropriate for the given vowel) at a fixed rate. If the vowel is reduced, the transitions are redirected toward the next consonant before reaching the vowel's target. If the redirection begins early enough, the shortened vowel is neutralized to *schwa*. "Since the speed of the articulatory movement is ... limited, the extent to which articulators reach their target positions depends on the relative timing of the excitation signals. If the signals are far apart in time, the response may become stationary at individual targets. If, on the other hand, instructions occur in close temporal succession, the system may be responding to several signals simultaneously and the result is coarticulation" (p. 1778).

More recently, Kozhevnikov and Chistovich report cases of *total* vowel reduction in Russian.[14] "From phonetics it is known that a vowel can disappear completely ... This occurs when the interval between syllables assigned in the program is too small in order to accomplish both the opening and closing of the organs which articulate the consonent in the case of a rapid rate of speech. As a result there is not sufficient time for the vowel" (p. 89).

In our laboratory we have observed this phenomenon in English. Especially interesting are cases permitting smooth transitions between sounds juxtaposed by the elimination of a vowel. Example are the words "psychiatric" and "station," which sound fluent and normal when uttered quickly as /say kyae tric/ and / stey šn/.

These coarticulatory findings can be tied together to form a more explicit and testable restatement of the stress-period isochrony hypothesis. Central to this restatement is the assumption that periodic pulses locate the onsets and establish the relative durations of stressed syllables according to a superordinate temporal structure of the preplanned type proposed by Martin; also, that the intervening articulations between the stressed ones are not under the automatic clock control of this central timing sequence, and so are subject to timing irregularities that are greater than those of the stress periods within which they occur. Unlike Lindblom's "excitation signals" or Kozhevnikov and Chistovich's "programmed assignments," the periodic pulses marking stress periods would not occur as often as each consonant, vowel, or syllable. Being separated by at least the time required for a stressed syllable, the interpulse period is necessarily at least long enough to permit any one fully executed CVC. Reductions and omissions of vowels, which are seen to occur only in unstressed segments, happen when addiional syllables are sandwiched into the stress period. Since the timing of the period is held to be unaffected by their inclusion, it is inferred that the accurate execution of unstressed syllables is subordinated to that of the stress period. Finally, since not all stressed syllables are of the same length (due to intrinsic differences in vowel quantity and the like), temporal compensation is predicted between stressed and unstressed portions of the period.

Testing this hypothesis requires the identification of the onsets of stressed syllables for a measure of the period, P, and a measure of stressed and unstressed segment durations. Support for it is indicated by a finding of a true negative correlation between durations of the two segment types in succession.

In the ideal case of perfect isochrony, the expected correlation between paired segment lengths is minus one, as the only timing variance is due to compensation between stressed, S, and unstressed, U:

$$r = \frac{\sigma_P^2 - (\sigma_S^2 + \sigma_U^2)}{2\,\sigma_S\sigma_U} = -1, \quad \text{where} \quad \sigma_P^2 = 0 \quad \text{and} \quad \sigma_S^2 = \sigma_U^2 = K.$$

In our laboratory, Podwall and I have analyzed five-minute samples of spontaneous monolog collected from ten normal male subjects. Syllable onsets and vowel durations were identified and measured by a PDP-12 computer, as described elsewhere.[18-20] For these subjects, vowels of 60 msec duration or less were identified as "unstressed." By Lehiste's definition, and perhaps by Abercrombie's, our criterion permitted the overcounting of stresses (although it should be noted that in casual speech style vowel durations are usually shorter than those measured during recitations in the phonetics laboratory).‡ The results are not yet fully analyzed, but estimates of the stress period based on average durations of stressed vowels and unstressed segments without regard to sequence and position effects resulted in negative correlations for nine of the ten normals.

It was first noted by Kozhevnikov and Chistovitch that measurement errors on adjacent segments sharing a common measured boundary will yield a spurious "compensatory" effect (Ref. 14, p. 102).

It can be shown that if measurement error constitutes proportion p of the common segment variance K, then under the null hypothesis the expected negative bias of the calculated r is equal to $-p/2$. We have estimated p to be about 0.05, and have corrected our calculations of r for the bias. Again, the same nine subjects yielded negative correlations—all were changed by the correction toward greater negativity.

Segment timing error experiments based on other segmentation criteria yield conflicting results. Ohala[21] reports no evidence for any rhythmic unit at all; Wright[22] found negative correlations between many segmentations ranging in length from consonant cluster to three word phrase. Consonant-vowel compensations, of course, have already been discussed.

Recently, Lindblom and Rapp have proposed a compensatory domain covering entire phases.[13] An equation is employed recursively to calculate the shortening of vowels as a direct function of the numbers of syllables and lexical stresses that precede and follow it in the phrase. "Anticipatory compensation" is their term for the shortening effect of following units, "backward compensation" for that of preceding units.

‡Nooteboom (see Ref. 23, p. 39) holds that the range for stressed vowel durations "in a normal speaking tempo" is 50–200 msec, at least for Dutch. Any vowel-length cutoff criterion can distinguish but two levels of stress, and ours was chosen to distinguish "unstressed" from the higher degrees. This distinction corresponds very closely to the "heavy-light" feature contrast of Vanderslice and Ladefoged (see Ref. 32, p. 820). I am indebted to George Allen for pointing out the similarity to me.

At all levels, the "anticipatory" effect is claimed to be the larger of the two. A vowel-length contour of similar configuration is proposed for Dutch by Nooteboom.[23] These considerations predict that the longest vowels will appear in final positions, a finding reported for English by Oller,[15] and by Lehiste.[6]§ In FIGURE 1 are segmentation patterns, exhibiting A) stress group isochrony with random vowel length, B) vowel-length contour with random stress period, and C) both isochrony and vowel-length contour, indicating compatibility between the two processes.

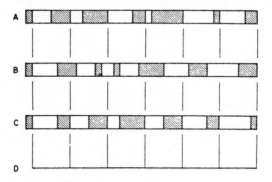

FIGURE 1. Stress-period configurations under three relative timing hypotheses. A: Random vowel length with periodic isochrony due to compensation between stress onsets; B: Vowel lengths follow compensatory contour, but with neither compensation nor isochrony over the stress period; C: Vowel-length contour as in B with stress-period compensation and isochrony as in A. Line D identifies the accent points for the isochronous periods of A and C. □ = stressed time; ▨ = unstressed time.

It is now time to refer back a hundred years to the quotation from Buhler with which this article began. Our reformulation of the isochronous stress group hypothesis requires a time schema like Buhler's, one that realizes a time program for stress pulses and *only* stress pulses in advance of the detailed articulation of individual speech sounds. We can find such a model in the work of Arnold Pick.[25]

As an aphasiologist, Pick found it important to try to distinguish carefully the order of events that must occur in the nervous system preparatory to speaking. The list of preparatory events begins unsurprisingly with a "thought pattern," which is unsuitable for expression until it is subjected to "linguistic formulation" (p. 31)—a process involving the following events: "First, an accentuation pattern (*Betonungsschema*) and then a sentence pattern (*Satzschema*) develop, which concern in their formation the topical sequence arising from the thought pattern (*Gedankenschema*) ..." (p. 32). The next step is word finding, which still acts independently of the ultimate sequence: content words are retrieved prior to "grammatical" (function) words. He says "The assumption of the conductance to the motor executive apparatus of more or less fixed engrams appears to be negated by the coming into play of parts of the intonational pattern ... showing the word to be a dynamic formation" (p. 33). Only at the very end of the linguistic formulation does speaking occur through "the sequential excitation ... via more or less automatized speech impulses (p. 33).

Since the notions of feedback and ballistic control processes in the nervous system were not developed in Pick's day, we may run the risk of retrospectively crediting

§Similar effects for English words are also reported by Abler.[24]

Pick unduly.[¶] In any case, it remains to be shown how the compensatory adjustment of a speech segment to the duration of its predecessor can be accomplished without external feedback: All that is necessary is a behavioral dominance of stressed articulations over unstressed, such that the onset of each stressed syllable can effectively interrupt any ongoing unstressed articulatory activity. Pulse-timed by their preplanned pattern, such a series of stresses will leave more or less time to be filled by their opposites according to their length—whether vowels be random or sequentially contoured. Of course, possibility of ballistic pacing is not proof. But there are two supporting arguments.

First is the direct evidence from vowel reduction, quantitatively a very large source of compensatory actions, in which it is seen that shorter vowels do not show the same degree of formant excursion as do long ones; that is, they are not long vowels "run off faster" but rather begin exactly as do long ones, being modified only at the end. This is consistent with shortening due to the arrival of an interrupting stress pulse, not with a speedup of the vowel program due to a late start forewarned by feedback from the preceding segment.

Second is the indirect finding of increasing evidence of neural "open loop" movement control for periods of about 100 msec (see Ref. 26), during which no feedback influences performance on tracking behavior. Since reduced vowels are probably shorter than this, feedback cannot be taken for granted and must be distinguished from corollary discharge. A feedback hypothesis, in Evarts words, "must meet two requirements:

1. It is necessary to specify the modality over which feedback is delivered to the system.
2. For a given modality, it is necessary to specify the particular feedback loop and the phase of the movement in which this particular loop is postulated to operate." (Ref. 26, p. 95.)

Finally, it should be remarked that nothing in this argument necessarily challenges familiar speculations about how feedback operates in speech control. Fairbanks, for example, says of the unit of feedback control: "Such a control unit should not be identified with any of the conventional units such as the phoneme the syllable, the word, or the word group . . . it is not theoretically necessary that the unit of control be any presently identified phonetic unit (Ref. 27, p. 138).

At this time, the weight of evidence seems to favor a ballistic explanation of rhythmic organization.

In conclusion, here are a few comments on the implications of this model for speech development.

McNeill[28] finds that the shortening of syllables as a function of organizing them into phrases is not automatic at age two, even when stringing as many as five syllables together, but matches the adult pattern by age four or five (see FIGURE 1, Ref. 28). He finds a similar shift for the speeding up of words in sentences, and cites other studies to further support the notion that the child's early multiple-word utterances acquire semantic appropriateness prior to organization into a time schema. He reports unpublished work of Rodgon showing that some polysyllabic utterances of 18-month-old children are temporally uncompressed while others are compressed into an adult time frame (p. 13). He finds that more abstract and grammatical utterances show the earliest tendency toward compression, supporting the view that the time

[¶]Nevertheless, Evarts[26] reports that Woodworth showed in 1899 that various kinds of movement "were not controlled by sensory inputs *during their execution"* [italics his]. (p. 94)

schema being acquired is that of a generative surface structure, the child having a prior knowledge of a slower underlying structure.

Unfortunately, McNeill does not report the phonological details, so we are unable to guess whether the process of compression is general, follows a vowel length contour, or is the result of a more sophisticated manipulation of stress contrasts. Much more work is needed in this domain.

Tingley and Allen[29] had children between the ages of five and eleven attempt to repeat a phrase thirty times at the same rate, and to tap their fingers for two minutes as steadily as possible. Findings were an improvement in timing accuracy over various speech segments and in tapping also, suggesting a "comon timing control mechanism."

Denckla and Rudel[30] found that normal children showed an increase in speed of naming series of pictured objects, colors, letters, and numbers between the ages of five and ten. Denckla[31] also found a slight speedup between ages five and seven for rapid finger movements, lending support to the common mechanism view of Tingley and Allen.

From Pick's notion that content words for speech are selected prior to grammatical words, we might infer, especially since few if any function words are stressed, that content word-finding is directly under the control of the stress-period schema, whether such words are utilized for sentence construction or only for naming. If so, we might expect that means and variances of *stress periods* would show a parallel reduction with age as a function of correspondingly lowered measures for rapid *naming* of objects, colors, and numbers, which have, of course, only content words for names. At this time, only the conjecture can be made, but the results I have reported point to a range of coarticulatory speech timing control that is at least as long as the syllable, and perhaps as long as the entire utterance. Possibly both ranges are correct, one in a cognitive sense, the other in an articulatory sense. It is evident that effective, normal speech requires that the nervous system apportion an appropriate timing for each of them.

REFERENCES

1. BUHLER, K. Quoted by CRITCHLEY, M. 1970. Aphasiology and Other Aspects of Language: 238. Arnold. London, England.
2. JAFFE, J. & S. FELDSTEIN. 1970. Rhythms of Dialogue. Academic Press, New York, N.Y.
3. MARTIN, J. G. 1972. Rhythmic (hierarchical) versus serial structure in speech and other behavior. Psychol. Rev. 79: 487–509.
4. LASHLEY, K. S. 1951. The problem of serial order in behavior. In Cerebral Mechanisms in Behavior. L. A. Jeffress, Ed.: 112–136. John Wiley & Sons. New York, N.Y.
5. CHOMSKY, N. & M HALLE. 1968. The Sound Pattern of English. Chap. 2. Harper & Row. New York, N.Y.
6. LEHISTE I. 1973. Rhythmic units and syntactic units in producton and perception. J. Acoust. Soc. Am. 54: 1228–1234.
7. CLASSE, A. 1939. The Rhythm of English Prose. Blackwell. Oxford, England.
8. ABERCROMBIE, D. 1964. Syllable quantity and enclitics in English. In In Honour of Daniel Jones. D. Abercrombie, et al., Eds. Longmans. London, England.
9. ALLEN, G. D. 1972. The location of rhythmic stress beats in English: An experimental Study. Lang. Speech. 15: 179–195.
10. RAPP, K. 1971. A study of syllable timing. Quart. Prog. Status Rept.: 14–19. Speech Transmission Lab. Stockhold Royal Inst. Technology. 1/1971.
11. HAGGARD, M. 1973. Abbreviation of consonants in English pre- and postvocalic clusters. J. Phonetics 1: 9–24.
12. HOUSE, A. S. 1961. On vowel duration in English. J. Acoust. Soc. Am. 33: 1174–1178.
13. LINDBLOM, B. & K. RAPP. 1973. Some temporal regularities of spoken Swedish. Papers from the Inst. of Linguistics 21: 1–58. Univ. Stockholm. Stockholm, Sweden.

14. KOZHEVNIKOV, V. A. & L. A. CHISTOVITCH. 1965. Speech Articulation and Perception. National Technical Information Service JPRS-30543. U.S. Dept. Commerce. Springfield, Va.

15. OLLER, D. K. 1973. The effect of position in utterance on speech segment duration in English. J. Acoust. Soc. Am. **54:** 1235–1247.

16. LEHISTE, I. 1970. Suprasegmentals. The MIT Press. Cambridge, Mass.

17. LINDBLOM, B. 1963. Spectrographic study of vowel reduction. J. Acoust. Soc. Am. **35:** 1773–1781.

18. ANDERSON, S. W. & J. JAFFE. 1972. The definition, detection and timing of vocalic syllables in speech signals. Sci. Rept. No. 12. Dept. Communication Sciences, New York Psychiat. Inst. New York, N.Y.

19. JAFFE, J., S. W. ANDERSON & R. W. RIEBER. 1973. Research and clinical approaches to disorders of speech rate. J. Communication Disorders **6:** 225–246.

20. PODWALL, F. N. How do speakers parse time? In preparation.

21. OHALA, J. J. 1970. Aspects of the control and production of speech. UCLA Working Papers in Phonetics No. 15. Univ. California. Los Angeles, Calif.

22. WRIGHT, T. W. 1974. Temporal interactions within a phrase and sentence context. J. Acoust. Soc. Am. **56:** 1258–1265.

23. NOOTEBOOM, S. G. 1973. The perceptual reality of some prosodic durations. J. Phonetics. **1:** 25–45.

24. ABLER, W. L. 1973. Speaking rate and the delivery of phonetic commands in Standard American English. J. Acoust. Soc. Am. **53:** 380.

25. PICK, A. 1973. Aphasia (trans. by Jason Brown). Charles C Thomas. Springfield, Ill.

26. EVARTS, E. V., E. BIZZI, R. E. BURKE, M. DELONG & W. T. THACH, JR. 1971. Feedback and corollary discharge: a merging of the concepts. In Central Control of Movement. Neurosciences Research Program Bulletin **9:** 86–112.

27. FAIRBANKS, G. 1954. Systematic research in experimental phonetics 1. A theory of the speech mechanism as a servosystem. J. Speech Hear. Disorders **19:** 133–139.

28. MCNEILL, D. 1972. The two-fold way for speech. Paper for the C.N.R.S. Conference on Psycholinguistics. Dec. 1971. Paris, France. Rev. 1972.

29. TINGLEY, B. M. & G. D. ALLEN. 1975. Development of speech timing control in children. Child Development **46:** 186–194.

30. DENCKLA, M. B. & R. RUDEL. 1974. Rapid 'automatized' naming of pictured objects, colors, letters and numbers by normal children. Cortex **10:** 186–202.

31. DENCKLA, M. B. 1973. Development of speed in repetitive and successive finger movements in normal children. Develop. Med. Child. Neurol. **15:** 635–645.

32. VANDERSLICE, R. & LADEFOGED, P. 1972. Binary suprasegmental features and transformational word-accentuation rules. Language **48:** 819–838.

THE ONTOGENY OF CEREBRAL DOMINANCE

Marcel Kinsbourne

Hospital for Sick Children
Toronto, Canada

It has long been known that in most people the language function depends on the activity of the left cerebral hemisphere. It is clear that language develops from a base state of no language. But does language lateralization analogously develop from a base state of no lateralization? It has been generally assumed that this is so. The child at the very beginning of language development is regarded as using both cerebral hemispheres for this purpose. Differences of opinion have related more to the time frame within which lateralization occurs[1,2] than to the question of whether lateralization develops at all.

Once progressive lateralization in childhood was assumed to occur, further assumptions seemed plausible to many. Two of these were that the rate of lateralization in some way represented the rate of language development and the ultimate extent of lateralization its ultimate level of excellence. It was then assumed that adults who were incompletely or anomalously lateralized for language would be found to be deficient in their verbal skills and, conversely, that children who were slow to develop language would be found to be relatively ill-lateralized for the age.[3-6] It was only one more, ostensibly easy, step to the enterprise of attempting to hasten lateralization in the hope of thereby accelerating the development of language skills.

Thus, on the narrow base of the assumption that lateralization develops *pari passu* with language behavior, there has been built a substantial edifice of further assumptions, culminating in elaborate remedial techniques. It is doubly crucial to determine whether the basic assumption is correct. This is so both for scientific reasons and because, if the basic assumption is incorrect, the great investment of time, effort, and expense in remedial techniques intended to modify lateralization woud be better spent in a manner more directly applicable to the interest of children with language disorder.

One might first ask whether the notion of developing lateralization is even plausible on general principles. One can then proceed to scrutinize the evidence that has been adduced in favor of the concept. This consists mainly of 1) an appraisal of the effect of early, lateralized brain damage on language, and 2) an interpretation of the life-span development of perceptual asymmetries for verbal material. We will then be in a position to decide whether the hypothesis of developing lateralization has face validity or whether the null hypothesis of lateralization as a stable and invariant characteristic of language development in the human should be regarded as not disconfirmed.

Two propositions can safely be made that contrast the immature and mature nervous system of any species. One is that the immature nervous system subserves a comparatively restricted behavioral repertoire. The other is that, when damaged in one of its parts, the immature nervous system exhibits a relatively high potential for compensation for that part's actual or potential function by the function of some other residual intact area. There are, then, two reasons why focal damage to the immature nervous system often results in less dramatic change in behavior than does comparable damage inflicted on the nature nervous system: 1) There is less behavioral versatility present to lose, and 2) any function that is lost is more readily compensated by other parts of the system. If one identifies a part of the adult brain that subserves a given function and then shows that destruction of a comparable section of the immature brain fails to disrupt that function, one has not thereby necessarily demonstrated a more widely spread localization for that function. The results could be accounted for by the well-known superior compensatory potential of the immature brain. Indeed, the concept that, in the course of maturation, the area of the brain involved with a given function progressively shrinks, is a curious one, for which there is no model whatever in the neurophysiological literature for any species. If, indeed, language representation in children retreats from a bilaterally based to a smaller, lateralized arena in the cerebrum, then this phenomenon is the first recognized of its type.

One source of evidence that has been related to the question under discussion is the difference in effect of lateralized cerebral lesions on language function depending on the time in the life span at which the damage occurs. The general proposition has been well validated; it is that damage to the left hemisphere at or around birth has only a minor effect on the rate and ultimate level of verbal development, whereas comparable damage in the fully mature brain may induce a language disability of great severity.[7-12] There is an intermediary period from the origins of language development to puberty, during which left-hemispheric damage does cause disruption of language behavior but also to a lesser extent and for a shorter period of time than one usually encounters in the adult aphasic.[1,2] There are two obvious ways in which such phenomena can be interpreted. It might be argued that the child in the left hemisphere is only part of a bilaterally distributed language area, and therefore, damage to it deprives the individual of only part of his language substrate. But one could more simply rely on the well-established principles of early plasticity and merely remark that, as might be expected, the opposite hemisphere compensates faster and better for damage to the language-relevant side of the brain the younger the individual when the damage occurs. Because of these two possible explanations, the sole fact that greater damage brings less language loss afterward cannot resolve the question of whether cerebral dominance develops as language develops.

Can we instead draw conclusions based on evidence relevant to the question of whether, as maturation progresses, language disorder is more or less likely to appear after selective injury to the ostensibly irrelevant right hemisphere? Lenneberg[1] has reviewed some reports in the neurological literature that discuss cases of children who were between the ages of two and five years at the time of an apparently right-sided brain injury which was said to have impaired some aspect of language function. We must ask ourselves two questions about these reports: Can they be trusted? If so, what can we then conclude?

In order to bear on the question of right-hemisphere language, the clinician who reports the case must show two things: 1) that the right hemisphere was selectively damaged, and 2) that language was thereby affected. Cases in the literature fall short on both these counts. It is at the best of times difficult to establish lateralization of brain damage in the absence of autopsy evidence or at least highly sophisticated neuroradiological or direct neurosurgical evidence. In fact, Lenneberg's reported cases[13-15] come nowhere near meeting adequate criteria for drawing such conclusions. With the exception of those in one particular series,[16] the reports of right-hemisphere lesion leave open the question of whether the left hemisphere was concurrently involved by the same pathological agent; such a situation would thereby disrupt language, to no one's surprise. Cases in which, perhaps after some virus infection or immunization, a child has one or more epileptic seizures, perhaps paralysis on one side of the body, and some changes in the EEG, cannot with validity be used to indicate a lesion confined to the hemisphere opposite the paralysis. Thus, the various case reports which in sum suggest an incidence of language problems nearly as great for right-sided as for left-sided disease in children under five[1,14] are, in fact, open to the criticism that in every single case any language deficit could have resulted from extension of the damage to the other side of the brain. Furthermore, in the one series in which evidence for right-sided lateralization of the insult in each case was unequivocal, there was not a single case in which that right-hemispheric damage affected language.[16]

The evidence in the other reports [13-15] that language was indeed interrupted is equally fragile. In no case are the results of speech and language testing reported, nor indeed is much heed paid to anything other than speech output. Usually the report amounts to no more than the observation that the child was not speaking to the clinician. There are, of course, a number of possible reasons for this.[17] A brain-based disorder of language cannot be assumed unless the nature of mistakes in language decoding and encoding can be shown to be consistent with this diagnosis and, if language function recovers, unless at recovery patients go through recognizable stages of decreasing aphasic deficit.

Were the evidence not so worthless, it might have been worthwhile adding that, in any case, it is not valid to contrast the relative frequency of a behavioral effect resulting from lesion A and lesion B on the basis of sporadic reports in the literature that one would assume to be biased towards publication of the less expected event. About one percent of aphasic syndromes in right-handed adults rise from lesions limited to the right hemisphere.[18] We must conclude that no acceptable evidence has been adduced for the proposition that the proportion is any different in children at any particular age.

There remains the theoretical question: What type of effect might one expect from unilateral damage to a bilaterally represented language system? The nature of the behavioral change would depend on the manner in which two sides of that language system interact to produce the total language skill. If each hemisphere contributed differently to that behavior, there would be qualitative differences in the aphasia produced by right-sided and left-sided damage. None such have been reported. One would then suppose that in some undefined way each hemisphere contributes some portion of total language facility, and damage to either would somewhat reduce it. Damage on one side would be expected to cause only a partial aphasia, rather than a complete loss of language skill. Suppose, however, one were to find such a case with right-sided damage; there would still be two possible explanations for the fact that the aphasia was partial rather than complete. The reason that language is partially spared might indeed be that the other hemisphere was continuing its normal function, but the reason could equally well be that the undamaged part of the same hemisphere was continuing its work. Thus, one might in fact be seeing not a case of bilateral but of right-hemisphere lateralization of language. In order to be sure that the residual language behavior comes from the other side, one would have to have a case in which the right hemisphere was abruptly totally destroyed, leaving language function *immediately* partially preserved (because merely a more rapid than expected recovery of language would only attest to plasticity of the residual young brain). Such cases have not been reported at any age.

Another type of lead on the question of progressive lateralization comes from observation of behavioral characteristics that appear to relate to lateralization of language in the individual. After all, the whole notion of progressive lateralization quite possibly arose from a very old line of speculation about relationships between left- and/or mixed-handedness and a variety of mental defects. Insofar as right-hand preference seems to indicate a left-hemisphere dominance for language, it has been thought that preference for left or neither hand would indicate some other lateralization or lack of lateralization of that function. In fact, the majority of left handers are right-lateralized for language. In any case, there is no convincing evidence that anomalous lateralization or incomplete lateralization of language in any way reflects the excellence of verbal skills except when the abnormal cerebral representation was the result of brain damage; in the latter case, the brain damage itself is sufficient cause for the cognitive deficit. Simply, anomalous handedness quite often is one consequence of damage to parts of the brain. Language delay is another consequence of such damage. These propositions do not imply a causal relationship between the hand preference and the state of the language function.

More recently a number of novel indicators in language lateralization have been developed. The earliest and best known of these are the hemifield asymmetry in visual recognition threshold for briefly presented verbal material, and the right-ear advantage for the report of two concurrent messages dichotically presented by earphones to the two ears.[19] The question has been repeatedly asked, as one tests children at a younger age: "Is the right-ear advantage to be found in dichotic listening, for instance, of dwindling magnitude?" It is assumed that if it were, this would indicate a lesser degree of lateralization in such individuals. In fact, this interpretation is unfounded, since it has never been shown that the degree of an ear advantage reflects the degree of lateralization on any test whatsoever. If anything, more likely it indicates the extent to which the subject found it necessary to enlist his verbal capabilities to solve the problem he has been set. This is not merely a function of the lateralization but of the extent to which he tries to perform on the task and uses a specifically verbal strategy to do so. These variables are not at the moment amenable to measurement. In any case, however, the evidence that asymmetries are less in younger children is equivocal, to say the least. In fact, most dichotic studies have shown no change in ear advantage even down to age four,[20,21] and several studies have shown that children as young as three years still as a group favor the right ear.[22-24] The point has been made in one study[25] that the younger the child, the more he tends to give primacy in his report to the right ear, whereas the older individual shows right-ear advantage even if directed to report the input to his left ear first. It is not clear what should be concluded from this. First of all, we have no way of knowing to which ear the subject initially attends; we merely know which material the subject in fact first reports. Secondly, it would appear that the fact that attention is biased is itself of fundamental importance.[26,27] A bias of attention to the right is a direct consequence of left lateralization of language in the context of a verbal task. With regard to this attentional bias, perhaps the most enormous right-ear asymmetry that has been found occurred in a yet unpublished study by Kinsbourne and Hoch, in which three-year-old children were asked selectively to report only the message coming into one ear, when a pair of dichotic digits was presented on each trial. Children found it easy to report one or both of the digit names represented at the trial. When asked to report from the right ear only, they did so with a good deal of accuracy. They scored very poorly when reporting from the left ear only, but an analysis of those responses showed that they were not failing to respond or responding with extraneous information. Rather, they were responding with the item that was presented to the right, unasked-for, channel. Their bias in attention to the right was far more extreme than it is in more mature individuals.

On general principles, this comes as no great surprise, because one would be quite ready to believe that any maladaptive or adaptively irrelevant biases in behavior would be less evident in the more versatile and flexible mature than the less subtly engineered immature organism. But for purposes of the present argument, at any rate, it is obvious that with respect to dichotic listening no case can be made for decreased lateralization at least down to age three years.

Two other newer techniques have been adapted to five-year-old children. One is the effect reported by Kinsbourne,[28] that verbal thinking induces momentary gaze shifts to the right in right-handed subjects. Kinsbourne attributed this to the left lateralization both of language and of the cerebral control center of rightward gaze, and a hypothesized intimate connection between the two. In an unpublished study by Kinsbourne and Jardno, a comparable finding was obtained for normal five-year-old children. Another paradigm used on a similar group was derived from a study that showed that, when right-handed subjects engaged in a unimanual performance, then in a condition in which they were asked simultaneously to speak, the unimanual performance was disrupted with respect to the right hand but not with respect to the left.[29] Kinsbourne and McMurray[30] adapted this to children by use of a finger-tapping technique. They found that whereas five-year-old children could tap, on the whole, more rapidly with their right than left index finger, when they were asked either to recite a nursery rhyme or to repeat the names of four animals, the tapping rate on the right suffered more than that on the left. The right-hand advantage disappeared and indeed was replaced by a trend in the opposite direction.

The effect is based on a hypothesized interference between the programming of two motor sequences, one for speech and one for hand movement in the same hemisphere. For purposes of the present argument it shows that a clear lateralization, in this case of verbal executive function, is easily demonstrable as early as five years of age.

The view that asymmetries extend down into infancy is interestingly supported by studies in very young babies both at the behavioral and the electrophysiological level. Newborn infants tend spontaneously to look to the right about four times as often as to the left.[31,32] Such a rightward preference of gaze certainly seems to arise earlier than right-hand preference, not to mention left-hemisphere lateralization of language. However, the generally held view that consistent right-hand preference, like the origins of language, is delayed until the second year of life has now been disconfirmed. Babies as young as three months of age maintain hold of a rattle far longer with their right hand than with their left.[33] Thus, an asymmetry of hand-use can be shown at a very early age, given that an age-appropriate test procedure is used. Related to this is the report of electrical cortical responses, i.e., that verbal stimuli caused a greater response over the left, and nonverbal stimuli over the right, convexity of the skull in newborns[34,35] long before any behavioral evidence of language skill appears.

Far from supporting the view that lateralization is a slowly emerging function that lags well behind the origins of language development, evidence suggests that some form of lateralization not only accompanies but even precedes the first traces of verbal behavior. The amount of lateralization as judged on behavioral grounds is no less and quite likely greater than that found in the mature organism. Of course, once one speaks of language-related lateralization that actually precedes language behavior, one needs to recast one's models of what left-hemisphere lateralization of language is all about. It could, on the one hand, be argued that language function is present on the left side of the brain long before this is shown in casually observable behavior. After all, Eimas' observation that very young infants could respond differentially to different phonemes would fit well with such a view. But perhaps the most promising, albeit speculative, interpretation might be one that gives priority in time to attentional biases released by specific materials or, more likely, to specific task orientations which form the substrate for the accumulation of experience on which subsequent language skill is based.

Cerebral dominance for language does not develop; it is there from the start. Thus, one could hardly relate the excellence of language behavior to such a development nor sensibly seek for measures which would accelerate that nonexistent process. It would seem advisable, in view of the evidence as summarized, to discontinue remedial therapies based on procedures that supposedly influence language lateralization in favor of procedures designed to act upon language behavior directly.

With references to the two main questions set for this conference:

1. The building up and the breakdown of language function takes place against an invariant background of cerebral dominance. However, under conditions of lateral brain damage the nondominant hemisphere can more readily compensate in the younger individual.
2. Rate of lateralization of the cerebral representation of language is not a significant dimension of individual difference, because language is lateralized from the start.

REFERENCES

1. LENNEBERG, E. 1967. Biological Foundations of Language. John Wiley & Son. New York, N.Y.
2. KRASHEN, S. 1972. Language and the left hemisphere. UCLA Working Papers in Phonetics **24:**.
3. EUSTIS, R. 1947. Specific reading disability: a familial syndrome associated with ambidexterity and speech defects and a frequent cause of problem behavior. New Eng. J. Med. **237:** 243–249.
4. ORTON, S. 1937. Reading, Writing and Speech Problems in Children. Norton. New York, N.Y.
5. SILVER, A. & R. HAGIN. 1964. Specific reading disability: Follow-up studies. Am. J. Orthopsychiatry **34:** 95–102.
6. ZANGWILL, O. L. 1960. Cerebral Dominance and its Relation to Psychological Function. Oliver and Boyd. Edinburgh, Scotland.
7. CARLSON, J., C. NETLEY, E. B. HENDRICK, & J. S. PRICHARD. 1968. A re-examination of intellectual disabilities in hemispherectomized patients. Trans. Am. Neurol. Assoc. **93:** 198–201.
8. KOHN, B. & M. DENNIS. 1974. Patterns of hemispheric specialization after hemidecortication for infantile hemiplegia. *In* Hemispheric Disconnection and Cerebral Function. M. Kinsbourne & W. L. Smith, Eds.: Charles C Thomas. Springfield, Ill. pages 39–47.
9. LANSDELL, H. 1969. Verbal and nonverbal factors in right-hemisphere speech: Relation to early neurological history. J. Comp. Physiol. Psychol. **69:** 734–738.
10. McFIE, J. 1961. The effects of hemispherectomy on intellectual functioning in cases of infantile hemiplegia. J. Neurol. Neurosurg. Psychiatry **24:** 240–249.
11. SMITH, A. 1974. Dominant and nondominant hemispherectomy. *In* Hemispheric Disconnection and Cerebral Function. M. Kinsbourne & W. L. Smith, Eds.: 5–33. Charles C Thomas, Springfield, Ill.
12. WILSON, P. J. E. 1970. Cerebral hemispherectomy for infantile hemiplegia. Brain **93:** 147–180.
13. ALAJOUANINE, T. & F. LHERMITTE. 1965. Acquired aphasia in children. Brain **88:** 653–662.
14. BASSER, L. 1962. Hemiplegia of early onset and the faculty of speech with special reference to the effects of hemispherectomy. Brain **85:** 427–460.
15. GUTTMANN, E. 1942. Aphasia in children. Brain **65:** 205–219.
16. BYERS, R. K. & W. T. McLEAN. 1962. Etiology and course of certain hemiplegias with aphasia in childhood. Pediatrics **129:** 367–383.
17. GESCHWIND, N. 1967. Neurological foundations of language. *In* Progress in Learning Disabilities. Vol. I. H. R. Myklebust, Ed. Grune and Stratton. New York, N.Y.
18. HECAEN, H. & J. AJURIAGUERRA. 1964. Left Handedness: Manual Superiority and Cerebral Dominance. Grune and Stratton. New York, N.Y.
19. KIMURA, D. 1963. Right temporal lobe damage. Arch. Neurol. **8:** 264–271.
20. BERLIN, C. I., S. S. LOWE-BELL, L. F. HUGHES & H. L. BERLIN. 1972. Dichotic right-ear

advantage in males and females—ages 5-13. Paper 84th mtg. Acoust. Soc. Am. Miami Beach, Fla.

21. KIMURA, D. 1963. Speech lateralization in young childen as determined by an auditory test. J. Comp. Physiol. Psychol. **56:** 899–902.

22. GEFNER, D. S. & I. HOCHBERG. 1971. Ear laterality preference of children from low and middle socio-economic levels on a verbal dichotic listening task. Cortex **7:** 193–203.

23. KINSBOURNE, M., D. HOCH & T. SESSIONS. 1975. In preparation.

24. NAGAFUCHI, M. 1970. Development of dichotic and monaural hearing abilities in young children. Acta Otolaryngol. **69:** 409–414.

25. BRYDEN, M. P. 1970. Laterality effect in dichotic listening: relations with handedness and reading ability in children. Neuropsychologia **8:** 443–450.

26. KINSBOURNE, M. 1974. The mechanisms of hemisphere asymmetry in man. *In* Hemispheric Disconnection and Cerebral Function. M. Kinsbourne & W. L. Smith, Eds. Charles C Thomas. Springfield, Ill.

27. KINSBOURNE, M. 1975. The interaction between cognitive process and the direction of attention. *In* Attention and Performance, V.P.M.A. Rabbitt & S. Dornic, Eds. In press. Academic Press. London, England., pages 81–97.

28. KINSBOURNE, M. 1972. Eye and head turning indicates cerebral lateralization. Science **176:** 539–541.

29. KINSBOURNE, M. & J. COOK. 1971. Generalized and lateralized effects of concurrent verbalization on a unimanual skill. Quart. J. Exp. Psychol. **23:** 341–345.

30. KINSBOURNE, M. & J. MCMURRAY. 1975. The effect of cerebral dominance on time sharing between speaking and tapping by preschool children. Child Dev. **46:** 240–242.

31. SIQUELAND, E. R. & L. P. LIPSITT. 1966. Conditioned head turning in human newborns. J. Exp. Child Psychol. **4:** 356–377.

32. TURKEWITZ, G., B. W. GORDON & M. G. BIRCH. 1968. Head turning in the human neonate: effect of prandial condition and lateral preference. J. Comp. Physiol. Psychol. **59:** 189–192.

33. CAPLAN, P. & M. KINSBOURNE. Baby drops the rattle. In preparation.

34. MOLFESE, D. L. 1973. Cerebral asymmetry in infants, children and adults: auditory evoked responses to speech and musical stimuli. J. Acoust. Soc. Am. **53:** 363 (A).

35. ENTUS, A. & M. CORBALLIS. 1975. In press.

CEREBRAL ASYMMETRIES IN HUMANS ARE DUE TO THE DIFFERENTIATION OF TWO INCOMPATIBLE PROCESSES: HOLISTIC AND ANALYTIC

Thomas G. Bever

Psycholinguistics Program
Departments of Psychology and Linguistics
Columbia University
New York, New York 10027

> Cerebral localization is determined by the separation of incompatible mechanisms.
> — Lashley[7]

Clinical and experimental evidence suggests that the left hemisphere of the brain is specialized for speech activity and the right hemisphere is specialized for many nonlinguistic functions. Jackson[1] related the hemispheric linguistic differences to differences in cognitive activity, suggesting that the left hemisphere is specialized for analytical organization, while the right hemisphere is adapted for "direct associations" among stimuli and responses. Modern researchers have substantially generalized this differentiation to encompass a wide range of behaviors in normal subjects. Experimental[2] and clinical[3] investigators of hemispheric asymmetry generally agree on the fundamental nature of the processing differences between the two sides of the brain: the left hemisphere is specialized for propositional, analytic, and serial processing of incoming information, while the right hemisphere is more adapted for the perception of appositional, holistic, and synthetic relations.

This asymmetry raises the question of whether there are essential differences in the way in which the two hemispheres organize behavior and process information. Several theories attribute hemispheric differences to a structural differentiation of some kind. Asymmetries might be due to differences intrinsic to each hemisphere: e. g., in the neurospatial organization of functions[4] or the existence of modality-specific differences in capacity,[5] or to some fundamental differences in the way the elementary neurological interactions occur. The structural difference might exist because of forces extrinsic to the brain, e. g., a muscular predisposition for handedness, asymmetries in sensory organs, or socially trained asymmetries in such observable traits as handedness and eyedness.

Each of these views supposes that there is some physical or social structure that specifically and directly causes functional asymmetry to occur; that is, these proposals are all extremely strong in that they make concrete claims about the nature of the phenomenon. Yet the apparent precision of each claim is of little use to us, since we do not know the relevant facts that would critically prove or disprove any of them.

I shall argue that unless we have evidence conclusively proving any of the more specific claims, we should view cerebral dominance as the result of certain general properties of the mind and of the relationship between the structures of the mind and the anatomy of the brain. The basic view underlying this proposal is that the mind is composed of a number of partially independent faculties, each of which has certain

251

unique properties.* On this view the nature and existence of cerebral asymmetries are predictable, if there is any difference at all in the neonatal adaptability of the hemispheres. I will also discuss a number of surprising experimental results that follow from this view.

There are four statements (two are primarily theoretical and two are more immediately substantive), which combine to predict that analytic activity will tend to be localized in the left hemisphere and holistic activity in the right hemisphere.

Statement 1

The mind is self-organizing. In particular, it differentiates in mental space the location of analytic modes of processing from holistic modes of processing. Often we may have available two ways of organizing our behavior in response to a stimulus: we may analyze the stimulus in terms of component parts, or we may respond to the stimulus if it triggers a holistic behavioral "template." Consider, for example, the perception of a square. It may be analyzed either as four equal-length lines at right angles enclosing a space, or it may be directly perceived by triggering a template that is set for a □. Analogously, we can listen to a syllable, e.g., "bik," either by recognizing it in terms of its constituent phonemes or by setting up a complete template that is sensitive to that particular acoustic object as a whole. Finally, we can listen to a melody in terms of the individual intervals formed by successive notes or we can listen to the melody in terms of its entire gestalt. Much of this may seem to be a matter of terminology without behavioral implications. However, I will show that there are behavioral differences that reflect the two different modes of processing a stimulus. For the moment, one must simply accept the claim that a complex stimulus can itself be processed as a primitive whole or be analyzed in terms of its constituent parts, and that those processes are incompatible; in general, they cannot occur simultaneously in the same place.

Statement 2

Analytic processing requires more mental activity than holistic processing. This point is essentially a necessary truth whenever it applies to a stimulus that offers both a holistic and analytical level of organization. There is a sense in which recognition of a figure through analysis of its constituent parts must include the recognition of the whole figure as well. For example, I may recognize the syllable sequence "bik" as "b," "i," "k," but in so doing I ordinarily will also perceive the stimulus sequence as the syllable "bik." There is a related substantive claim, namely, that when instructed to perceive analytically, subjects nevertheless tend to start by perceiving a stimulus as a whole and then use additional processing to break the whole into constituent parts. This latter result is not itself the only possible consequence of the relative difficulty of analytic processing, but it does seem to be true. For example, suppose we ask a listener to respond as soon as he hears the syllable "bik" in a list of syllables presented one per second. The listener does so considerably faster than if he is listening for a syllable that begins in the sound "b" (even though he knows that the first such syllable *is* "bik").[6]

Statement 3

The dynamic mapping of mental processes onto functional brain structures is maximally simple. This is a substantive point, claiming that mental activities of the same kind tend to be represented anatomically in the same part of the brain. For

---

*See my discussion paper in this annal for a fuller presentation of this view. If the reader is concerned about the use of the word "mind," it may be glossed as "higher integrative functions." See the discussion of Statement 3 in this paper.

the purposes of this discussion I do not need to specify how this occurs, in particular, whether the higher order functions have this effect on the brain or vice versa. All I must claim is that there is some flexibility in the neurological localization of function that allows for maximal localization in the same area of the brain of similar mental functions.

This view may appear to be dualistic, in the sense that it distinguishes the operation of "the brain" from that of "the mind." The distinction, however, does not render the notion of "mind" mystical or unscientific. The model that sets the framework for this discussion is the following:

(A) Physiological properties of the brain make possible certain fundamental operations, and combinations of those operations.

(B) These operations organize modality-specific activities (e.g., audition, vocalization. . .) integrating receptive and productive behavior in response to limits set by other physiological structures (e.g., the ear, the mouth). Such kinds of activities differentiate into modality systems. An independent differentiation occurs in terms of the organization of the capacities (e.g., "language", "music". . .).

(C) The representation of these higher-order functions segregates in the brain according to similarity of function, *and* according to adaptation of the particular brain structures for that kind of function. (Note that such "adaptation" can be due to intrinsic properties of a brain structure or to its anatomical connectedness to the stimulus-response organs that ordinarily carry out the activities.)

There is nothing magical about this view, nor does it strike me as particularly novel. It is a commonplace that mechanistic systems combine to produce functions that no system alone could serve. Futhermore, it is a commonplace in biology that the operations of individual systems are phylo- and ontogenetically shaped by the larger functions in which those systems participate. The view presented here simply combines these two simple notions, as part of the explanation of cerebral localization of function in general and hemispheric dominance in particular.

An explicit example of the sort of view I have in mind is discussed by Lashley.[7] He argues that fundamental properties of brain systems make it impossible for the same neurological area to serve different kinds of functions. Separate localization of functions is determined by the existence of diverse kinds of integrative mechanism that cannot function in the same nerve field without interference. For example, neurological "fields in which [temporal order] is dominant cannot also serve in other space systems." Lashley gave special attention to potential physiological morphogenesis of functional localization. However, he also emphasized the need to understand any brain area in relation to the entire brain. "On anatomical grounds alone there is no assurance that cerebral localization is anything but an accident of growth."

Statement 4

The left hemisphere is more "adaptable" at birth. This principle is not intended to mean that the left hemisphere is either more or less "mature," since relative maturity might predict greater capacity, but it also might predict less flexibility. There is evidence that certain anatomical areas of the left hemisphere are, in fact, larger at birth.[8] It would be premature, however, to rest this part of my syllogism on the functional relevance of that fact. Furthermore, there are alternate claims that the right hemisphere functionally matures earlier than the left.[9] Notice that this claim is not a claim about the nature of the organization of activities in the left hemisphere, nor is it a claim about the specific neurochemical interactions in the left hemisphere. Rather, it simply proposes that at birth the left hemisphere is more able to deal with and to develop mastery over mental activity. The reason for that might be an intrinsic property of differing maturation rates, or an extrinsically imposed asymmetry (e.g., asymmetric pressure *in utero*).†

Conclusion

The mentally more demanding kind of activity (analytic) will become localized in the more adaptable hemisphere (the left hemisphere). This conclusion involves no claim about the relative frequency of holistic and analytic processing in the child. All it claims is that proportionately more of the analytic processing will be taken over by the left hemisphere and proportionately more of the holistic processing will be left to the right hemisphere.

It should be clear that the statements in this argument are constructed to be either logically true or consistent with known or testable phenomena. On this view behavioral asymmetries emerge as a dynamic function of the self-organizing properties of the mind and the brain in differentiating the mental activities and segregating them neurophysiologically. The further question is whether this way of interpreting cerebral asymmetries makes predictions beyond the claim that the right hemisphere is dominant for those activities that involve holistic processing (e.g., perception of simple visual figures) and the left for analytic tasks (e.g., language).

My proposal argues that asymmetries result from a *process* of mental and neurological differentiation that operates initially at the highest and most central levels. A general prediction from this interpretation is that lateral asymmetries should occur with unilateral stimulation, rather than requiring bilateral sensory inhibition at the peripheral sense-organ level. Unilateral asymmetries have usually been found in visual studies, in which the stimuli are characteristically presented only to one visual field. In auditory studies, however, most researchers present their stimuli dichotically; in fact, some argue that it is only with dichotic presentation that asymmetries should occur.[10] Nevertheless, a growing number of experiments have found monaural differences,[11] and I shall review several others. (All experiments in the present paper used right-handed subjects.)

Consider as a simple example the fact that if a list of random words is followed by a three-second interference task, the right and left ears perform identically. However, when those same random words are respliced into a sentence order, then sequences presented to the right ear are recalled significantly better than sequences presented to the left ear (TABLE 1). In the general view outlined above, the processing asymmetry in this paradigm occurred only when the sequences had syntactic structures, because it is the syntactic structures that make possible processing the word sequences in an analytic mode.[12]

In addition to the general prediction that monaural asymmetries should occur, the nature of asymmetry sketched above makes other somewhat surprising predictions, which turn out to be true.

Prediction 1

The kind of processing that subjects are asked to perform should determine which side is dominant in processing a stimulus. This would be the strongest way of testing the claim that indeed it is the *kind* of processing that determines behavioral asymmetry, not the modality in which the processing is categorized (e.g., language, music, vision, etc.). To show this, Richard Hurtig, Ann Handel, and I ran monaurally the initial-phoneme vs. syllable-recognition experiment described in *Statement 2.*[13] We

---

†Of course, such externally imposed asymmetries might trigger early structural differentiation as well.

TABLE 1

RESULTS OF IMMEDIATE RECALL OF WORDS IN ARRANGED SENTENCE ORDER AND IN RANDOM ORDER*

	Words in Sentence Order		Words in Random Order	
	% sequences totally correct	% words correct	% sequences totally correct	% words correct
Sequence heard in				
Left ear	54	94	4	57
Right ear	65	96	4	57

*From Bever,[2] Table II.

found that the time taken to recognize a syllable beginning in "b" is shortest when the materials are presented to the right ear and the subject responds with the right hand compared with other hand/ear configurations. There was no difference in amount of time to recognize the entire syllable, e. g. "bik." We checked this result in two ways; we alternated whether listeners were listening for an entire syllable, target, or an initial phoneme target, and in a second group of subjects we held the task constant but alternated the ear to which the stimulus was presented. Both experiments gave the same results. (See TABLE 2). This investigation shows that the same stimulus can be differentiated according to the kind of processing the subject must carry out on the stimulus. If the subject must analyze the stimulus internally, then the condition in which only the hemisphere is involved (right-ear/right-hand) is more facilitating than the other conditions. The task in which the subject listens holistically shows no overall differences in this case. (It remains to be seen whether one can show a statistically reliable favoring of right-ear input with a linguistic stimulus.)

A second experiment of this type has been done by Victor Krynicki at Columbia University.[14] Characteristically, previous studies have shown that the recognition of nonlinguistic visual stimuli is best when the stimuli are presented to the left visual field. Since visual stimuli must be presented off the fovea to be completely lateralized anatomically, these experiments characteristically use simple visual stimuli which can be differentiated in the visual periphery (e.g., angle of line, recognition of a face, recognition of a simple geometric figure.) Overall performance on complex stimuli in the periphery can be so low that laterality differences might not be meaningful. Consequently, the experimental requirement that the visual discrimination task must be simple when stimuli are in the visual periphery may account for the apparent right-hemisphere dominance vision that is claimed in the literature.

To test this, Krynicki used a figure-recognition task with brief presentations of irregular eight- and sixteen-sided geometric figures. In one situation the subjects had to recognize rapidly presented stimulus figures from a target set of twenty (20 msec, 2°

TABLE 2

MEAN RT (msec) TO IDENTIFY A SYLLABLE IN TERMS OF THE INITIAL PHONE, OR THE WHOLE SYLLABLE*

	Left Hand			Right Hand		
	Left Ear	Right Ear	Difference	Left Ear	Right Ear	Difference
Initial Phone	360	354	6	377	342	35
Syllable	257	254	3	261	262	−1

*From Bever et al.,[13] combining experiments 1 and 2.

off fovea; a nonius fixation task and EOG monitoring ensured correct fixation). Although the success rate was low, the sixteen-sided figures were identified better in the right visual field (the eight-sided figures showed no differences). Krynicki suggests that the subjects must recognize the complex figures in terms of isolated configurational features (e.g., a jagged edge), thus leading to a left-hemisphere superiority. The basis for this assumption is that a large number of complex and similar figures would be easiest to differentiate, identify, and recognize in terms of some criterial visual feature that distinguishes it from the others in the target set. In a second task the stimulus figures were always rotated 90° or 180°. This task was even more difficult. Nevertheless, there was a left visual field superiority for both eight- and sixteen-sided figures. This result was predicted by the view that holistic processing is relegated to the right hemisphere and the assumption that recognizing a figural rotation is a holistic task that can operate on the gross contour of the stimulus. It is an important fact that in this condition *both* eight-and sixteen-sided figures showed a left visual field superiority, suggesting that figure complexity was not an effective variable. If these results hold up in other paradigms, they will show that the frequent claim that *vision* (of nonlinguistic stimuli) is dominant in the right hemisphere was based on research that involved holistic processing; analytic processing can stimulate left-hemisphere dominance in visual recognition of nonlinguistic stimuli.

Prediction 2

If one shifts ontogenetically from holistic to analytical ways of perceiving a stimulus, one should also shift from being right-hemisphere dominant to being left-hemisphere dominant for that stimulus. Up to now, the perception of music has been a well-documented exception to the differentiation of the hemispheres according to analytic vs. holistic processing. Melodies are composed of an ordered series of pitches, and hence should be processed analytically by the left hemisphere, rather than the right. Yet the recognition of simple melodies has usually been reported to be better in the left ear than the right.[15] This finding is *prima facie* evidence against the functional differentiation of the hemispheres proposed by Jackson; rather, it seems to support the view that the hemispheres are specialized according to stimulus-response modality, with speech in the left, vision and music in the right, and so forth.[16] Such conclusions however, are simplistic, since they do not consider the different kinds of processing strategies that listeners use as a function of their musical experience.[17]

Psychological and musicological analysis of processing strategies resolves the difficulty for a general theory of hemispheric differentiation posed by music perception. It has long been recognized that the perception of melodies can be a "gestalt" phenomenon. That is, that fact that a melody is composed of a series of isolated tones is not relevant for naive listeners—rather, they focus on the overall melodic contour.[18] The view that musically experienced listeners have learned to perceive a melody as an articulated set of relations among components rather than as a whole is suggested directly by Werner.[19] "In advanced musical apprehension a melody is understood to be made up of single tonal motifs and tones which are distinct elements of the whole construction." This is consistent with Meyer's[20] view that recognition of "meaning" in music is a function not only of perception of whole melodic forms but also of concurrent appreciation of the way in which the analyzable components of the whole forms are combined. If a melody is normally treated as a gestalt by musically naive listeners, then the functional account of the difference between the two hemispheres predicts that melodies will be processed predominantly in the right hemisphere for such subjects. It is significant that the one investigator who failed to find a superiority of the left ear for melody recognition used college musicians as subjects,[21] the subjects in other studies were musically naive (or unclassified).

If music perception is dominant in the right hemisphere only insofar as musical form is treated holistically by naive listeners, then the generalization of Jackson's proposals about the differential functioning of the two hemispheres can be maintained. To establish this we conducted a study with subjects of varied levels of musical sophistication that required them to attend to both the internal structure of a tone sequence and its overall melodic contour.[22] The listener's task is sketched below:

| hear melody | 2 sec pause | hear excerpt | say if excerpt was from melody | say if melody was heard before in the experiment |

We found that musically sophisticated listeners could accurately recognize isolated excerpts from a tone sequence, whereas musically naive listeners could not. However, musically naive people could recognize the entire tone sequences, and did so better when the stimuli were presented in the left ear; musically experienced people recognized the entire sequence better in the right ear (TABLE 3). This demonstration of the

TABLE 3

PERCENTAGE CORRECT ON RECOGNITION OF WHOLE AND OF EXCEPTS FROM THE MELODIES*

	Relative Percentage Correct			
	Musically naive subjects		Musically experienced subjects	
	Left ear	Right ear	Left ear	Right ear
Excerpt recognition	−7	−22	27	31
Melody recognition	54	36	44	57

*Percentages are corrected for guessing, from Bever & Chiarello,[20] Table 1.

superiority of the right ear for music shows that it depends on the listener's being musically experienced; it explains the previously reported superiority of the left ear as being due to the use of musically naive subjects, who treat simple melodies as unanalyzed wholes.

We also compared the performance of a group of choir boys with nonmusical boys from the same school on a similar task.‡ Here, too, the choirboys performed more effectively on stimuli presented to the right ear, while the musically naive boys performed better on the left-ear stimuli. Since half the choir boys cannot read music (they memorize their parts), this could not be due to mapping the music onto a score or note-names. It is also possible, in principle, that developing musical ability is not the cause of left-hemisphere dominance but its result: it might be that those boys who are *already* left-hemisphered for music are thereby more musical, and that is why they sign up for the choir. This is inconsistent with several facts. First, the boys join the choir for a mixture of social and financial reasons (choirboys receive a scholarship to their schools). Second, the longer a boy was in the choir, the more pronounced his right-ear dominance (compared with non-choirboys in the same age and grade). Recently, a similar relation between the musical ability of the subject and right-ear superiority was confirmed by Gordon,[23] who reanalyzed data from an experiment on melody and chord recognition. He found that listeners who recognized more melodies overall tended to be more right-eared.

‡We used a "yoked subject" design: for every choirboy there was a corresponding non-choirboy (who was also not studying an instrument) of the same age and grade.

Our interpretation is that musically sophisticated subjects can organize a melodic sequence in terms of the internal relation of its components. This is supported by the fact that only the experienced listeners could accurately recognize the two-note excerpts as part of the complete stimuli. Dominance of the left hemisphere for such analytic functions would explain dominance of the right ear for melody recognition in experienced listeners; as their capacity for musical analysis increases, the left hemisphere becomes increasingly involved in the processing of music.

The shift to left-hemisphere processing does not occur for all aspects of music perception. For example, musically sophisticated listeners continue to show left-ear superiority for recognition of chords (also found by Gordon[21]). Recently L. Kellar and I tested this on our adult population by asking listeners to identify a two-note chord as a musical fourth, augmented fourth, or a fifth:§ we presented musically naive and sophisticated listeners with two-note intervals that were acoustically intermediate between the musical intervals. There is an overall left-ear superiority for all subjects in the consistency of judging intermediate intervals; this tendency was even stronger in musicians.¶ Thus, being musically sophisticated does not involve shifting *all* music processing to the left hemisphere, but only these aspects that require analytic processing.

Prediction 3

Variation in the complexity of syntactic structures should stimulate greater correlations in behavioral complexity when heard in the right ear than in the left. This prediction follows from the view that if the left hemisphere carries out analytic processing, the perceptual strategies that listeners use to analyze relations among the words in sentences will be indigenous to the left hemisphere. A common strategy of speech perception is one that maps an "NVN" sequence onto the grammatical relations "actor, action, object."[24] This strategy accounts for the fact that a sentence like (A) is easier to compare with a picture than sentence (B).[25] In sentence (A) the NVN pattern conforms

(A) They are fixing benches. (Progressive construction.)
(B) They are performing monkeys. (Participial construction.)

to the expectation expressed by the strategy, whereas in (B) it does not. We tested the comprehension of these sentences monaurally to see if the comprehension time between sentences like (A) and sentences like (B) would differ more in the right ear than in the left (listeners heard five sentences structurally like (A) or five sentences like (B); and matched each one to a picture; the sentences were always presented to the same ear for a particular subject). The results are summarized in TABLE 4. The predicted differences occurred for sentences heard in the right ear, but the results were actually the reverse, numerically, for those heard in the left ear.[26] It should be noticed that the average comprehension time for the two constructions together was similar in the two ears; however, the right ear presentation differentiated the constructions according to their conformity with the perceptual strategy, while the left ear presentation did not.

If the left-ear presentation does not show evidence of perceptual strategies, how are the sentences understood at all? One possibilty is that the information is transmitted to the left hemisphere via the callosum, thus circumventing the application of the strat-

§The notes were pure sine waves lasting for one second. Listeners were first presented a reference set (pure fifth, augmented fourth, pure fourth) and then a series of intermediate cases.

¶A puzzling fact is that right-handed subjects who reported left-handers in their family appeared to differ on these tasks from other subjects.

TABLE 4

MEAN LATENCY (sec) TO MATCH PICTURES TO PROGRESSIVE AND PARTICIPIAL SENTENCES IN
LISTENERS WITHOUT EXPERIENCE AT THE TASK*

	Left Ear	Right Ear
Participial	.98	1.29
Progressive	.96	.79
Difference	.02	.50

*From Carey et al.,[23] Table 2.

egies but leaving intact other mechanisms of perception. A second possibility is that
the monotony of the task of hearing the same construction type repeatedly allows for
the formation of a holistic *schema* in the right hemisphere. (The results in Prediction 4
are consistent with this interpretation.)

Prediction 4

*It should be possible to shift analytical processing to the right hemisphere, at least
temporarily.* This follows from the view that cerebral asymmetry is maintained in part
by the dynamic self-organizing properties of the mind and brain.[27] In particular, it is
presupposed that the right hemisphere *can* carry out analytic processing at birth, but
that it does not ordinarily do so during development (and perhaps cannot readapt to
do so after adolescence). If one forces the left ear to continue processing, then it is at
least possible on this view of asymmetries that continued monaural stimulation would
shift some analytical processing to the right hemisphere and predicts that the left ear
would start to show responses with the same pattern as the right ear. This was in fact
observed in the experiment involving the two types of sentences, (A) and (B). TABLE 5
presents the mean reaction time for the two constructions in the second half of the experiment. In this task listeners continued to hear the sentences in the same ear as before, but now heard the set of five sentences that they had *not* heard in the first half of
the experiment. (The delay between the first and second half was less than a minute.)
Listeners continue to find construction (B) more difficult than construction (A) in the
right-ear presentation, although the difference is reduced from the first half. What is
striking is that the left-ear presentation now shows the relative complexity of
construction (B).

It might be that this result occurs because information is now being transmitted
from the left ear directly to the left hemisphere, in such a way that the left-hemisphere
perceptual strategies can apply. However, this would predict that during the second
half of the experiment the differences between the two sentence constructions should
be the same in the right and left ear (or should be less in the left ear than the right, on
the assumption that the information transfer or unaccustomed application of the
strategies is imperfect). The fact is, however, that the left-ear difference in the second

TABLE 5

MEAN LATENCY (SECONDS) TO MATCH PICTURES TO PROGRESSIVE AND PARTICIPIAL SENTENCES IN
LISTENERS WITH EXPERIENCE AT THE TASK*

	Left Ear	Right Ear
Participial	1.27	1.08
Progressive	.72	.91
Difference	.55	.17

*From Carey et al.,[23] Table 2.

half of the experiment is *larger* (significantly) than the right-ear difference in the second half of the experiment.

Prediction 5

Attention should be shifted laterally as a function of the kind of processing that subjects use. This prediction also follows from the claim that asymmetries emerge from self-organizing properties of mind and brain. If sensory information is routed to the left hemisphere during analytical processing, this will have the consequence of giving relative priority to information from all the right sensory organs. This prediction has been confirmed by a number of experiments[28] showing that attention to the right side of the body is enhanced during speech processing. We have extended this in our laboratory** to the finding that during dichotic stimulation, speech sounds presented to the right ear are perceived as *physically* louder than those presented to the left ear. That is, even a simple *sensory* judgment about the speech stimuli is affected by the processing asymmetries.

If the asymmetry emerges in part as a function of self-organizing *functional* properties as opposed to isolated neurological ones, then we would also predict that any stimulus perceived by the subject to be to the right would be treated differentially. This should occur even if both ears are receiving the input, as is the case when a listener hears two signals from two loudspeakers, one to the left and one to the right. Morais and Bertelson have confirmed this prediction (1974).[29] They showed that verbal material presented from a right loudspeaker is recalled better than verbal material presented simultaneously to a left loudspeaker. Morais[30] has extended this finding by showing that the lateral position of a dummy loudspeaker (which the listener *thinks* he is hearing) can influence the recall of verbal material actually presented from a central speaker. That is, it is not the lateral sensory organ of input alone that determines asymmetry, but also the perceived location of input. We tested this kind of finding in an experiment similar to the preceding one on perceived loudness, except that the different diotic words were presented over speakers to the subjects left and right. In this study, the words coming from the right loudspeaker were perceived as louder than those from a left loudspeaker.

These results are crucial to our general view because they invalidate the claim that asymmetries result from a low-level neurologically based routing of information to one hemisphere or the other. Rather, the proposed process must be something like the following: input stimulus information is routed to the left or right hemisphere for initial processing according to its perceived relative location. Once the sensory information is routed in this way, the intrinsic advantages (or disadvantages) of the specific hemisphere determines the results.

Conclusion

I have argued that organizational processes account for the existence of functional hemispheric asymmetries in humans. The substantive claim is that the left hemisphere becomes the locus for analytic processing because it is more flexible during childhood. This is the weakest claim that is compatible with the facts we currently have. The general view I have sketched also predicts facts about asymmetry that would be surprising on more structural theories of its basis.

Part of the difficulty in isolating an ultimate cause for such a complex phenomenon is that it is embedded in many manifestations of human psychology and culture. The

---

**The listener's task was to adjust the loudness of a word in one earphone to be equally loud to a different word in the other earphone (both earphones were adjusted in different phases of the experiment).

result of this is that the emergence of cerebral asymmetry in an individual is overdetermined. Whatever its "original" biological basis, it is shaped by explicit social patterns and artifacts, as well as by implicit patterns of thought. In order to disentangle the problem it is necessary to apply logical principles to isolate the minimum substantive claims.

The most general reason to study asymmetries is that brain structures are generally symmetrical in animals except for the higher functions in humans. This could lead to speculation about the ultimate evolutionary "advantage" of asymmetric function. The near universality of symmetry in nature suggests that asymmetry is *disadvantageous*, given that it makes any difference at all. If the present discussion is correct, asymmetries emerge because of the human ability to differentiate holistic and analytic processing: the advantage of that implicit differentiation seems intuitively clear, although its evolutionary and ontogenetic cause is obscure. Nevertheless, the present formulation of the problem argues that hemispheric asymmetry is the *result* of the evolution of a general mental capacity, not the cause.

NOTES AND REFERENCES

1. TAYLOR, J., Ed. 1932. Selected Writings of JOHN HUGHLINGS JACKSON. Vol. 2: 130 ff. Hodder and Stoughton. London, England.
2. Perception of patterns: KIMURA, D. 1966. Neurophychologia 4: 273. Letter arrays: COHEN, G. 1973. J. Exp. Psychol. 97: 349. Face recognition: LEVY, J., C. TREVARTHEN & R. W. SPERRY. 1972. Brain 95: (61). G. RISZZOLATI, C. GEFFEN, J. L. BRADSHAW & G. WALLACE. 1971. J. Exp. Psychol. 87: 415. Spatial configurations: KIMURA, D. 1969. Can. J. Psychol. 23: 445; DURNFORD, M. & D. KIMURA. 1971. Nature (Lond.) 231: 394. Chords: GORDON, H. W. 1970. Cortex 6: 387. MOLFESE, D. 1972. Paper presented at 84th mtg. Acoustical Soc. Amer. Miami Beach, Fla. Dec. 1. Environmental Sounds: KING, F. L. & KIMURA, D. 1972. Can. J. Psychol. 26: 2. Pitch and intensity: DOEHRING, D. C. 1972. Can. J. Psychol. 26: 106. Emotional tone of voice: HAGGARD, M. P. 1971. Quart. J. Exp. Psychol. 23: 168. Also, recalled words ordered in sentences show right-ear dominance, and unordered word strings do not: BAKKER, D. 1969. Cortex 5: 36; BEVER, T. G. 1971. *In* Biological and Social Factors in Psycholinguistics. J. Morton, Ed. Univ. Illinois Press. Urbana, Ill.; FRANKFURTER, A. & R. P. HONECK. 1973. Quart J. Exp. Psychol. 25: 138; LEVY, J., C. TREVARTHEN & R. W. SPERRY. 1972. Brain 95: 61; GORDON, H. W. 1970. Cortex 6: 387.
3. SHANKWEILER, D. 1966. J. Comp. Physiol. Psychol. 62: 115; GAZZAGNIGA & R. W. SPERRY. 1967. Brain 90: 131; BOGEN, J. E. 1969. Bull. Los Angeles Neurol. Soc. 34: 135; LEVY-AGRESTI & R. W. SPERRY. 1968. Proc. Nat. Acad. Sci. USA 61: 1151; MILNER, B. & L. TAYLOR. 1972. Neuropsychologia 10: 1; BOGEN, J. 1972. *In* Drugs and Cerebral Function. W. L. SMITH, Ed.: 36–37. Charles C Thomas. Springfield, Ill. MILNER, B. 1961. *In* Interhemispheric Relations and Cerebral Dominance. V. B. Mountcastle, Ed. Johns Hopkins Univ. Press. Baltimore, Md.
4. e. g. SEMMES, J. 1968. Neuropsychologia 6: 11.
5. e. g. KIMURA, D. 1973. Sci. Amer. March: 70.
6. SAVIN, H. & T. G. BEVER. 1970. The nonperceptual reality of the phoneme. J. Verbal Learning Verbal Behav. 9: 295–302.
7. LASHLEY, K. S. 1937. Functional determinants of cerebral localization. Arch. Neurol. Psychiat. 38: 371–387.
8. WADA. J. 1972. Morphological hemispheric asymmetry and cerebral speech lateralization. Quoted in L'asymmetrie droit-gauche de *planum temporale*. D. Teszner, A. Tzavaras, J. Gruner & H. Hecaen. Eds. Rev. Neurol. 126: 444–449.
9. e. g. SETH, G. 1973. Eye-hand coordination and handedness: a developmental study of visuomotor behaviour in infancy. Brit. J. Educ. Psychol. 43: 35-49; CROWELL, D., J. JONES. L. KAPUNAI & J. NAKAGAWA. 1973. Unilateral cortical activity in newborn humans. Science 180: 205-208.
10. KIMURA, D. 1969. Can. J. Psychol. 23: 445.

11. Cf. BAKKER, D. 1969. Cortex **5**: 36; SPRINGER, S. 1971. Percept. Psychophys. **10**: 239-241; SPRINGER, S. 1973. Hemispheric Specialization for speech opposed by contralateral noise. Percept. Psychophys. **13**: 3, 391–393. BEVER, T. G., R. KIRK & J. LACKNER. 1969. An autonomic reflection of syntactic structure. Neuropsychologia **7**: 23-28.

12. See BEVER.[2] This result was replicated in FRANKFURTER & HONECK.[2] See also JARVELLA, R. J. & S. J. HERMAN. 1973. J. Exp. Psychol. **79**: 1, 111–113.

13. BEVER, T. G., R. HURTIG & A. HANDEL. 1975. Analytic processing elicits right-ear superiority in monaurally presented speech. Neuropsychologia. In press.

14. KRYNICKI, V. 1974. Hemispheric differences in the recognition of and evoked potential to random sided forms. Unpublished dissertation research.

15. KIMURA, D. 1964. Quart. J. Exp. Psychol. **16**: 355; DARWIN, C. F. 1971. Quart. J. Exp. Psychol. **23**: 46; SPELLACY, F. J. & BLUMSTEIN. 1971. J. Acoust. Soc. Am. **49**: 87; SPREEN, O., F. SPELLACY & J. REID. 1970. Neuropsychologia **8**: 243; KIMURA, D. 1967. Cortex **3**: 163. See also BOGEN, J. & H. GORDON. 1971. Nature (Lond.) **230**: 524 for clinical evidence for the involvement of right-hemisphere functioning in singing.

16. KIMURA, D. 1973. Scientific American **229**: 70.

17. For a similar differentiation of hemispheric function in vision and language, see LEVY, J., C. TREVARTHEN & R. W. SPERRY. 1972. Brain **95**: (61); MILNER, B. 1971. Brit. Med. Bull. **27**: 272.

18. Melody perception is a classic gestalt demonstration. VON EHRENFELS, C. 1890. Vierteljahrsschr. Wiss. Philos. Vol. 14; WERNER, H. 1917. Leistungsknechte **4**: 182; 1926. Z. angew. Psychol. **26**: 101; MEISSNER, H. 1914. Zur Entwicklung Des Musikalischen Sinns Beim Kind Waehrend Des Schulalters. Trorvitzsch. Berlin, Germany; BREHMER, F. 1925. Beih. Z. Angew Psychol. (monograph) 36–37; WERNER, J. 1940. Psychol. **10**: 149. For recent investigations, see DOWLING, W. J. 1971. Percept. Psychophys. **9**: 348; DEUTSCH, D. 1972. Percept. Psychophys. **11**: 411.

19. WERNER, H. 1948. Comparative Psychology of Mental Development: 54. International Universities Press. New York. N. Y.

20. MEYER, L. 1956. Emotion and Meaning in Music. Univ. Chicago Press. Chicago, Ill.

21. GORDON, H. W. 1970. Cortex **6**: 387. The subjects in this study were probably intermediate in musical sophistication; accordingly, they did not show a consistent left- or right-ear superiority. We would expect individual differences in such a population to be quite large.

22. See BEVER, T. G. & R. J. CHIARELLO. 1974. Cerebral dominance in musicians and nonmusicians. Science **185**: 137–139.

23. GORDON, H. W. Science. In preparation.

24. Such strategies are a component of a general model of speech perception. See BEVER, T. G. 1970. The cognitive basis for linguistic structures. *In* Cognition and Language Development. R. Hayes, Ed.: 277–360. John Wiley & Sons, Inc. New York, N.Y.; FODOR, I. A., T. G. BEVER & M. F. GARRETT. 1974. The Psychology of Language. McGraw-Hill Inc. New York, N.Y.

25. Cf. CAREY, P., J. MEHLER & T. G. BEVER. 1970. Judging the veracity of ambiguous sentences. J. Verbal Learn. Verbal Behav. **9** (2): 243–254.

26. The constructions in the left ear did not differ significantly. For a complete statistical analysis of these results, see CAREY *et. al.*,[23] BEVER.[2]

27. See BROWN, J. W. & J. JAFFE. 1975. Note: hypothesis on cerebral dominance. Neuropsychologia **13**: 107–110, for a review of clinical evidence bearing on this point of view.

28. See KINSBOURNE, M. 1970. The cerebral basis of lateral asymmetries in attention. Acta Psychologica **33**: 193–201. Also, KINSBOURNE, M. 1971. The minor cerebral hemisphere as a source of aphasic speech. Arch. Neurol. **25**: 302–306.

29. MORAIS, J. & P. BERTELSON. 1973. Laterality effects in diotic listening. Perception **2** (1): 107–111.

30. MORAIS, J. Cognition **3**: (1). In press.

LINGUISTIC COMPETENCE IN APHASIA

Herman Buschke

*The Saul R. Korey Department of Neurology
and Rose F. Kennedy Center for
Research in Mental Retardation and Human Development
and the Department of Neuroscience
Albert Einstein College of Medicine, Bronx, New York 10461*

The traditional evaluation of aphasia has been more concerned with reading, writing, speaking, and listening to speech than with central linguistic processing. In order to increase our understanding of language impairment in aphasia, we are trying to assess language competence in aphasic patients by asking them to make simple discriminations that show their lexical, semantic, syntactic, and cognitive competence. Since these discriminations require only simple "yes" or "no" responses, they permit evaluation of at least some important aspects of linguistic competence without extensive production by aphasic patients. The necessary evaluation of competence as well as performance should increase our appreciation of the language impairment in aphasia.

Since linguistic behavior is rule-governed behavior,[1] and since it is reasonable to regard a language as a set of elements together with rules for combining such elements into acceptable sentences,[2] it seems reasonable to begin evaluation of linguistic competence in aphasia by trying to determine if aphasic patients can discriminate real words that belong to the language (English) from paralogs that do not, meaningful sentences from grammatical but nonsensical anomalous strings, grammatical from ungrammatical strings, and true from false sentences. These four kinds of discrimination should provide at least some initial evaluation of lexical, semantic, syntactic, and cognitive competence. Evaluation of other aspects of linguistic competence will be considered later. This attempt to evaluate linguistic competence in aphasia is intended to determine whether the patient can appreciate elements of his language and correct use of the rules to relate such elements to each other, when the semantic, syntactic, and cognitive constraints involved in linguistic processing are varied appropriately.

LINGUISTIC COMPETENCE OF A CHILD

For this evaluation of linguistic competence we have used materials that seem simple enough to be used for evaluating children as well as adults. The idea is simple to keep the processing sufficiently elementary, so that any adult with normal linguistic competence would make these discriminations without error. This evaluation of lexical, semantic, syntactic, and cognitive competence is illustrated by the following results obtained from a normal four-year-old boy.

FIGURE 1 shows his lexical competence in discriminating between real English words and paralogs.[3] Each of the ten words and paralogs was read aloud to him, so that he could decide whether each was a real English word or not. He was instructed to say yes only when he was *positive* that the item is a real English word which he already knows, and otherwise to say no. These constraints were imposed on his response bias to limit errors to failure to recognize real English words by minimizing false alarms. He

This work is supported by USPHS grants MH-17733 from NIMH, NS-03356 from NIMS, and HT-01799 from NICHD.

263

A. DISTINGUISHING REAL ENGLISH WORDS FROM PARALOGS (LEXICAL COMPETENCE)

The patient is simply asked to say "yes" whenever he is absolutely **positive** that the item read to him is a real English word; otherwise the patient should say "no." This minimizes false alarms (gue-sing that a paralog is a real word which he does not know), so that errors will be restricted to failure to recognize real English words. The words and paralogs are:

		YES (words)	NO (non-words)
1.	HOTEL	⊕	-
2.	VUMAC	-	⊕
3.	LATUK	-	⊕
4.	BAKER	⊕	-
5.	ZUBER	-	⊕
6.	TOPIC	+	⊖
7.	RIVER	⊕	-
8.	GORAL	-	⊕
9.	COKEM	-	⊕
10.	POWER	⊕	-
		4	5

FIGURE 1. Real English words; four-year-old.

B. (Optional) DISTINGUISHING SYNONYMS FROM UNRELATED WORDS (APPRECIATING SAME MEANING)

The patient is asked to indicate "yes" when the two words "have the same meaning," and "no" when the two do not have the same meaning.

		YES (synonyms)	NO (unrelated)
1.	NOISY - LOUD	⊕	-
2.	SAD - LARGE	-	⊕
3.	BRIGHT - HOLLOW	-	⊕
4.	QUICK - FAST	⊕	-
5.	CORRECT - RIGHT	⊕	-
6.	NEW - CLOUDY	-	⊕
7.	SWEET - EASY	-	⊕
8.	STRONG - POWERFUL	⊕	-
9.	BEAUTIFUL - PRETTY	⊕	-
10.	BRAVE - EMPTY	-	⊕
		5	5

FIGURE 2. Synonyms; four-year-old.

correctly rejected all five paralogs and failed to identify only one of the real English words ("topic"), which he had probably not yet learned. FIGURE 2 shows how the discrimination of synonyms can be used to evaluate semantic competence in terms of words. He was asked to say yes when the two words in each pair read to him both "have the same meaning" and to say no when the two words do not have the same meaning. He correctly rejected all pairs that were not synonyms, and correctly identified all pairs of synonyms.

FIGURE 3 shows his discrimination of meaningful sentences from nonsensical but

I.   DISTINGUISHING MEANINGFUL SENTENCES FROM NONSENSICAL BUT
     GRAMMATICAL STRINGS OF WORDS
     (SEMANTIC COMPETENCE)

     All of these strings have acceptable grammatic structure, but
     only half of them make sense. The patient is asked to indi-
     cate "yes" if the strings make sense, and "no" if the string
     does not make sense. The strings are:

                                           YES   NO
                                        (sentence) (anomalous)

     1. BLACK CLOUDS MEAN SUDDEN STORMS.   (+)   -

     2. WILD ANIMALS BITE STRANGE PERSONS.   (+)   -

     3. RICH CLOUDS HAVE IMPORTANT PERSONS.   -   (+)

     4. PLEASANT SOLDIERS BITE BEAUTIFUL
         STORMS.   -   (+)

     5. PLEASANT AFTERNOONS HAVE CLEAR SKIES. (+)   -

     6. FAMOUS ANIMALS BUY SUDDEN SKIES.   -   (+)

     7. FAMOUS SOLDIERS FIGHT IMPORTANT
         BATTLES.   (+)   -

     8. BLACK AFTERNOONS FIGHT STRANGE CLOTHES. -   (+)

     9. WILD GENTLEMEN MEAN CLEAR BATTLES.   -   (+)

     10. RICH GENTLEMEN BUY BEAUTIFUL CLOTHES. (+)   -

                                               [5]   [5]

FIGURE 3. Meaningful sentences; four-year-old.

grammatical strings of words. These meaningful and anomalous sentences were patterned after those described by Miller and Isard. [4,5] He was told that only half of the sentences "make sense" while the others do not, and was asked to say yes when a sentence makes sense ("Black clouds mean sudden storms.") and to say no when a sentence does not make sense ("Rich clouds have important persons.") He was able to discriminate meaningful from anomalous sentences without any errors.

FIGURE 4 shows the evaluation of his syntactic competence by discrimination of anomalous sentences with grammatical structure from random word lists without grammatical structure. He was told that none of these strings make sense, but that half of them sound like sentences because "the right kinds of words are in the right kind of order," and was asked to discriminate such grammatical strings by saying yes. He was able correctly to reject all five of the random word strings ("Pleasant beautiful bite soldiers storms.") as ungrammatical and to identify correctly four of the five grammatical strings ("Rich clouds have important persons.").

K. DISTINGUISHING GRAMMATICAL STRINGS FROM RANDOM WORD STRINGS
(SYNTACTIC COMPETENCE)

None of these strings makes sense, but half of them have acceptable grammatical form, while the rest do not because they are simply strings of unrelated, randomly ordered words. The patient is asked to indicate "yes" if the string sounds like a sentence because "the right kinds of words are in the right kind of order" (i.e., the string is grammatical), and "no" if the string simply sounds like a string of unrelated words. The strings are:

		YES (gram.)	NO (random)
1.	RICH CLOUDS HAVE IMPORTANT PERSONS.	(+)	-
2.	PLEASANT BEAUTIFUL BITE SOLDIERS STORMS.	-	(+)
3.	ANIMALS SKIES FAMOUS SUDDEN BUY.	-	(+)
4.	MEAN BATTLES GENTLEMEN WILD CLEAR	-	(+)
5.	WILD GENTLEMEN MEAN CLEAR BATTLES.	(+)	-
6.	PLEASANT SOLDIERS BITE BEAUTIFUL STORMS.	+	(-)
7.	IMPORTANT RICH HAVE PERSONS CLOUDS.	-	(+)
8.	RICH CLOUDS HAVE IMPORTANT PERSONS.	(+)	-
9.	FAMOUS ANIMALS BUY SUDDEN SKIES.	(+)	-
10.	CLOTHES STRANGE BLACK FIGHT AFTERNOONS.	-	(+)

$\boxed{4}$ $\boxed{5}$

FIGURE 4. Grammatical strings; four-year-old.

FIGURE 5 shows the evaluation of his cognitive competence by discriminating between true and false sentences. He was told that only half these sentences were true, and that he should say yes if the sentence was true and no if the sentence was not true. He correctly discriminated all five of the true sentences and correctly rejected four of the five false sentences.

The performance of this four-year-old boy seems good enough to suggest that these particular tasks should not present any problem for adults with normal linguistic competence, and that this kind of evaluation might possibly be useful in studies of language development.

LINGUISTIC COMPETENCE OF AN APHASIC PATIENT

Evaluation of lexical, semantic, syntactic, and cognitive competence in aphasia is illustrated by the evaluation of a 62-year-old man with aphasia due to recurrence of tumor two months after left occipital lobectomy for glioblastoma. He was readmitted because of difficulty in communicating, in reading, and in recognizing words, objects, and faces. He was alert, oriented, and cooperative. He spoke fluently but with dysnomia, paraphasia and circumlocution, and occasional neologisms. He could read letters but not words. He could not copy words but could write from dictation, and could repeat dictated words. His other neurological findings were restricted to a right Babinski sign and a right homonymous hemianopsia. He is a native English speaker with a high school education.

FIGURES 6 and 7 show intact lexical and semantic competence by this evaluation. FIGURE 8 shows gross impairment of syntactic competence. Even though he was essentially unable to discriminate grammatical from nongrammatical strings (FIGURE 8), he was able to distinguish meaningful sentences from nonsensical but grammatical strings of words (FIGURE 7). He showed fairly intact cognitive competence by discriminating true from false sentences (FIGURE 9), correctly rejecting all five false sentences and incorrectly rejecting only one of the five true sentences. Such intact semantic competence despite impaired syntactic competence, as judged by failure to distinguish grammatical from ungrammatical strings, suggests that syntactic processing may not always be necessary to extract linguistic meaning. Such selective impairment of syntactic competence has been found in other aphasic patients who also have shown good appreciation of meaning.

LINGUISTIC COMPETENCE IN A SECOND LANGUAGE

A similar finding of intact semantic processing despite impaired syntactic processing in the second language of a normal adult is illustrated by the following evaluation of the linguistic competence of a normal 27-year-old woman whose first language was Spanish. She learned English at age ten, after coming to the United States from Puerto Rico.

L.   DISTINGUISHING TRUE FROM FALSE SENTENCES
       (COGNITIVE COMPETENCE)

All of these sentences are meaningful and have acceptable grammatical structure, but only half of them are true while the rest are false. The patient is asked to indicate "yes" when the sentence is true, and to indicate "no" when the sentence is false. The sentences are:

		YES (true)	NO (false)
1.	SMALL CHILDREN LOVE SWEET CANDY.	⊕	–
2.	SOME DOGS HAVE SHORT TAILS.	⊕	–
3.	BROWN BEARS SING FUNNY SONGS.	–	⊕
4.	SMALL CHILDREN DRIVE FAST CARS.	–	⊕
5.	LARGE MICE CHASE SMALL CATS.	⊖	+
6.	BROWN BEARS EAT SWEET HONEY.	⊕	–
7.	SNOW IS SOFT AND COLD.	⊕	–
8.	ALL DOGS HAVE SHORT TAILS.	–	⊕
9.	LARGE CATS CHASE SMALL MICE.	⊕	–
10.	SNOW IS SOFT AND WARM.	–	⊕

$$\boxed{5} \qquad \boxed{4}$$

FIGURE 5. True sentences; four-year-old.

A. DISTINGUISHING REAL ENGLISH WORDS FROM PARALOGS
(LEXICAL COMPETENCE)

The patient is simply asked to say "yes" whenever he is absolutely <u>positive</u> that the item read to him is a real English word; otherwise the patient should say "no." This minimizes false alarms (gue-sing that a paralog is a real word which he does not know), so that errors will be restricted to failure to recognize real English words. The words and paralogs are:

		YES (words)	NO (non-words)
1.	HOTEL	⊕	-
2.	VUMAC	-	⊕
3.	LATUK	-	⊕
4.	BAKER	⊕	-
5.	ZUBER	-	⊕
6.	TOPIC	⊕	-
7.	RIVER	⊕	-
8.	GORAL	-	⊕
9.	COKEM	-	⊕
10.	POWER	⊕	-
		5	5

FIGURE 6. Real English words; aphasic patient.

I. DISTINGUISHING MEANINGFUL SENTENCES FROM NONSENSICAL BUT GRAMMATICAL STRINGS OF WORDS
(SEMANTIC COMPETENCE)

<u>All</u> of these strings have acceptable grammatic structure, but only half of them make sense. The patient is asked to indicate "yes" if the strings make sense, and "no" if the string does not make sense. The strings are:

		YES (sentence)	NO (anomalous)
1.	BLACK CLOUDS MEAN SUDDEN STORMS.	⊕	-
2.	WILD ANIMALS BITE STRANGE PERSONS.	⊕	-
3.	RICH CLOUDS HAVE IMPORTANT PERSONS.	-	⊕
4.	PLEASANT SOLDIERS BITE BEAUTIFUL STORMS.	-	⊕
5.	PLEASANT AFTERNOONS HAVE CLEAR SKIES.	⊕	-
6.	FAMOUS ANIMALS BUY SUDDEN SKIES.	-	⊕
7.	FAMOUS SOLDIERS FIGHT IMPORTANT BATTLES.	⊕	-
8.	BLACK AFTERNOONS FIGHT STRANGE CLOTHES.	-	⊕
9.	WILD GENTLEMEN MEAN CLEAR BATTLES.	-	⊕
10.	RICH GENTLEMEN BUY BEAUTIFUL CLOTHES.	⊕	-
		5	5

FIGURE 7. Meaningful sentences; aphasic patient.

K. __DISTINGUISHING GRAMMATICAL STRINGS FROM RANDOM WORD STRINGS__
(SYNTACTIC COMPETENCE)

None of these strings makes sense, but half of them have
acceptable grammatical form, while the rest do not because
they are simply strings of unrelated, randomly ordered words.
The patient is asked to indicate "yes" if the string sounds
like a sentence because "the right kinds of words are in the
right kind of order" (i.e., the string is grammatical), and
"no" if the string simply sounds like a string of unrelated
words. The strings are:

		YES (gram.)	NO (random)
1.	RICH CLOUDS HAVE IMPORTANT PERSONS.	+	(−)
2.	PLEASANT BEAUTIFUL BITE SOLDIERS STORMS.	−	(+)
3.	ANIMALS SKIES FAMOUS SUDDEN BUY.	(−)	+
4.	MEAN BATTLES GENTLEMEN WILD CLEAR	(−)	+
5.	WILD GENTLEMEN MEAN CLEAR BATTLES.	+	(−)
6.	PLEASANT SOLDIERS BITE BEAUTIFUL STORMS.	+	(−)
7.	IMPORTANT RICH HAVE PERSONS CLOUDS.	(−)	+
8.	RICH CLOUDS HAVE IMPORTANT PERSONS.	(+)	−
9.	FAMOUS ANIMALS BUY SUDDEN SKIES.	+	(−)
10.	CLOTHES STRANGE BLACK FIGHT AFTERNOONS.	−	(+)

$$\boxed{1} \qquad \boxed{2}$$

FIGURE 8. Grammatical strings; aphasic patient.

L. __DISTINGUISHING TRUE FROM FALSE SENTENCES__
(COGNITIVE COMPETENCE)

All of these sentences are meaningful and have acceptable
grammatical structure, but only half of them are true while
the rest are false. The patient is asked to indicate "yes"
when the sentence is true, and to indicate "no" when the
sentence is false. The sentences are:

		YES (true)	NO (false)
1.	SMALL CHILDREN LOVE SWEET CANDY.	(+)	−
2.	SOME DOGS HAVE SHORT TAILS.	(+)	−
3.	BROWN BEARS SING FUNNY SONGS.	−	(+)
4.	SMALL CHILDREN DRIVE FAST CARS.	−	(+)
5.	LARGE MICE CHASE SMALL CATS.	−	(+)
6.	BROWN BEARS EAT SWEET HONEY.	(+)	−
7.	SNOW IS SOFT AND COLD.	(+)	−
8.	ALL DOGS HAVE SHORT TAILS.	−	(+)
9.	LARGE CATS CHASE SMALL MICE.	+	(−)
10.	SNOW IS SOFT AND WARM.	−	(+)

$$\boxed{4} \qquad \boxed{5}$$

FIGURE 9. True sentences; aphasic patient.

FIGURE 10 (*top*) shows intact word recognition and appreciation of equivalent meaning (*bottom*). FIGURE 11 (*top*) shows that she could also discrimination antonyms from unrelated pairs of words. FIGURE 11 (bottom) shows good discrimination of homophones from unambiguous words with only one meaning. She was asked to say yes if the single word read aloud has more than one meaning or referent ("beat," "beet") and to say no if the word has only one basic meaning ("melt"). This kind of "search for word meanings" is the reverse of the more conventional "word finding" in the traditional aphasia examination.

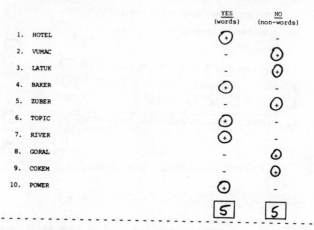

<u>A</u>.   REAL WORDS/PARALOGS (word recognition)

The patient is simply asked to say "yes" whenever he is <u>positive</u> that the item read to him is a real English word; otherwise the patient should say "no."

		YES (words)	NO (non-words)
1.	HOTEL	⊕	-
2.	VUMAC	-	⊕
3.	LATUK	-	⊕
4.	BAKER	⊕	-
5.	ZUBER	-	⊕
6.	TOPIC	⊕	-
7.	RIVER	⊕	-
8.	GORAL	-	⊕
9.	COKEM	-	⊕
10.	POWER	⊕	-
		5	5

B.   SYNONYMS/UNRELATED WORDS (appreciating same meaning)

The patient is asked to indicate "yes" when the two words "have the same meaning," and "no" when the two do not have the same meaning.

		YES (synonyms)	NO (unrelated)
1.	NOISY - LOUD	⊕	-
2.	SAD - LARGE	-	⊕
3.	BRIGHT - HOLLOW	-	⊕
4.	QUICK - FAST	⊕	-
5.	CORRECT - RIGHT	⊕	-
6.	NEW - CLOUDY	-	⊕
7.	SWEET - EASY	-	⊕
8.	STRONG - POWERFUL	⊕	-
9.	BEAUTIFUL - PRETTY	⊕	-
10.	BRAVE - EMPTY	-	⊕
		5	5

FIGURE 10. Real English words (*top*) and synonyms (*bottom*); second language.

C.   ANTONYMS/UNRELATED WORDS (appreciating opposite meaning)

The patient is asked to indicate "yes" when the two words are opposites, and "no" when the two words are unrelated.

		YES (antonyms)	NO (unrelated)
1.	STRONG - WEAK	⊕	-
2.	CHEAP - CLEAN	-	⊕
3.	THIN - NEAT	-	⊕
4.	BEAUTIFUL - UGLY	⊕	-
5.	SHORT - SMART	-	⊕
6.	QUICK - SLOW	⊕	-
7.	NOISY - QUIET	⊕	-
8.	FULL - RICH	-	⊕
9.	CORRECT - WRONG	⊕	-
10.	COLD - DRY	-	⊕
		5	**5**

- -

D.   HOMOPHONES/UNAMBIGUOUS WORDS (search for word meanings)

The patient is asked to indicate "yes" when the single word read aloud sounds like another, different word which means or refers to something completely different, and to indicate "no" when the single word read aloud has only one clear meaning or referent.

		YES (more than one meaning)	NO (only one meaning)
1.	BEAT (BEET)	⊕	-
2.	MADE (MAID)	⊕	-
3.	WEEK (WEAK)	+	⊖
4.	MELT	-	⊕
5.	MAP	-	⊕
6.	STEAL (STEEL)	⊕	-
7.	DAY	-	⊕
8.	BOAT	-	⊕
9.	FLOWER (FLOUR)	⊕	-
10.	BROOM	-	⊖
		4	**5**

FIGURE 11. Antonyms (*top*) and homophones (*bottom*); second language.

FIGURE 12 (*top*) shows that she was able to categorize words semantically, since she correctly discriminated sets of four words in the same semantic category from sets of four words containing three words from the same category and one word from another category. FIGURE 12 (*bottom*) showed that she had difficulty in categorizing grammatically, since she could not discriminate between sets of four words having the same grammatical form and sets of four words in which only three of the four words have the same grammatical form.

E. SAME WORD TYPE/DIFFERENT (categorizing words by meaning)

The patient is asked to indicate "yes" if all of words in each group
are the same in some sense (e.g., belong to the same category, because
"they are the same kind of thing"), and to indicate "no" if all of the
words in each group are not the same. Use all 4 words or only last 2
words as appropriate.

		YES (all same)	NO
1.	dog - cat - elephant - rabbit	(+)	-
2.	potato - beets - corn - chair	-	(+)
3.	hand - foot - nose - mile	-	(+)
4.	spider - moth - bee - cabbage	-	(+)
5.	Nancy - Jane - Susan - Alice	(+)	-
6.	shoes - boots - slippers - sandals	(+)	-
7.	bowling - baseball - golf - football	(+)	-
8.	diamond - ruby - emerald - book	-	(+)
9.	green - blue - red - banana	-	(+)
10.	uncle - daughter - mother - sister	(+)	-

YES: [5]   NO: [5]

- -

F. SAME WORD TYPE/DIFFERENT (categorizing words by grammatical function)

The patient is asked to indicate "yes" if all of words in each group are
the same kind of words (e.g., all nouns), and to indicate "no" if all of
the words in each group are not the same. Use all 4 words or only last
2 words as appropriate.

		YES (all same)	NO
1.	table - car - cheese - school	+	(-)
2.	run - eat - swim - listen	+	(-)
3.	hold - sell - drop - apple	-	(+)
4.	sold - heard - took - carry	-	(+)
5.	loud - sad - rich - shoe	-	(+)
6.	gave - told - bought - found	(+)	-
7.	unless - or - but - since	(+)	-
8.	radio - minor - rabbit - sing	-	(+)
9.	happy - fast - wet - sweet	(+)	-
10.	either - never - if - quiet	(-)	+

YES: [3]   NO: [4]

FIGURE 12. Categorizing words semantically (*top*) and categorizing words grammatically (*bottom*); second language.

(optional)

G.   MEANINGFUL PHRASES/NONSENSE (appreciating phrase meaning)

The patient is asked to indicate "yes" if the phrase makes sense and
to indicate "no" if the phrase does not make sense.

		YES	NO
1.	TALL TREES	⊕	-
2.	DRINK WATER	⊕	-
3.	READ CHAIRS	-	⊕
4.	BLUE SHIRT	⊕	-
5.	SOUR TREES	-	⊕
6.	PEOPLE LAUGH	⊕	-
7.	DRINK BREAD	-	⊕
8.	SLOW SHIRT	-	⊕
9.	PEOPLE BLOOM	-	⊕
10.	READ BOOKS	⊕	-
		$\boxed{5}$	$\boxed{5}$

- -

(optional)

H.   GRAMMATICAL PHRASES/NON-GRAMMATIC (appreciating phrase syntax)

The patient is asked to indicate "yes" if the phrases "sound like
English because the words are in the right order," and "no" if the
phrase just sounds like two unrelated words.

		YES	NO
1.	SOUR TREES	⊕	-
2.	DRINK BREAD	+	⊖
3.	READ CHAIRS	+	⊘
4.	SLOW SHIRT	-	⊕
5.	TREES SOUR	⊖	+
6.	PEOPLE BLOOM	+	⊖
7.	HEAD DRINK	-	⊕
8.	SHIRT SLOW	-	⊕
9.	BLOOM PEOPLE	-	⊕
10.	CHAIRS READ	⊕	-
		$\boxed{2}$	$\boxed{4}$

FIGURE 13. Meaningful phrases (*top*) and grammatical phrases (*bottom*); second language.

FIGURE 13 (*top*) shows that she could discriminate correctly between meaningful phrases and nonsensical but grammatical phrases, even though she could not discriminate between gramatical and nongrammatical phrases (*bottom*).

FIGURE 14 (*top*) shows that she could correctly discriminate meaningful sentences from anomalous strings of grammatical nonsense, even though she could not discriminate between grammatical strings and anagrammatic strings without grammatical structure. Such anagrammatic strings ("Beautiful rich buy clothes gentlemen.") were

I.   MEANINGFUL SENTENCES/ANOMALOUS (appreciating meaning)

The patient is asked to indicate "yes" if the strings make sense, and "no" if the string does not make sense.

		YES (sentence)	NO (anomalous)
1.	BLACK CLOUDS MEAN SUDDEN STORMS.	(+)	-
2.	WILD ANIMALS BITE STRANGE PERSONS.	(+)	-
3.	RICH CLOUDS HAVE IMPORTANT PERSONS.	-	(+)
4.	PLEASANT SOLDIERS BITE BEAUTIFUL STORMS.	-	(+)
5.	PLEASANT AFTERNOONS HAVE CLEAR SKIES.	(+)	-
6.	FAMOUS ANIMALS BUY SUDDEN SKIES.	-	(+)
7.	FAMOUS SOLDIERS FIGHT IMPORTANT BATTLES.	(+)	-
8.	BLACK AFTERNOONS FIGHT STRANGE CLOTHES.	-	(+)
9.	WILD GENTLEMEN MEAN CLEAR BATTLES.	-	(+)
10.	RICH GENTLEMEN BUY BEAUTIFUL CLOTHES.	(+)	-

YES: 5   NO: 5

- -

(optional)

J.   GRAMMATICAL STRINGS/ANAGRAMMATIC (appreciating syntax-1)

The patient is asked to indicate "yes" if the string sounds like a sentence because the right kinds of words are in the right kind of order, and to indicate "no" if the string sounds like the words are out of order.

		YES (grammatical)	NO (anagrammatical)
1.	PLEASANT SOLDIERS BITE BEAUTIFUL STORMS.	(+)	-
2.	WILD GENTLEMEN MEAN CLEAR BATTLES.	(+)	-
3.	SOLDIERS BATTLES FAMOUS IMPORTANT FIGHT.	(-)	+
4.	BEAUTIFUL RICH BUY CLOTHES GENTLEMEN.	(-)	+
5.	RICH CLOUDS HAVE IMPORTANT PERSONS.	+	(-)
6.	PLEASANT HAVE SKIES AFTERNOONS CLEAR.	(-)	+
7.	STORMS SUDDEN BLACK MEAN CLOUDS.	(-)	+
8.	BLACK AFTERNOONS FIGHT STRANGE CLOTHES.	+	(-)
9.	BITE PERSONS ANIMALS WILD STRANGE.	-	(+)
10.	FAMOUS ANIMALS BUY SUDDEN SKIES.	+	(-)

YES: 2   NO: 1

FIGURE 14. Meaningful sentences (*top*) and grammatical strings (*bottom*); second language.

generated by randomizing the words in meaningful sentences. FIGURE 15 (*top*) shows that she also could not discriminate between grammatical strings and random word lists ("Pleasant beautiful bite soldiers storms."), in which the words are not related to each other. FIGURE 15 (*bottom*) shows good discrimination of true from false sentences.

This evaluation of linguistic competence is a second language (FIGURE 16) shows intact semantic processing despite poor syntactic competence, consistent with similar findings in some aphasic patients. It also illustrates how such simple discriminations can be used to evaluate additional aspects of linguistic competence.

K.   GRAMMATICAL STRINGS/RANDOM WORDS (appreciating syntax-2)

The patient is asked to indicate "yes" if the string sounds like a sentence because "the right kinds of words are in the right kind of order" and "no" if the string simply sounds like a string of unrelated words.

		YES (grammatical)	NO (random)
1.	RICH CLOUDS HAVE IMPORTANT PERSONS.	+	⊖
2.	PLEASANT BEAUTIFUL BITE SOLDIERS STORMS.	−	⊕
3.	ANIMALS SKIES FAMOUS SUDDEN BUY.	−	⊕
4.	MEAN BATTLES GENTLEMEN WILD CLEAR.	⊖	+
5.	WILD GENTLEMEN MEAN CLEAR BATTLES.	⊕	−
6.	PLEASANT SOLDIERS BITE BEAUTIFUL STORMS.	+	⊖
7.	IMPORTANT RICH HAVE PERSONS CLOUDS.	−	⊕
8.	RICH CLOUDS HAVE IMPORTANT PERSONS.	+	⊖
9.	FAMOUS ANIMALS BUY SUDDEN SKIES.	+	⊖
10.	CLOTHES STRANGE BLACK FIGHT AFTERNOONS.	−	⊕

1   4

- -

L.   TRUE SENTENCES/FALSE (evaluating semantic content)

The patient is asked to indicate "yes" when the sentence is true, and to indicate "no" when the sentence is false.

		YES (true)	NO (false)
1.	SMALL CHILDREN LOVE SWEET CANDY.	⊕	−
2.	SOME DOGS HAVE SHORT TAILS.	⊕	−
3.	BROWN BEARS SING FUNNY SONGS.	−	⊕
4.	SMALL CHILDREN DRIVE FAST CARS.	−	⊕
5.	LARGE MICE CHASE SMALL CATS.	⊖	+
6.	BROWN BEARS EAT SWEET HONEY.	⊕	−
7.	SNOW IS SOFT AND COLD.	⊕	−
8.	ALL DOGS HAVE SHORT TAILS.	−	⊕
9.	LARGE CATS CHASE SMALL MICE.	⊕	−
10.	SNOW IS SOFT AND WARM.	−	⊕

5   4

FIGURE 15. Grammatical strings (*top*) and true sentences (*bottom*); second language.

Name: __A. M.__   Date: __6/6/74__

Age: __27__   Sex: __F__   Hosp.# _____

Diagnosis: __NORMAL: ENGLISH SECOND, SPANISH FIRST LANGUAGE__

		YES	NO	%
A.	REAL WORDS/PARALOGS (word recognition)	5	5	100
B.	SYNONYMS/UNRELATED WORDS (appreciating same meaning)	5	5	100
C.	ANTONYMS/UNRELATED WORDS (appreciating opposite meaning)	5	5	100
D.	HOMOPHONES/UNAMBIGUOUS WORDS (search for word meaning)	4	5	90
E.	SAME WORD TYPE/DIFFERENT (categorizing words by meaning)	5	5	100
F.	SAME WORD TYPE/DIFFERENT (categorizing words by grammatical function)	3	4	70
G.	MEANINGFUL PHRASES/NONSENSE (appreciation of meaning)	5	5	100
H.	GRAMMATICAL PHRASES/NON-GRAMMATIC (appreciating syntax)	2	4	60
I.	MEANINGFUL SENTENCES/ANOMALOUS (appreciating meaning)	5	5	100
J.	GRAMMATICAL STRINGS/ANAGRAMMATIC (appreciating syntax-1)	2	1	30
K.	GRAMMATICAL STRINGS/RANDOM WORDS (appreciating syntax-2)	1	4	50
L.	TRUE SENTENCES/FALSE (evaluating semantic content)	5	4	90

FIGURE 16. Evaluation of second-language competence.

DISCUSSION

Evaluation of lexical, semantic, syntactic, and cognitive competence in linguistic processing has been illustrated by evaluation of the linguistic competence of a normal 4-year-old boy, a 62-year-old man with aphasia, and a normal 27-year-old woman who learned English as a second language at age ten. The evaluation of this four-year-old suggests that such evaluation of language competence might be useful in studies of the development of language, and that these tasks are probably well within the linguistic competence of normal adults.

The evaluation of this aphasic patient suggests that the addition of such an evaluation of linguistic competence might enhance the more traditional aphasia examination.[6,7] Since impaired use of language does not necessarily indicate decreased linguistic competence, some such analysis of linguistic competence in aphasia seems necessary if analysis of aphasia is to contribute to our understanding of the neurological bases of language perception and production. This aphasic patient showed good semantic competence despite impaired grammatical competence.

The evaluation of the second-language competence of this normal adult bilingual also showed good semantic competence without effective grammatical competence. The intact semantic processing despite impaired or poorly developed syntactic competence shown by this aphasic patient and this normal bilingual suggests that the extraction of meaning may not always involve extensive syntactic analysis (or perhaps that syntactic analysis may operate in conjunction with semantic analysis). This does not seem too surprising, since a good deal of meaning seems to be extracted from grammatically awkward or incomplete linguistic communications in the course of ordinary conversation. This preliminary analysis of language competence by discrimination of acceptable elements and combinations of elements that conform to the rules of the language illustrates its relevance for studies of language impairment and bilingualism, as well as for studies of normal linguistic competence.

ACKNOWLEDGMENT

I thank Christine Sinclair-Prince for experimental assistance.

REFERENCES

1. MILLER G. A. 1965. Some preliminaries to psycholinguistics. Amer. Psychol. **20:** 15–20.
2. CHOMSKY, N. 1964. Syntactic structures. Mouton & Co. The Hague, The Netherlands.
3. TAYLOR, J. D. & G. A. KIMBLE. 1967. The association value of 320 selected words and paralogs. J. Verb. Learn. Verb. Behav. **6:** 744–752.
4. MILLER, G. A. & S. ISARD. 1963. Some perceptual consequences of linguistic rules. J. Verb. Learn. Verb. Behav. **2:** 217–228.
5. MARKS, L. E. & G. A. MILLER. 1964. The role of semantic and syntactic constraints in the memorization of English sentenes. J. Verb. Learn. Verb. Behav. **3:** 1–5.
6. BOLLER, F. & E. GREEN. 1972. Comprehension in severe aphasics. Cortex **8:** 382–394.
7. ZURIF, E. B., A. CARAMAZZA & R. MYERSON. 1972. Grammatical judgments of agrammatic aphasics. Neuropsychologia **10:** 405–417.

DISCUSSION

Louis Gerstman, *Chairperson*

City College
The City University of New York
New York, New York 10009

Ms. ELAINE KAUFMAN: I've had a lot of experience teaching foreign languages to American students both on an adolescent and an adult level. Dr. Krashen, I was wondering, in terms of your experience in English as the second language, did you group all your foreign language people together? Were your students Spanish, or were they, let's say, Israeli, or Russian, or whatever, or all grouped together?

DR. KRASHEN: For practical reasons, they're all grouped together. There are not usually enough from one language group to justify a separate class. It's an open question whether it's better that way or not.

Ms. KAUFMAN: It seems to me that the phonic problems would be very different for the different groups. For example, the Spanish person cannot ever pronounce the word "street" without saying "estreet," and that simple thing would not be the same for a Hebrew or a Russian speaker. Second, the method used today in most schools is an audiolingual one; is that true?

DR. KRASHEN: No, I don't think there's a single teacher in the whole staff at Queens College who uses audiolingual in its pure form.

DR. BLANK: I have two comments. First, I think that any conclusion about English as a second rather than a first language, has to be very cautious. Any comparison must acknowledge the fact that first-language acquisition occurs with an intensive exchange between the mother and the child, hours and hours of it.

DR. KRASHEN: Not necessarily. How about orphans?

DR. BLANK: I'm not saying "necessarily." But, first of all, in orphanages, children's language learning is seriously delayed when they don't have this kind of very carefully matched feedback. The role of the feedback is unclear; but clearly no English-as-a-second-language program that I know gives this kind of really intensive, immediate, correct feedback to the person. So the person's learning capacity is totally different, because he's got a mess to figure out, compared with the young child, who has a much easier task, in a sense.

The second issue I'd like to raise is that the idea of formal operations is a very difficult one, because most people never attain formal operations and most people can learn a second language past twelve years of age. There's a correlation there, I think; it's a very tenuous one, at best.

DR. KRASHEN: Okay. Let me respond to both those points. With respect to how we teach adults second languages and the role of feedback, my impression is that not only is feedback present but that it's an integral part of all systems that teach adults a second language. It may not always take the same form. It may simply be the teacher asking you to repeat, it may simply be a note of disapproval, but in all successful systems, it's there all the time. In fact, one of the most successful systems, not popular in New York City, is one that seems to be producing results far outstripping other systems. It is called "Silent Way," and is basically nothing but error correction from the very beginning.

With respect to formal operations, I'll ask Dr. Furth to comment on that. Is it true that most people don't attain them?

278

DR. FURTH: Our knowledge of formal operations is very inadequate, and therefore Dr. Krashen can use the term, just like Piaget or anybody else; and that's about all you can say.

DR. KRASHEN: Thanks a lot.

DR. PHILLIP DALE (*University of Washington, Seattle, Wash.*): I wonder if it's true that the critical-period hypothesis must depend on the claim that the sequence of acquisition is the same in second- as in first-language acquisition. It seems to me we're learning that with children, the sequence of development is a function both of cognitive and linguistic factors. Mastering an aspect of language means mastering the concept and mastering the linguistic means of expression. At various times, either one or the other may be the factor that holds up the acquisition. I take that to be Slobin's point.

If a child is learning a second language, he's starting at a point somewhat older, so that his cognitive development is likely to be ahead. Therefore, even if he's using the same strategies for mastering the linguistic means of expression, the sequence may be different because it won't have certain cognitive problem.

DR. KRASHEN: All I can say is that I agree. What is important is determining whether the same strategies are being used by all learners.

DR. SANDRA BEN-ZEEV (*Bilingual Education Service Center, Mt. Prospect, Ill.*): Bruner and his people have found that formal ways of thinking don't come into certain cultures. For example, in primitive Mexican villages, adults never develop to that formal level. I would think that a way of testing the theory would be to try to teach a second language to people in that sort of culture and see what happens.

DR. KRASHEN: I would predict, if that is correct, that they would be able to "acquire" language, and they would be much more successful at it at age 19 and 20. That would be a good demonstration.

DR. BEN-ZEEV: Another possibility is that it's not a matter of formal operations, but that the interference from the first structure is simply keeping the person from second-language learning.

DR. KRASHEN: Interference. I've a theory about what might be causing interference—not a very good theory, but it predicts the data. David Elkins has some ideas that certain personality changes that happen at around adolesence are the results of formal operations. His theory goes like this: First, what happens in formal operations is that the adolescent can think about thought, or he can take thought as an object of thought.

Once he does that, he begins to think about what other people are thinking, the very fact that they're thinking. He then assumes they're thinking about him. Not only are they thinking about him, but they're thinking about his acne and all the things that he is sensitive about. This makes him reluctant to reveal himself and results in a loss of self-confidence. Now, if this is a general thing that pervades the entire personality, it also may affect language learning. The loss of self-confidence may result in an unwillingness to test out linguistic rules or to try new hypotheses. He may rely more on what he feels to be right and natural, mainly the rules of his first language.

For example, when I speak French, I speak French with an accent that sounds absolutely correct to me, the American accent, because I don't (at some level) perceive it as an error. That is a theory of where interference comes from. It is interesting that we find interference only in adults. Dulay and Burt (1973) have shown in the area of syntax that except for an initial stage, children generally don't have interference errors in English as a second language. All the work on accent, our work, the work of Asher and Garcia, and Susan Oyama's work, has shown that the same thing is true in the realm of phonology.

DR. GLUCKSBERG: I have two comments to make. First, it seems to me that there are two issues here. One has to do with the best or most optimal techniques for teaching second languages to both children and adults; the second has to do with the concept of the critical period itself. I would like to ask two questions. First, I would suggest that field studies of the kind you're doing are highly suggestive, but are inextrably confounded, so we cannot make serious interpretations of the critical-period hypothesis or of the nature of that hypothesis because of those confoundings. For example, you find that instruction is not particularly useful for children, yet it is useful for adults. One obvious confounding is that children are usually forced to take language classes; usually, adults take them voluntarily. So we have a simple confounding there.

Second, with respect to the notion of critical periods, it seems to me that a strong critical-period hypothesis could not allow for a single counterexample, and there are clearly many counterexamples to all of the data that you've talked about; namely, that there are adults who acquire a second language in their late twenties and thirties without any trace of accent at all. In fact if we couldn't do that, we couldn't possibly have an efficient spy system. I would like you to comment primarily on how strong you take the critical-period hypothesis to be.

DR. KRASHEN: Let me comment with respect to the exceptions. First of all, most of the spies I know were bilingual from before age twelve or so. Another interesting thing is that people always come and say "I know so-and-so, who speaks a certain language without an accent and he learned it at twenty. It's always a language that nobody else in the room knows. The number of adults that I've met in my life who speak English convincingly and who learned it after puberty are zero. If you have these people, bring them around to Queens College. I'd love to tape-record them and give them our whole battery of English tests. With respect to the first comment, all I can say is that it is a problem. There are a few studies in the English-as-a-second-language literature that conclude by saying that exposure is better than instruction, by taking, say, two groups of foreign students. One group has to attend ESL classes (English as a second language). Group two is told that they can postpone ESL classes for a semester. English tests are administered before and after, and the group that was out of class does just as well or better. All I can say is that, I'd like to know what these people are doing out of class. In many cases, the people outside of classes are getting for themselves what we call the "essential characteristics" of formal instruction. They're getting rule isolation from grammar books or friends. They're getting feedback via error correction. The ones who must go to class may not even be especially motivated. The problem with children, though, is a real one.

DR. RIEBER: Dr. Klima, if I understood you correctly, you and Dr. Bellugi said that the visual was the simultaneous language and the auditory was the sequential language. I wonder what the rationale for that is. I don't quite see why that necessarily has to be the case. If by the "sequential" you mean the integration of the parts into a whole, rather than breaking them up, it seems to me perfectly reasonable that one can do that in either modality.

DR. KLIMA: It is interesting to compare the organization and modulation of words in spoken languages and in sign. In spoken language there is a sequential arrangement of the constituent elements. For example, "cats" consists of a $/k/$ segment, followed by an $/a/$ segment, followed by a $/t/$ segment, followed by an $/s/$ segment. These could be rearranged in any number of ways, six that I can think of: tacks, ax, stack, what-have-you. Spoken languages also have some simultaneous modification—tone, for example—but more typical overall is the sequential organization. Typical in modulation of meaning in spoken language is a sequential addition of some morpheme. In spoken language we have something like "blue," and then we make a sequential modulation to give "bluish."

Now, what is the case in sign? Certainly not segments at any level of the analysis. Rather, we have the simultaneous occurrence of certain primaries. You can perhaps see some of them. What is this? [Dr. Klima signs.] This turns out to be a location, a specific location. It occurs in many signs; in fact, it also occurs in "noon," one of the errors on our test. Typical hand configurations, this one [sign] and this [sign] occur in many other signs, and this one [sign] and the hand movement during signing. Now, what interested us here was that, typically, modulations and meaning, the sort of thing we do in derivation in spoken language, rather than being sequential, rather than being a segment passed on, was some simultaneous change in a parameter, in movement, for example. Blue like this [sign] and bluish like this [sign]. Again, simultaneous.

The next observation is this: how interesting it would be if the langauge made use completely of this simultaneity to its fullest logical possibility. For example, there are two hands, but many signs are made with one hand alone. How interesting it would be if the language expressed the subject of a verb with one hand, and the verb itself simultaneously with the other hand!

Let's take "bird" and "sleeping." Let's say it did this, a logical possibility [sign]. Here we find that a general linguistic faculty takes over. Here you get sequentiality because there is segmentation. But it's at a level different from the individual sign, as our words are strung one after the other.

Dr. PAULA STARKS WILSON (*O.M.R. Developmental Team, Connecticut State Department of Health, Hartford, Conn.*): My question regards your last discussion of changes in signs. Leard has mentioned many examples of English spoken words that change over a period of time; that is, say, over 50 years the pronouncations of some words change. I'm wondering if any of these changes in signs as you have described, could be attributed to a general change in language; that is, as people use a symbol, they change it systematically, rather than possibly going from iconic to arbitrary, as you indicated.

Dr. KLIMA: Changes from the iconic to the arbitrary are just one sort of example. In a film we have from 1913, we've observed that signs have changed from more or less transparent to more or less systematic. Also, some of the signs have been made more and more like other signs, so that there are fewer parameters being used. Specifically, it seems that the signs have a tendency to be concentrated within a very restricted signing space, articulation around the face. Pat Siple has done some work on where the gaze tends to be when two signers are communicating. There is less specificity around the body. There is more of a tendency for both hands to be used lower down here, and single hands up here. So one might suggest that certain perceptual factors are involved.

Dr. PAULA WILSON: Are you aware of any studies which have made any attempt to compare the changes in signs over a period of time with the changes in words over a period of time?

Dr. KLIMA: Yes, two of our students are working on that. The changes are in terms of general principles, like assimilation and so on. At that level of abstraction, I'm not sure how much you're really comparing. For example, if a sign begins in two elements that have a difference in hand configuration, there will tend to be a simplification of that hand configuration.

Dr. HENRY M. TRUBY (*Mailman Center for Child Development, University of Miami, Miami, Fla.*): Dr. Anderson, I'm naturally very much interested in your ballistic model postulate. These types of measurements and observations are the bases of research that I and my colleagues, including Dr. Gerstman, at Haskins Laboratories, carried out in the early 1950's. I believe they form the basis for resolving the existing controversy about voice printing. Individual ballistic rhythms, lengths, and temporal compensations, such as you mentioned, are apparent on spectrograms and are in fact the essence of voice-printing. They can be substantiated by measurements to provide a basis for speaker identification, e.g., in the courtroom. The advantage of this approach is that it focuses on the physical properties of voice, rather than on the phonological or linguistic properties of what is said, such as whether "tree" rhymes with "ski." The essence of voice-printing and voice-print identification is voice, not speech.

DR. ANDERSON: I was not aware that the voice-printing controversy had such a long history, but I agree with your general remark; in fact, I have a report on this matter in preparation. At the Psychiatric Institute, Dr. Joseph Jaffe and I are now looking at pathological variations in speech rhythm.

DR. TRUBY: There are two, and each is pathological in its way, and they show up in the voice-print.

DR. ANDERSON: We have found more than two, but there are two principle ones which I unfortunately don't have time to go into in detail. They represent, I think, the disruption of the stress-period rhythm on the one hand, and the disruption of the independently timed microarticulatory process for individual syllables on the other. I would like to talk with you further about the ones that you found.

DR. D. KIMBROUGH OLLER (*University of Washington, Seattle, Wash.*): My question concerns your discussion of isochrony and your own data on the question. You made it clear that the notion of isochrony could be operationalized in any number of ways, but it wasn't quite clear from what you said, how you had operationalized it in your own experiment. I wonder, for instance, whether or not you did anything to control the final-syllable effect. A great deal of information has been collected to support the claim that isochrony exists in English, but much of it rests on a fallacious assumption. There is a large final-syllable effect that turns out to be virtually the only basis for isochrony. Have you controlled for this?

DR. ANDERSON: I read your article in JASA, and I am aware that you have a very good point. I realize that it will be necessary to deal with the question of syllable-position dependencies, which I have not yet done. But since I am finding stress periodic rather than syllabic indicators of isochrony, I don't think your criticism applies, unless you would propose a final *stress-period* effect. I suppose if the lengthening of the final vowel is great enough to make the final period monosyllabic, then the two effects would tend to coincide, as the final period would *become* the final syllable. But it is not yet known whether this happens often enough to explain my effect in that way to any significant extent.

I might add that the average spontaneous utterance is only two or three periods long and the distribution is heavily skewed, so that eliminating the final period from the analysis would result in taking away almost half of the speaking time that most people produce. I am reluctant to throw away that much of the data, but I agree that syllable-position dependencies should be looked at.

DR. TRUBY: Dr. Kinsbourne, the lateralization phenomenon might very well be manifested already very early, in fact, prenatally, for a very simple reason. In a paper that I gave a few years ago, which I daringly called "Prenatal Speech," I first of all redefined speech to include that aspect of speech which is the input end. Then I reported some experiments they were doing in Sweden at the time to detect congenital deafness in the fetus, or no deafness at all. Those experiments do indicate that the newborn infant, whether he's a premie or term baby or whatever, is a very competent hearer and has been for a long time. Analogously, a baby is able to cry at birth, and therefore he's been preparing to cry for a long time, fetally. It is possible to indicate that the baby is detecting sound on one side or the other. I would venture to say, especially in light of what you're saying that this detection has more to do with lateralization than with unilateral deafness.

DR. KINSBOURNE: I think that the observation, if documented, is a very interesting one. Of course, the baby's position in the uterus is not symmetrical but more to one side than the other, and that might either be a confounding or a self-relevant phenomenon. But I appreciate your comment.

DR. MARTIN GARDNER, (*Childrens' Hospital, Boston, Mass.*): I published some research, some of which I think you heard in Montreal, that confirms what you have said. So far, we have continued to show physiological evidence from continuous EGG recordings during speech, that in six-month-old babies you can get a very nice left-hemisphere effect to speech, as compared to music. In fact it's cleaner in the young babies than you can get in adults. I suspect it has to do with attentional factors. You get these data clearer at times when you can believe that the baby is paying attention to the stimulus, in the sense that it has been moving around, suddenly freezes, and does something which can be called "orienting-quiet." The baby just stops and becomes amazed for maybe 30 or 40 seconds, and at that time the data become cleanest and nicest in relation to what you would want to see if it were lateralized.

DR. KINSBOURNE: That's beautiful. I always thought babies were the best people.

DR. MENYUK: I recently heard results of a study that was carried out by I believe, Kurseo, Rosen, and Macabee, in which they did both digit listening and sentence listening. Interestingly, their data indicated that as the child developed and got older, the right-ear advantage became less, because correct responses increased from both right ear and left ear. The data also indicate that the eight-year-old child with reading difficulty performs, in terms of right-ear advantage, very similarly to a younger child. Would you respond to this? Also, I'm not sure that you explained to us why, after a certain period, you got aphasia with left-handed hemisphere damage. Lateralization alone is not going to account for it.

DR. KINSBOURNE: I think any finding suggesting that an older disordered reader is like a younger normal or immature reader is very acceptable, because that's what learning disability is. It refers to children who, although of normal general intelligence, are cognitively, in certain respects, relatively immature, and comparable to younger children who are normal. Why might a right-ear advantage in dichotic listening get less with increasing age? Because adults use different strategies in listening. Perhaps, for example, you're an adult who's missing input on the left side. You notice this and switch your attention. A child might not use such a compensatory strategy, and so would show greater dichotic asymmetry. The younger the aphasic child at the time of damage (especially for extensive damage that inactivates the left hemisphere), the better and quicker the right hemisphere is able to take over and do the language work instead. In an adult, quite often the right hemisphere still takes over. Many aphasics, in fact, talk by virtue of the activity of the right hemisphere. But there's a ceiling on their performance, and it falls short of excellence. This, one could explain on the general biological principle of decreased plasticity, or the ability to rearrange circuitry as the brain gets older. Now, the details of this, of course, I don't know any more than anybody else does.

DR. LLOYD KAUFMAN (*New York University, New York, N.Y.*): My name is Wilhelm Wundt, I'm from the University of Leipsig. Tom Bever, why, why do you have to insist or claim that there is something simpler about glump or gestalt-type stimulation, because there's really not; they're very complicated. We don't understand them very well. The best evidence we have today, the so-called "simple" gestalt laws, are highly derivative, and indeed many aspects of "gestalt" pattern perception are in fact sequential. I want to ask you this question. What would be inconsistent between what you've been saying and the proposition that the real difference of hemispheric functions is on the response side, i.e., what the hemisphere wants to do in response to the stimulus.

For example, in response to language, I can imagine shadowing. I can imagine sequential, highly complicated, articulated behavior, rather than analysis. In response to pattern, I think in terms of even equally complicated analyses, for example, enormously complicated analyses associated with integrating the two eyes or views of a million random dots in a Julez pattern. But I want to do something different in response to that. My behavior is different. The efferent program I'm calling up is different, and perhaps the hemispheres are specialized in terms of the efferent programs of activity aroused by the stimuli, rather than in terms of what the stimuli are per se. How do you react to that?

DR. BEVER: In English? I would say two things about that. One is that it seems to me to be simply retreating in the face of my apparent onslaught into the perceptual world and saying; "Well, really, we don't understand any of the differences in the perceptual world: it must be in the response, and in the organization of the response." But I don't see that as any more than a retreat at face value.

But, as to your point that the gestalt way of perceiving things is itself very complex, I think that's true. I think that what is in fact at issue is a counterpoint. During perceptual development, and so-called "cognitive development," more gestalten or more complex gestalten are formed out of simpler elements. Once formed, they may thereafter be deployed by the mind as within a gestalt mode, although in their formation and in their analysis in the formative stages, they may have undergone a good deal of construction. One would predict, with respect to certain kinds of perceptual activities, an oscillation between whether the activity is in the left hemisphere or in the right hemisphere. So, I suggest that certain kinds of gestalten are themselves very elaborate in their internal structure, and at the same time I maintain the distinction in terms of the kind of activities that the brain, the mind, carries out at a given time.

MR. DARIUS KLEIN, (*Columbia Univ., New York, N.Y.*): I was wondering if laterality would affect the way you picked up the telephone. In your experiments, did motor control of right-handedness versus left-handedness affect the hemispheric laterality separation? Can we take a poll here on people who hold the telephone more preferentially to their left or right ear?

DR. GERSTMAN: I always wondered about that. Left-hand phone holders do it so they can write with their right. Those are all left-handed people.

DR. AARONSON: Raise your hand if you are right-handed and hold the phone in your left hand.

DR. GERSTMAN: It looks like 60% up here.

DR. AARONSON: All right, the other side, right-handed people, who hold the phone in your right hand. It looks like 40%.

DR. BEVER: That answers the questions much better than I could.

MR. KLEIN: It looks about half and half, doesn't it? Forty-sixty. I have a personal story about holding a telephone and applying for a job. A friend told me where they were going to need me during the course of the conversation, and I answered him. After the phone conversation, I had no idea of where he had said I should meet them. He was talking to my left ear.

DR. BEVER: Let me just say something about this. Most people walking around, most of the time, are reasonably coherent organisms—I don't mean coherent linguistically, but coherent organismically. The left hemisphere is connected to the right hemisphere. Except under experimental conditions, I would expect that in an integrated organism these effects would be quite variable. They might indeed crop up at times and the kind of experience you're talking about might be related to this, but it would be very hard to know.

DR. GERSTMAN: May I direct a question to Dr. Kinsbourne on this? Is there any evidence that in a monotic situation, the left brain gets any poorer informaton from the right ear?

DR. KINSBOURNE: None at all, I don't think there's any evidence that either brain gets poorer information from either ear at any time. I think that what's important is the following: given competing source-information, which source the particular half-brain attends to first. I'd like to say also that the subject of hemispheric asymmetry does tend to generate the kind of question that you ask. All I can say in answer to the questions is, wow!

MR. KLEIN: The last point that Dr. Bever made was an interesting one. You attempted to bring in the possibility of experimental operations. Even though one side had dominance at any time, it may be that the sides change during the course of an analysis. I was wondering if, in your experiments, at some point the subjects chose one side to respond to rather than the other.

DR. BEVER: Dr. Kinsbourne is the expert on turning the hemispheres on and off.

DR. KURT HAMMERY, (Northern Michigan University, Marquette, Mich.): I'd like to direct a question to Tom Bever. Studdert-Kennedy reported that his subjects identified consonants more accurately in the left hemisphere, and vowels in the right hemisphere. I can't give you the methodology, I can't recall it. He found associate consonant identification with the "categorical" kind of function and vowels with "non-categorical." Is that consistent with your "analytic-synthetic" theory?

DR. BEVER: Sure. The argument with respect to that paper specifically is that vowels that could be steady-state are, in effect, treatable as musical stimuli, if the subject wishes. In other experiments, if vowels are more heavily encoded, that is, more transitional although perfectly perceivable, more transitional in movement of the formant, then the right-ear effect emerges for vowels as well.

DR. RIEBER: In defense of Dr. Wundt i.e., L. Kaufman, I am neither his student nor his follower. I simply wear his button, but I do believe that Dr. Kaufman has made a necessary request for clarity. This was not a retreat. In fairness to gestalt psychology, if one is going to use their terminology one should use it in an appropiate manner. If you can't do that, then it is better not to use this terminology at all.

DR. GARDNER: I just thought I'd mention to you another physiological study that speaks to what you said today, which is in press, and was done by Linda Rogers, Warren Tenousan, Charles Kaplan, and me at UCLA. We studied speech by the same methods I used with babies. We compared EEG recordings from Hopi children while listening to English language and Hopi language. Now, Hopi is their first language, and English their second; English turns out to be less lateralized, but more in the left-brain than Hopi. So, the study indicates some caution in assigning language to just the left hemisphere. In that sense, it's comparable to what you reported with music. However, it would seem that your hypothesis that the first language goes to the left hemisphere doesn't quite match these data, the first language being, in this case, the Hopi. If the left brain were more developed, there should be more Hopi in the left than in the right. In fact, there are many good reasons why the Hopi language should be more right, have more right hemisphere components in it.

DR. KINSBOURNE: I think this gives an opportunity for a methodological point. It is not justified to assume a one-to-one correspondence with the degree of an ill effect and the degree of lateralization of a function. Suppose the Hopi kids were better at Hopi than at English, which is at least possible. They might then have to switch on their language processor harder and tougher for English than for Hopi and thereby get more attention for the right-brain with English than for Hopi although both of them were left-lateralized. Now I'm not saying it's the case, but I think that unless you deal with these mediating variables, you cannot yet make the leap from the behavior to the structure.

DR. STERN: Is there any evidence on asymmetrical processing of visual information—information coming in from the left visual field versus the right.

DR. BEVER: There's a lot. Most of the studies use nonfoveal stimulus displays in order to increase the hemispheric separation. But with nonfoveal stimuli, one can't use visually complex figures, for example, linguistic stimuli. So the usual result is a left visual-field dominance. We don't know what happens with complex stimuli.

DR. FISHER (*City College, CUNY, New York, N.Y.*): Dr. Buschke, would it be helpful to consider the effects in terms of paradigmatic versus syntagmatic units? Would it be helpful to think about people forming meanings in terms of word units versus meanings in terms of sentence units, rather than get into a hassle over the difference between semantics and syntax?

DR. BUSCHKE: I can't answer that question in the time allotted. I'd rather answer those questions later, I think, because it's so terribly late now and in fairness to the rest of the panel, I think we should have open questions. My anwer to your question is no. I'll defend it later.

DR. MENYUK: I assume that since it's open question period now, Dr. Buschke, you *will* answer my question. I'm interested in the presentation of the stimuli because, obviously, this kind of experiment has been run fairly frequently with youngsters who are developing language. When you present your semantically anomalous, grammatically intact stimuli versus both semantically and grammatically distorted, how is the material being presented? Does your patient read this material or is it presented orally, and if orally, is it under some kind of notion of sentence, intonational contour, and so on?

DR. BUSCHKE: Yes. It's obviously read, and read aloud because the four-year-old couldn't read. We just read it aloud to try to make life simple, and we try to read it like a sentence. There are some obvious problems and you're right about pointing them out.

DR. DAVE RIKER (*Children's Hospital, Los Angeles, Calif.*): Dr. Kinsbourne, my question concerns the developmental progression that you postulated in terms of hemispheric development. What are the implications of this for the critical-period hypothesis as it concerns primary language learning? There is a notion, (Lenneberg and others) that primary language learning is limited to the time before the full development of lateralization. Now, if lateralization takes place at a very early point, and if that lateralization is a function of the more mature, better developed hemisphere from this very point, what are the implications of this for the inability to acquire primary language at some given critical period in life?

DR. KINSBOURNE: The hypothetical variable of rate of lateralization of cerebral function can no longer be used as an explanatory principle for language learning or for anything else, for that matter. But that is not to say that there mightn't be some other organizing principle related to hemisphere development that could serve in its stead. I might add that earlier on we had some specific examples of the ability of adults to learn a second language. They can provide a counterexample. When I was seven years old, the CIA taught me English, and I still talk with a German accent. So, you know, you can never be sure about these things. [Editor's note: Dr. Kinsbourne's first language is, very obviously, French.]

DR. RICKER: I would think that the principle of decreasing plasticity would certainly be invoked.

DR. KINSBOURNE: At any rate it's not a dichotomous matter. It's not a step function; it's a continous function over the whole of life. Decreasing plasticity would generate a diminishing capability that perhaps does not peter out completely until one has one foot in the grave.

DR. RICKER: That would certainly raise questions about the viability of a critical-period hypothesis. Dr. Bever, you commented on changes that might take place in test-related performance with respect to hemispheric processing: the task might shift from right hemisphere to left. Do you have any examples of whether the shift would go in the other direction, or is it always to the left hemisphere?

DR. BEVER: No, I think that we have no experimentally verified examples, but in principle, the answer that I gave to a question earlier articulates what one would look for. If there are stages in which the construction of a patterned perception of a well-ingrained, habitually perceived form of one kind or another is itself constructive, then there might be a point in which that pattern actually would be better handled ultimately by the otherwise coherent "subject" in the right hemisphere. But we have no such examples. I think that the development of that kind of case, and it's the unexpected case, will require a lot of very careful work and thought about how the more elaborate gestalten are themselves constructed out of the more primitive.

DR. RICKER: It is at least plausible that an alternative interpretation of your facts, as you presented them, is that the shift is always to the left hemisphere. Given that kind of situation, there might be a developmental relationship in terms of how a task is mastered.

DR. BEVER: That's possible. I don't believe it, but it's possible.

401. 1
D48

622-1
5-39

LINCOLN CHRISTIAN COLLEGE